# Teeth and Anthropology

edited by

E. Cruwys and R. A. Foley

BAR International Series 291
1986

# B.A.R.

5, Centremead, Osney Mead, Oxford OX2 0DQ, England.



B.A.R. -S291, 1986: 'Teeth and Anthropology'

Price £17.00 post free throughout the world. Payments made in dollars must be calculated at the current rate of exchange and $8.00 added to cover exchange charges. Cheques should be made payable to B.A.R. and sent to the above address.



ISBN 0 86054 373 0

For details of all new B.A.R. publications in print please write to the above address. Information on new titles is sent regularly on request, with no obligation to purchase.

Volumes are distributed from the publisher. All B.A.R. prices are inclusive of postage by surface mail anywhere in the world.

Printed in Great Britain

## CONTENTS

# PREFACE

The overlap between dentistry and anthropology in relation to dental research has long been recognized. Since teeth constitute the most enduring component in the body, they frequently provide the only frame of reference in which the anthropologists working with skeletal material can operate. Knowledge of the biochemistry, structure and function of teeth is therefore essential to the paleoanthropologist. By examing the intra- and inter-population variability of human teeth - in both living populations from diverse environments and in prehistoric and extinct hominids - deductions can be made regarding the origins and development of particular human traits or functions. These in turn may be of use to the oral biologist in defining treatments or understanding the aetiology of dental disease or abnormalities.

This volume aims to bring together some of the areas of common interest between anthropology and dentistry, including analysis of dental structures, biochemical status, methodology of research, tooth wear studies of normal and pathological conditions, periodontal disease, and analysis of past populations which have recently been undertaken. It arises out of a one day conference held at the University of Durham in March 1985, under the auspices of the Department of Anthropology. This conference had as its objective the presentation of papers dealing with work in progress, rather than broader scale review papers. In this way it was hoped to communicate to each other, and in this volume to a wider audience, the current concerns and interests of workers in this field. It does not, therefore, set out to be comprehensive, but instead to give a flavour of an expanding and active research field.

Because the conference arose out of anthropological interests, this volume is concerned mainly with anthropological issues, rather than oral biology as a whole, and aims to provide an identification of current and further directions of research in dental anthropology.

We should like to thank Dr. Robert Layton, Chairman of the Board of Studies in Anthropology at the University of Durham and Professor Alan Bilsborough for their support and help. Dr. Sarah Atkinson was one of the conference organisers, and Sally Sherren and Moustapha Ibrahim provided considerable help in running the conference. We are grateful to all of these people, and also the many people who participated in and contributed to a most enjoyable and profitable, if extremely wintry, day at Durham.

## LIST OF CONTRIBUTORS

Robert Foley
Elizabeth Cruwys
Department of Physical Anthropology,
Downing Street,
Cambridge CB2 3DZ

A.D. Benyon
The Dental School,
Framlington Place,
Newcastle-upon-Tyne NE2 4BW

C. Robinson
J. Kirkham
J.A. Weatherell
M. Strong
School of Dentistry,
Department of Oral Biology,
Clarendon Way,
Leeds LS2 9LU

Keith Dobney
Don Brothwell
Institute of Archaeology,
31-34, Gordon Square,
London WC1H OPY

J.F. Cross
M.F. Bruce
Department of Anatomy,
Marischal College,
Aberdeen AB9 1AS

N.W. Kerr
Department of Dental Surgery,
Aberdeen Royal Infirmary,
Foresterhill,
Aberdeen AB9 2ZB

D.R. Williams
C.M. Woodhead
Department of Prosthetic Medicine
The Dental School,
Lower Maudlin Street,
Bristol BS1 2LY

Patricia Watson
Department of Prosthetic Dentistry,
School of Dentistry,
Clarendon Way,
Leeds LS2 9LU

Simone K. Bullion
Department of Classics and Archaeology,
University of Lancaster,
Lonsdale College,
Bailrigg,
Lancaster LA1 4YN

Charlotte Roberts
Calvin Wells Laboratory,
School of Archaeological Sciences,
Bradford,
West Yorkshire BD7 1DP

D. James Rackham
Department of Archaeology,
46 Sadler Street,
Durham DH1 3NU

M.V. Stack
The Dental School,
Lower Maudlin Street,
Bristol BS1 2LY

D.K. Whittaker
Department of Oral Biology,
The Dental School,
Hetah Park,
Cardiff CF4 4XY

Sonia A. Williams
Department of Child Dental Health,
School of Dentistry,
Clarendon Way,
Leeds LS2 9LU

Dorothy Lunt
Department of Oral Biology,
University of Glasgow Dental Studies,
378, Sauciehall Stereet,
Glasgow G2 3JZ

# INTRODUCTION

Chapter 1

# DENTAL ANTHROPOLOGY: PROBLEMS AND PERSPECTIVES

Robert Foley and Elizabeth Cruwys

Department of Physical Anthropology
University of Cambridge

## The Anatomy and Biology of Teeth

Teeth constitute the hardest tissue in the human body. Each tooth is made up of three basic components - enamel, which forms the hard outer surface of the crown; dentine, a partly organic tissue that lies under the enamel; and cementum, a highly inorganic substance that surrounds the root. The core of the tooth is the pulp cavity, consisting of minute blood vessels, nerves, cells and fibres. Teeth are usually taken to have two anatomical parts - the crown, which is covered in enamel, and the root, which is composed of cementum and dentine (Figure 1.1). The strength of teeth derives from their chemical and physical structure. They are largely inorganic, made up of calcium salts and an organic matrix.

The principal function of teeth is the mastication of food. Their morphology reflects the various demands made by different food types - shearing, chopping, and grinding. Several basic tooth forms have evolved among mammals that reflect these basic activities - incisors, canines, premolars and molars; the sizes and numbers of these reflect the functional requirements. Teeth may also have a secondary function analagous to tool use - grooming, food preparation, preparing and manufacturing artefacts and material items, and they may also have social significance - acts or threats of aggression, status and dominance.

Among mammals two sets of teeth develop - the deciduous, which are "temporary" teeth that occur during infancy and juvenile stages to allow the jaw to reach adult size, and the permanent dentition which must last the full adult life span. Constant attrition occurs throughout life, and the complete wearing down of teeth may be said to represent thelimit of longevity in most species. Rates and sequences of tooth eruption vary within and between species, but are known in broad outline (Table 1.1).

Teeth have long been a source of information in anthropology and a focus for research. Their durability has meant that teeth form a large component of the hominoid fossil record, while their clear functional importance has attracted workers interested in comparative functional anatomy, leading to conclusions regarding social and ecological behaviour. Furthermore, tooth form varies with taxonomy and phylogeny and so can be used to reconstruct evolutionary patterns. Among living populations dental morphology and health are known to vary considerably and so have attracted the interest of biological anthropologists as well as dental clinicians.

In view of the importance of teeth in anthropology, and the crucial need to bring together anthropologists and oral biologists, this volume has been comprised in order to discuss issues of mutual interest; to make available for anthropologists recent developments in oral biology, and to present the

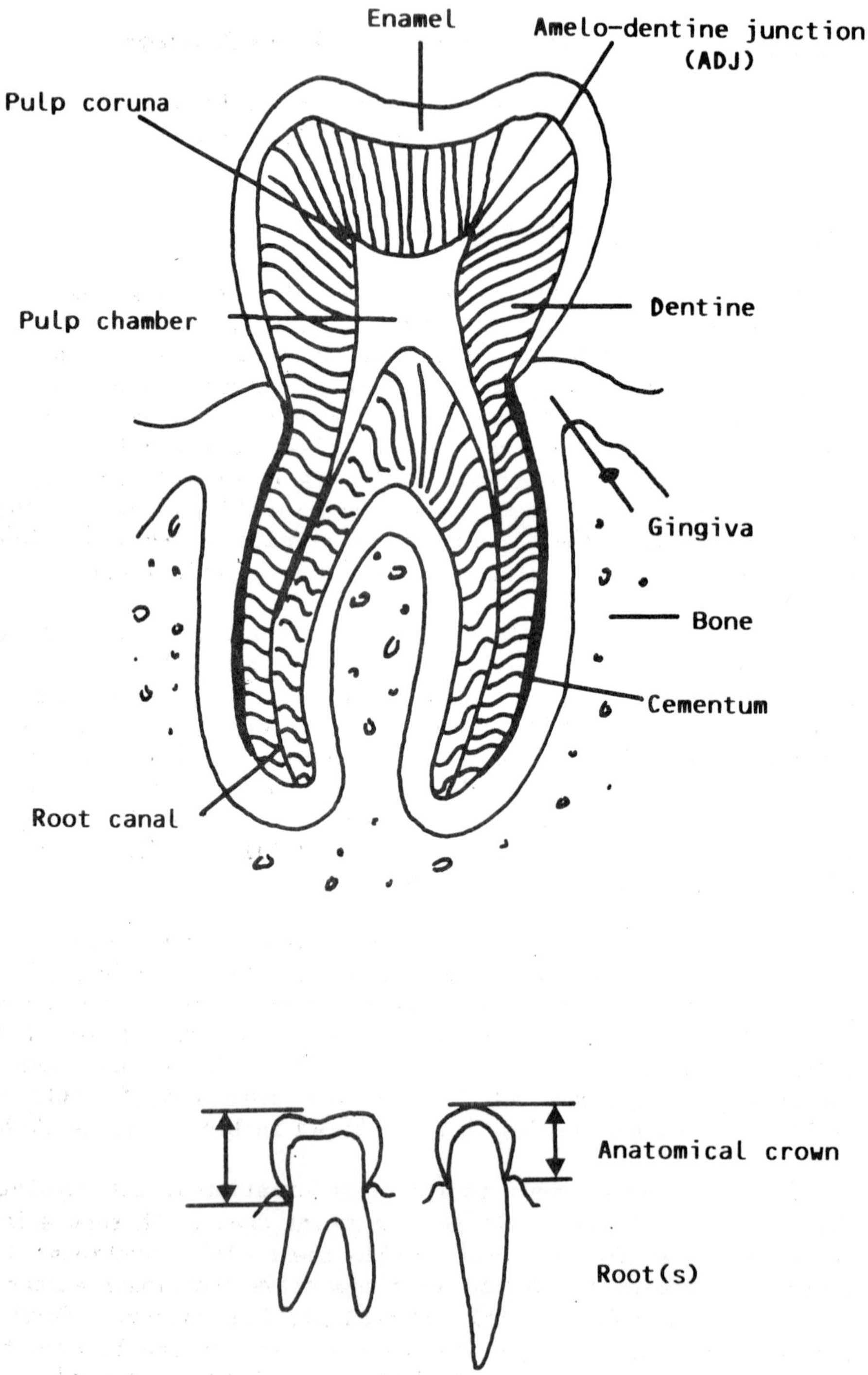


Figure 1.1. The basic anatomy of a tooth.

TABLE 1.1: AGE IN YEARS OF PERMANENT TOOTH ERUPTION IN DIFFERENT POPULATIONS (sexes combined).

| | Danes | W.Gd.[1] | S. Chin.[2] | Pima | Iceland | Gorilla | Pan |
|---|---|---|---|---|---|---|---|
| Maxilla | | | | | | | |
| I2 | 8.0 | 7.9 | 8.6 | 8.5 | 7.95 | 6.5 | 6.73 |
| C | 11.25 | 10.75 | 10.1 | 11.3 | 11.1 | 7.7 | 8.97 |
| Pm1 | 10.35 | 9.6 | 9.65 | 9.85 | 10.2 | | |
| Pm2 | 11.2 | 10.9 | 10.75 | 11.0 | 11.1 | 6.95 | 7.47 |
| M2 | 12.15 | 11.65 | 12.35 | 11.55 | 12.15 | 6.77 | 6.79 |
| Mandible | | | | | | | |
| C | 10.1 | 9.5 | 10.1 | 10.25 | 10.1 | 8.9 | 8.99 |
| Pm1 | 10.35 | 10.15 | 10.15 | 10.25 | 10.3 | 7.32 | 7.35 |
| Pm2 | 11.25 | 11.25 | 10.9 | 11.1 | 11.2 | 7.14 | 7.35 |
| M2 | 11.65 | 11.25 | 11.65 | 11.1 | 11.65 | 6.58 | 6.45 |

[1] West Greenland
[2] South China
Modified from Boesen _et al_ (1976) and Biegert (1981).

anthropological prespective to oral biologists. This paper sets out to review recent advances in anthropology in relation to oral biology.

## Teeth in Anthropology

The role that teeth have played in anthropological research can be thought of in terms of three complimentary frameworks.

1. Dental tissues: as stated above, teeth consist of several different components. Research has tended to focus on particular tissues, and so it will be necessary to review recent developments within each of these areas.

2. Approaches: recent methodologies have employed a variety of techniques, odontometry, macro- and micro-wear, biochemical analysis, and comparative anatomy at individual and population levels, as well as scanning and optical microscopy of dental structure. Each of these has yielded a wealth of new information.

3. Anthropological Issues: the study of teeth involves a wide range of disciplines, each with its own aims and objectives. This paper, and indeed the volume as a whole, is concerned primarily with anthropological issues, rather than those of oral biology as a whole. Consequently in this paper we shall look at some of the current issues in the anthropological study of teeth to provide an indication of the future direction of research.

Dental Tissue Enamel: owing to its high levels of phosphate and calcium, enamel is the hardest material in the body. It is translucent, which gives variations in colour depending on the quality of mineralisation (hypoplasia/hyperplasia) and how effectively light is reflected from the underlying dentine. Salivary and bacterial deposits may also discolour enamel. Microscopically, enamel is made up of prisms or rods running from the surface to the amelo-dentinal junction (ADJ). In cross section the rods have a variable appearance (Boyde 1976), which has recently been employed for phylogenetic analysis of the Hominoidea (Gantt *et al.* 1977).

Gantt (1977) claimed that it was possible to distinguish hominids from other members of the Hominoidea on the basis of their enamel prisms. According to him, hominids possessed a "keyhole" prismatic structure, where the living apes had a circular or hexagonal one. On this basis it seemed possible to identify the earliest fossils within the hominid clade from analysis of the microscopic structure of their enamel. Gantt's analysis suggested that the australopithecines possessed the keyhole structure, but that *Ramapithecus* did not.

These results have been criticised by Vrba and Grine (1978a and b) and by Boyde and Martin (1984). All these authors have suggested that different hominoids cannot be distinguished on the basis of general differences in enamel structure. This difference of opinion arose partly from methodological problems. The degree and nature of prism packing varies with depth within the enamel. Surface enamel should therefore be removed through acid etching, and differences in the depth and extent of the etching can produce different results. More extensive sampling by Boyde and Martin (1984) has shown that prism pattern may vary within a single species and within a single tooth. Observation of a single pattern consequently cannot be used for phylogenetic differentiation.

Unlike Vrba and Grine (1978a and b), however, Boyde and Martin (1984) claim that phylogenetic information can be extracted from enamel ultrastructure. Higher taxa among the primates (Strepsirhini, Platyrrhini, Cercopithecoidea and Hominoidea) may be distinguished by the relative frequencies of different prism patterns, and by the extent of decussation - that is, the degree to which the enamel prisms pursue a wavy or straight-line path from surface to amelo-dentinal junction. Extension of this more detailed and quantitative analysis should make it possible to distinguish some of the Hominoidea. However, it is very likely that these differences in enamel structure affect biomechanical properties, and may thus arise independently and recurrently in relation to selective pressures and the character of the diet.

Apart from prism structure, other microscopic aspects of enamel have potential for anthropological investigation. The prisms of enamel are threadlike bundles that traverse from the tooth surface to the junction with the dentine. Where they reach the surface they may, on eruption, form a pattern of ridges and grooves, known as perikymata. These eventually wear down. Along the length of the enamel prisms are striations known as the brown striae of Retzius. These are indicative of the incremental growth patterns of the enamel, and may be used as chronological indicators of development.

The brown striae of Retzius have recently been studied in fossil hominid populations. Bromage and Dean (1985) examined the relationship between the number of striae of Retzius (which indicates actual age in days from birth) and dental eruption ages of deciduous teeth. Such a relationship should calibrate dental age with actual age. The results of their analysis showed that the early hominids were developing at a rate more consistent with the pattern known in pongids than that of modern humans. For example, the assigned specimen Sts24a from Sterkfontein, assigned to Australopithecus africanus had a dental age of 6.05 years based on a modern human analogue, but an actual age of only 3.3 years on the basis of enamel incremental lines. The same pattern held true for specimens of robust australopithecines and early genus Homo. Although this technique is still at an early stage of development, it has the potential of radically improving our understanding of changes in patterns of development during the course of human evolution.

Further information may be obtained from biochemical anaylsis of dental enamel. The uptake of specific chemical components may provide further information as to the living conditions of a population or a group. The chemistry of human dental enamel and the distribution of chemical components has been analysed by Robinson et al., (Chapter 3 of this volume) in order to offer a basis for distinguishing between normal and pathological tissue, to assess prenatal nutrition affecting tooth formation, and to examine post-mortem changes which may occur. Fluoride levels and other enamel defects, such as hypoplasia, may also provide information as to the environmental or dietary conditions of populations. For example, the teeth of Inuit living on traditional diets of raw sea mammals, which have very high natural fluorine levels, have few defects in their enamel and a high level of dental health.

Enamel may further aid anthropological investigations in terms of its thickness (Kay 1981). Thickened enamel was once regarded as a distinctive hominid trait (Pilbeam 1979) (an evolutionarily derived (synapomorphic) condition relative to the other hominoids). Its presence in certain fossils was therefore used as a basis for assigning them to the Hominidae. This was particularly the case with Ramapithecus, which possessed thick tooth enamel. However, further analysis showed that thin tooth enamel was confined to the African great apes among the living hominoids, and was therefore unlikely to be a simple primitive condition, and furthermore that other, particularly Asian, Miocene hominoids, had thickened tooth enamel. As a result of the work by Martin (1985), tooth enamel thickness on its own does not give straightforward phylogenetic information, but rather seems to have evolved independently in different hominoid groups. However, it may still be a useful indicator of diet. Furthermore, it is necessary to extend work on enamel prism structure and thickness to studies of variability in modern human populations.

Dentine: the intertubular nature of dentine is similar histologically to bone, containing collagen and an inorganic component - mainly hydroxyapatite. The dentinal tubules run parallel to each other, and fibres perpendicular to the tubules form a collagen matrix. Predentine is found at the pulp cavity-dentine interface and makes up the matrix continaully formed by odontoblasts throughout dental life.

With age, dentine becomes less sensitive, thicker and more brittle. The roots also become schlerosed (i.e. translucent) as the linings of the dentinal tubules become more calcified. The extent to which the roots become transparent with increasing age is important for forensic and anthropological purposes.

Although dentine may be of value to anthropological studies in terms of structural and biochemical analysis, research is still at a very early stage. With regard to tooth wear, very little can be ascertained from examination of wear facets of dentine under the SEM, although the position and shapes of these facets can provide an index for assessing and measuring wear (Brothwell 1965).

Throughout the life of an individual, new dentine (reparative or secondary dentine) is formed near the pulp. This can be identified by its darker colour. Thus, as the enamel is worn away, reparative dentine prevents the exposure of the pulp in cases of extreme attrition. This dentine is deposited in incremental lines which could be under similar controls to those of the striae of Retzius, but other factors seem to be influential in this deposition thus making the interpretation of any banding rather difficult (Morris 1978). Dentine form and structure may be used to provide information on the development of the individual, but this has yet to be developed as an area of anthropological research, and little can be ascertained until the exact nature and mechanisms of these processes are better understood.

Cementum: the roots of teeth are covered with cementum, which is deposited throughout life. The thickness of the cementum and the rate of deposition varies from species to species, but in many animals it occurs on a regular annual or seasonal basis, and has thus been used as an ageing technique (Laws, 1952; Klevezal & Kleinenberg 1967). Deposition seems to be affected by nutritional conditions, such that for many animals, especially sea mammals and for herbivores, annual banded increments can be observed in dental sections. Apart from wildlife applications this characteristic has been employed in the analysis of palaeontological and archaeological samples.

The underlying causes of cementum deposition are still not fully understood. The pattern of deposition has been ascribed to both environmental conditions, such that banding indicates seasonality, and also to reproductive behaviour ('rutting lines'). For both humans and other animals this needs further research, so that cementum banding can be intepreted, as it should be, in terms of an individual's life history, rather than general external conditions. This theme is pursued in this volume by Foley (Chapter 5).

Calculus is formed from plaque, which absorbs minerals and becomes hard around the neck of the tooth. Whilst this can cause gingival or periodontal disease, it can also be interesting for anthropological purposes since food debris and micro-organisms may become trapped within the calculus, providing an insight into diet and habitat. Studies have been conducted by Dobney and Brothwell (Chapter 4, this volume) to analyse some of the extraneous materials found in the calculus of skeletal populations. Critical in these investigations must be the analysis of material incorporated in calculus of animals whose diets and environments are well-known, prior to application to the anthropologically and archaeologically unknown.

To date the findings of Dobney and Brothwell have included observation of the presence of particles of cereal chaff epidermis, opal phylotyiths, charcoal particles and other food fragments. As with the studies of other dental tissues, analysis of calculus composition may provide insights into the variability between individuals that must form the basis for a broader understanding of human dental variation.

## Approaches to Dental Anthropology

Morphometrics: one of the oldest traditions in biological anthropology is that of anthropometry - the metrical study of human physical characteristics - and this is equally applicable to teeth. Dental morphometrics can provide excellent information on the evolutionary, ecological and anatomical nature of humans and hominids.

Many studies have been conducted to establish the size and shape of teeth in populations of both living (for example East Greenland Inuit (Pedersen 1949); the Aleut (Moorrees 1957); American Indians (Dahlberg 1963) and extinct hominids (for example Wolpoff, 1971 and 1978; Wood and Abbott, 1983). Various anthropological issues have arisen from these findings.

One of the most important issues has been the pattern of change in hominid and human tooth size. The earliest hominids are characterised by an enlargement of their posterior tooth row and reduction of the anterior teeth, particularly the canine. Indeed, Darwin (1871) was the first to recognise that this was an important element of human evolution. Identification of these dental changes has been critical in the recognition of the earliest hominids in the fossil record, and was a significant reason for considering Miocene hominoids such as *Ramapithecus* and *Gigantopithecus* as possible hominid progenitors. However, it is now clear that dental enlargement, probably in response to a drier climate and a harder and more seasonally variable diet, may have led to complex patterns of parallel evolution among the hominoids, similar to those seen in changes in enamel thickness. Attention is now focussed on the functional anatomy of dental enlargement, particularly the explanation of the trend towards megadonty seen in the evolution of the robust members of the genus Australopithecus (Paranthropus), which display this feature.

The evolution of the robust australopithecines was contrary to the trend of reduction in the size of the teeth and jaws seen in the genus Homo from the Plio-Pleistocene to the present day. Reasons for this decrease are uncertain, although several theories have been put forward. Brace (1962) proposed that dietary factors, particularly the introduction of softer foods, decreased the need for a large gnathosthomatic system. Particularly important, although still poorly understood, is the introduction of food preparation techniques, especially cooking. Others (i.e. Y'edynak, 1978) have suggested that with a more complex technology and material culture, hominoid teeth and jaws were released from other, non-dietary selective pressures, and so reduced in size and robusticity.

Tooth size is also important in the anthropology of more recent populations, as they show a continuation of the trend towards smaller teeth and jaws, and also a reduction in the number of teeth, particularly the third molars. However, it does not necessarily follow that the reasons underlying dental reduction in the earlier hominoids were the same as those which contribute to dental reduction, loss and crowding in modern human populations. One particular problem is the extent to which dental changes occurring over very short timescales are comparable with longer term evolutionary ones observable in the fossil record. Here the study of more recent historic and prehistoric populations from archaeological excavations may be critical in reducing the gap between evolutionary, essentially palaeontological approaches, and more modern biological studies.

With more recent populations dental crowding and malocclusion has been a focus of research, and one that links directly with problems of health in living peoples. For example, we have analysed toothsize in relation to dental arch dimensions for various modern British populations (Cruwys and Foley, 1986). Intuitively, it might have been expected that there would be a correlation between the size of the jaw, its constituent teeth, and various forms of malpositioning. Figures 1.2 a to d show the poor relationship which exists between malpositioning of teeth (for example, crowding, impaction and rotation) in two genetically separate populations. Clearly, other factors are involved in the build up of malocclusion in modern human teeth than size alone.

In all thse studies of tooth size, whether of fossil or modern populations it is increasingly clear that absolute size is of less significance than size relative to other aspects of body size. Modern biologists, especially those concerned with evolutionary patterns have recently focused on body size differences, and argue strongly that all studies of anatomical dimensions must be corrected to take into account the overall body size of the organism. This has had an important effect on studies of early hominoid populations, but has yet to be pursued in detail for anatomically modern humans.

Apart from the biological issues raised by dental morphometrics, it should be remembered that there are also technical problems related to the measurement of teeth and jaws. First, there is a lack of easily defined datum points, and second confusion exists in the literature in nomenclature,

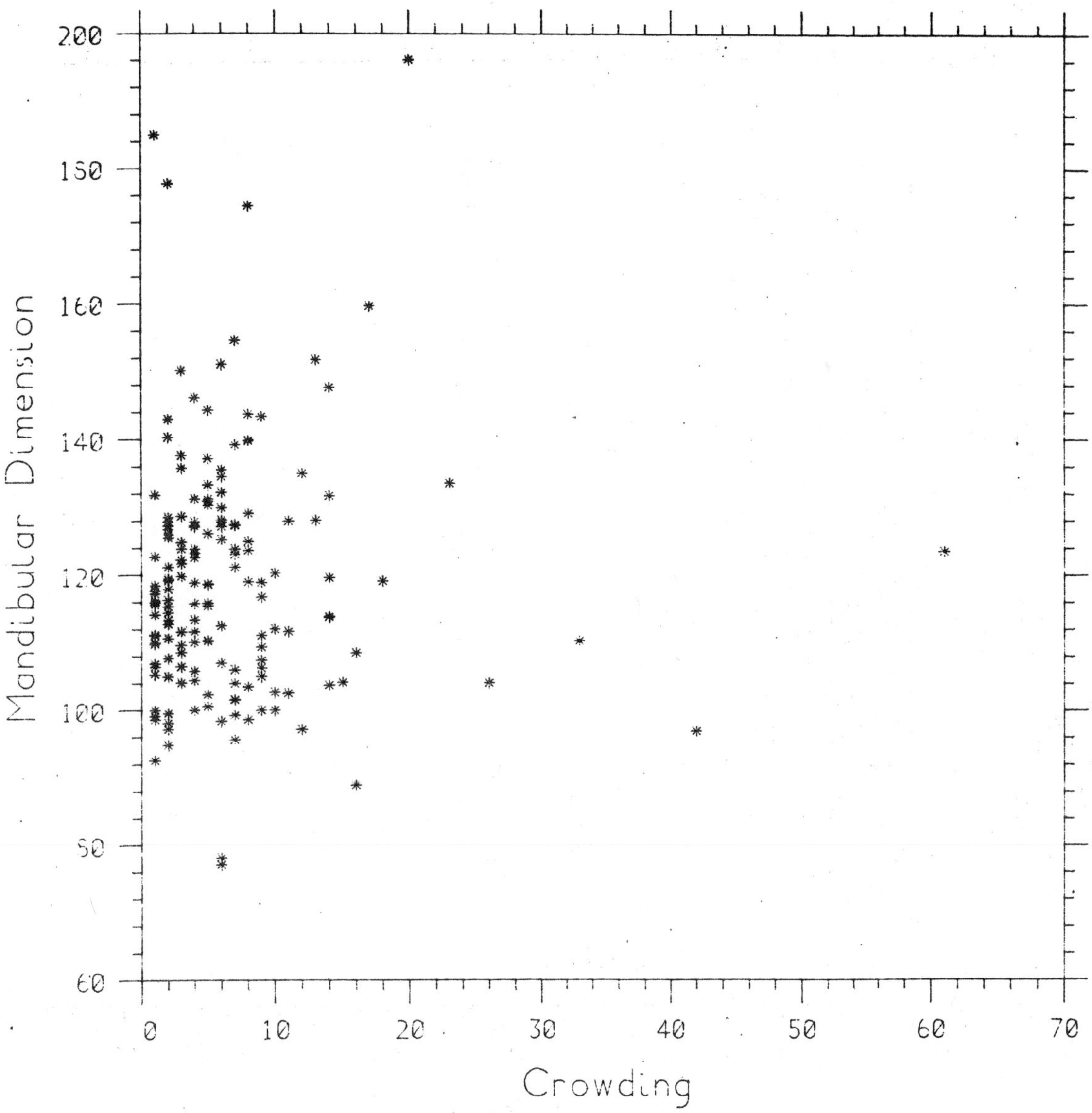


Figure 1.2a. The relationship between crowding and arch dimension in the mandibles of British patients.

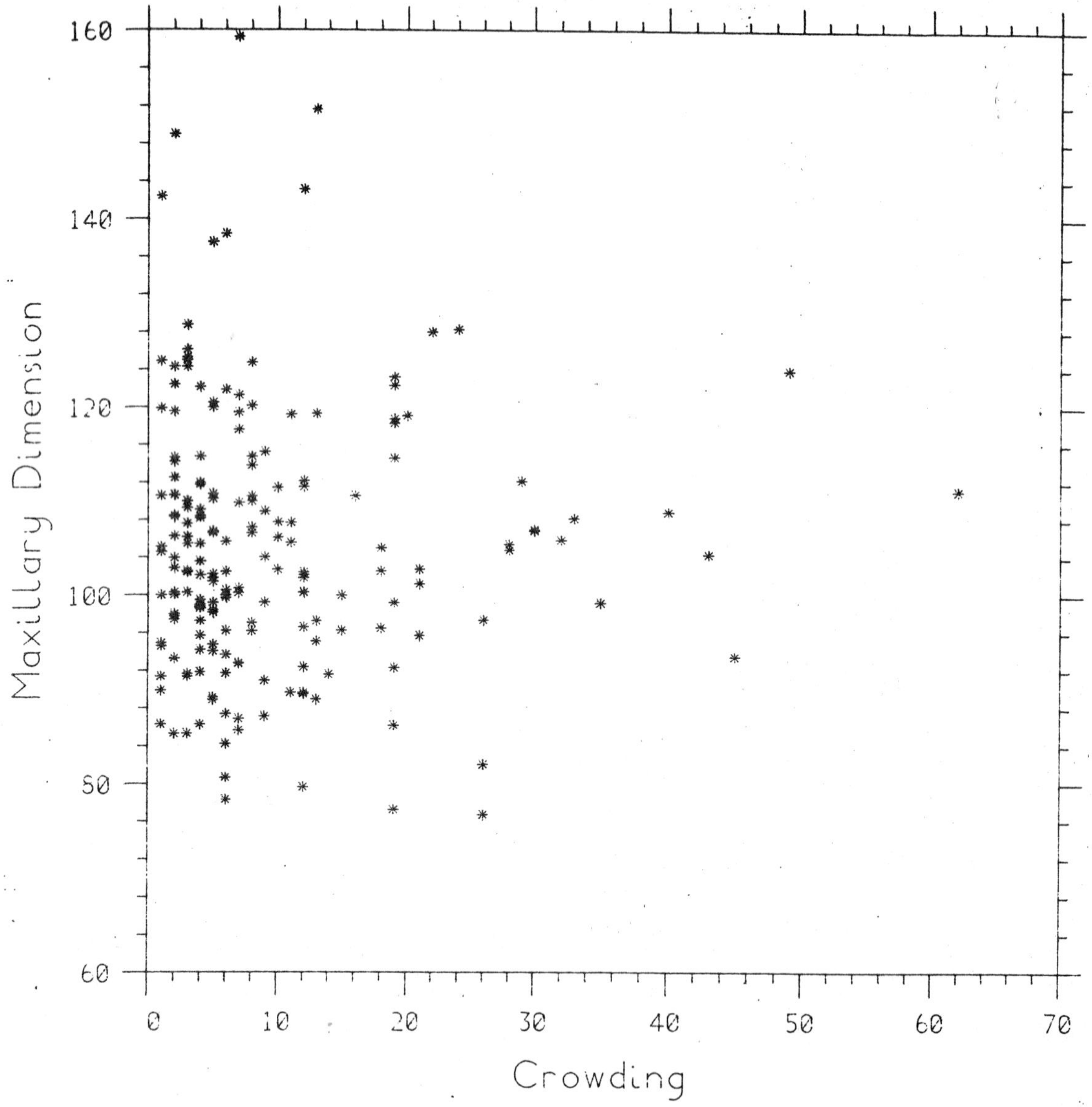


Figure 1.2b. The relationship between crowding and arch dimension in the maxillas of British patients.

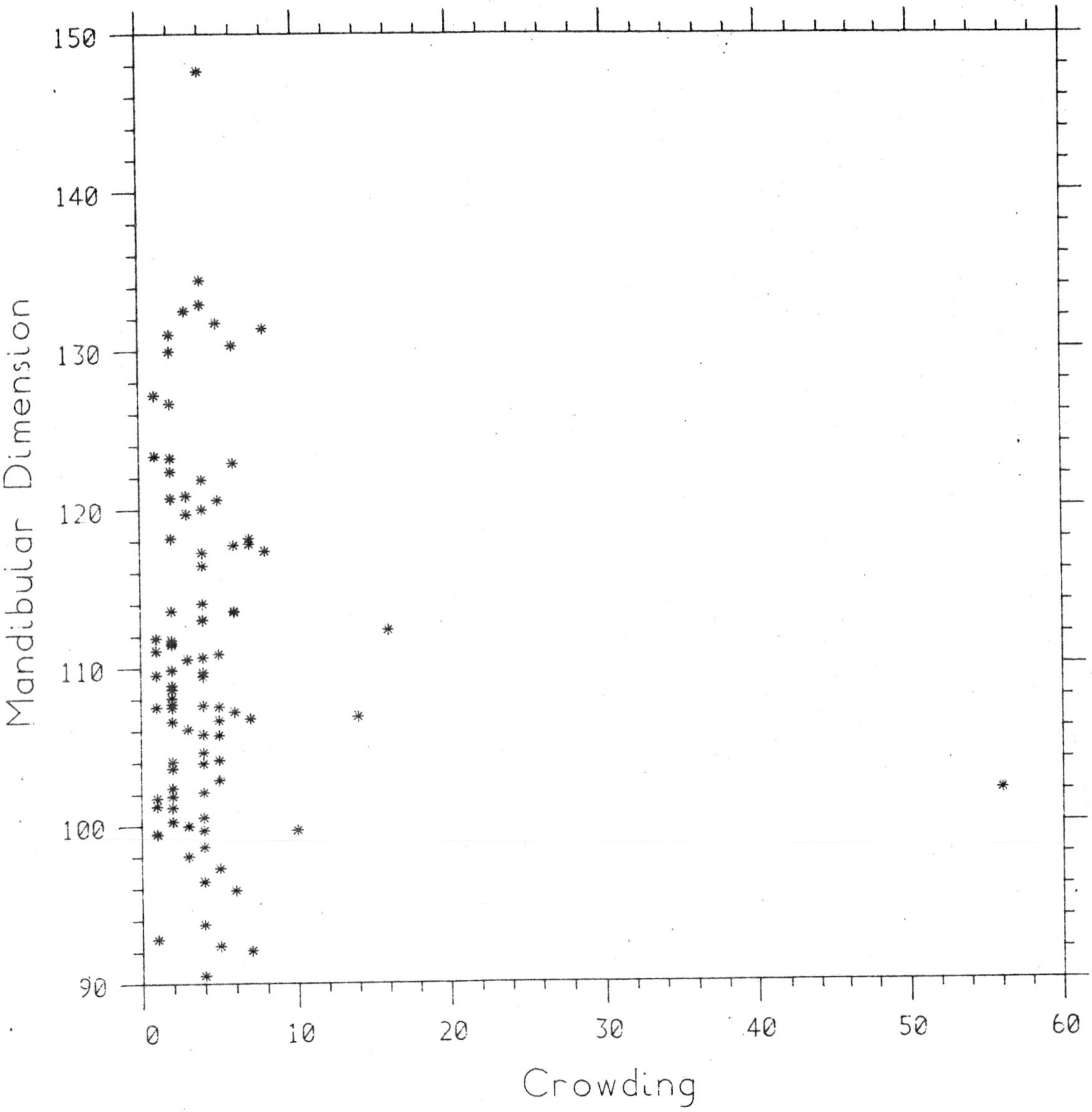


Figure 1.2c. The relationship between crowding and arch dimension in the mandibles of British Asian patients.

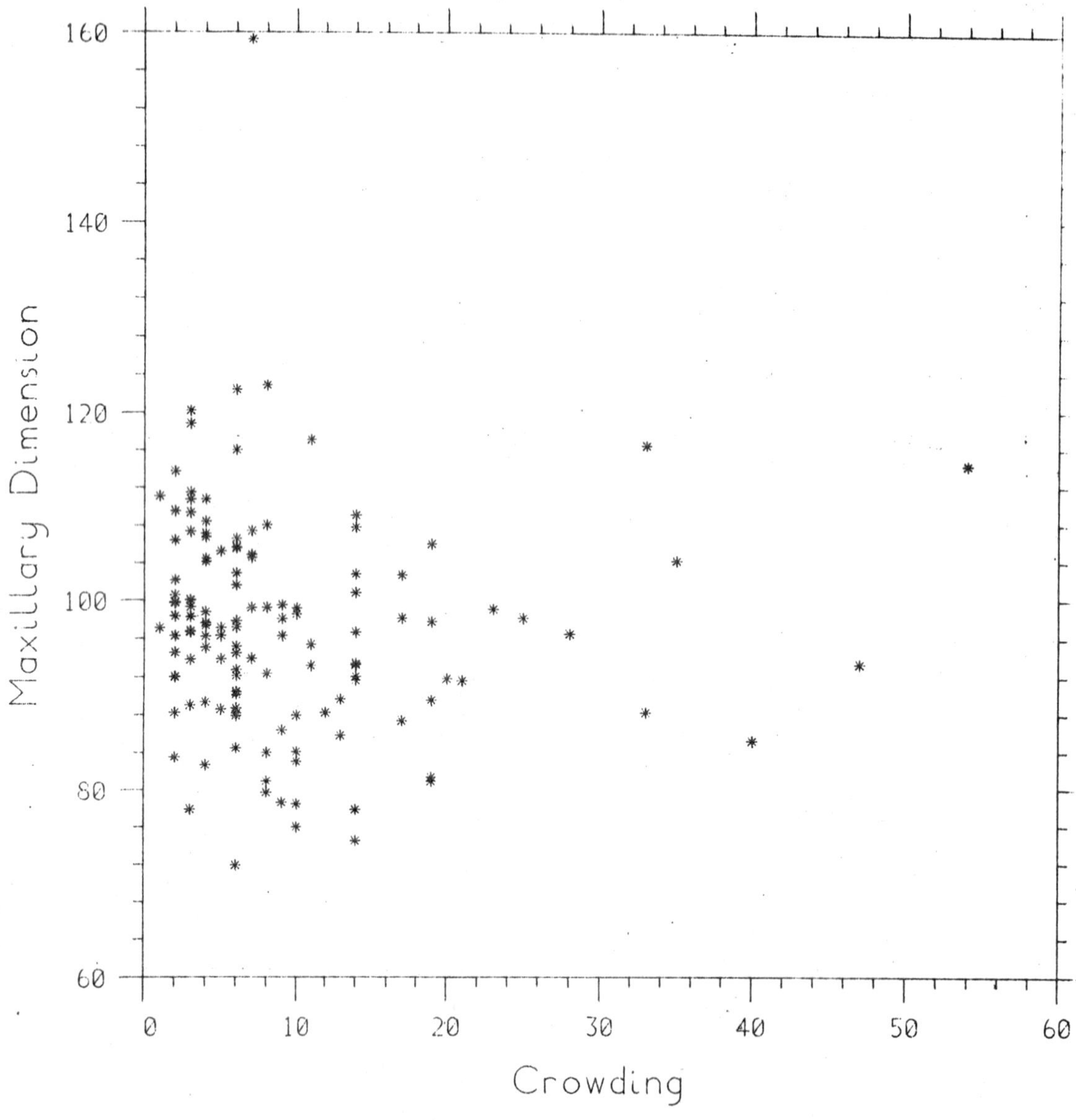


Figure 1.2d. The relationship between crowding and arch dimension in the maxillas of British Asian patients.

making cross-population analysis difficult. Odontometrics is further complicated by the non-uniform shape of the tooth, and therefore any measurement will not be indicative of shape and vice versa. Furthermore, teeth, despite their appearance of permanence and hardness, change dimensionally during life - for example changing dimensions of surface area as a result of wear, or the movement of teeth within their bony matrix. Until these methdological problems are solved comparisons between studies and between population measurements may be fraught with difficulties.

One further area of current research is the genetics of tooth and jaw size. It would seem fairly certain that tooth size is controlled to some extent by the X and perhaps the Y chromosome (Garn et al., 1965, 1966). The degree that tooth size is determined by environmental factors if at all, is still disputed.

## Gross Comparative Anatomy

Not all biologically or anthropologically significant characteristics of teeth are metrical in nature. It has been observed by many researchers that specific morphological traits occur with greater frequency in some populations than in others. Variability in characteristics such as shovel-shaped incisors, the Carabelli complex and the protostylid has been measured in many living populations (for example Carbonell, 1963; Dahlberg, 1963).

Although it is not possible to take an isolated tooth or dentition and ascribe it to a particular group or population on the basis of morphology, it may be possible to assign probabilities concerning the population from which it was drawn. Identification of isolated skeletal or fossil specimens, whilst not absolute, occasionally can be inferred.

The range of variation in the human dentition is immense. Variation can occur between population and population, individuals within the population and between teeth in a series in an individual, causing the dentition to be almost as unique as fingerprints. This variation can be attributed to many factors - most importantly genetic, although the role played by hereditary factors has not been determined conclusively in many cases. Other factors include sexual dimorphism, which affects the size and robusticity of a dentition, diet, age and cultural context.

In general anthropologists have concentrated upon specific traits that are immeditely discernable, such as the cusp of Carabelli, and the shovel-shaped anterior teeth characteristic in populations with Mongoloid affinities. Hrdlicka (1920) found an incidence of 62.5% and 75.0% shovel-shaping in Chinese central and lateral incisors respectively. This can be compared to the much lower percentages in non-Mongoloid groups - 3.8% and 2.9% in central and lateral incisors of Finns (Koski and Hautala, 1952) and 8% in American whites (Lasker, 1950). The functional significance of this trait is uncertain. Hrdlicka (1920) maintains that the shovel-shaped form provides a much stronger structure less likely to fracture or chip. Shovel-shaping frequency is high among the Inuit who exert considerable pressure on the anterior teeth in dietary and cultural practices. It is probably also significant that the Inuit possess one of the highest bite forces known in living populations (Hylander, 1977). In a recent study, conducted by Cruwys, of British and British Asian populations, shovel shaping reached frequencies of 21.1% and 14.8% respectively. The different frequencies in various populations would seem to indicate that some degree of heritability is at work, although it is not known whether the trait is polygenic.

The Carabelli complex, occurrring on the maxillary molars, is more frequent in Caucasian populations, than in populations with Mongoloid affinities. Studies of British patients in Newcastle showed that there was an overall percentage of 47.1% maxillary first molars with some incidence of the trait. In British Asians the percentage of affected teeth was 48.5%. Again, the functional significance is obscure, although it may be that the extra cusp enlarges the occlusal surface of the tooth for mastication, and may therefore have conferred a selective advantage over smaller teeth.

This is of relevance anthropologically, since it can assist in assessing the origins of certain populations - the low incidence of cusps of Carabelli and the extent of shovel-shaping in Inuit populations would therefore be indicative that their roots lie in Central Asia, with the North American Indians and other Mongoloid peoples.

Further traits analysed include incidence of the protostylid complex, various extra ridges, cusplets, occlusal pitting and wrinkling, taurodontism, dental tubercles and enamel crown extensions. Cusp number variation and occlusal groove configuration have also been examined. It is thought, for example, that the 'Dryopithecus' pattern of five cusps and a Y-shaped groove (Y5) is more ancient than the anatomically advanced +4 pattern.

Dental variation in living populations indicates the genetic relationships between populations and groups. Since the morphological variants were probably maintained by the selective advantages conferred from the functional capacities of these characteristics, their incidence in modern populations may provide clues to the dental history of the human species.

Microwear: recent studies involving dental microwear have centred on two main fields of interest - information about diet; and what may be deduced in terms of masticatory movement. Several papers have also been written developing the methodology of microwear analysis and suggesting means of quantification and qualification of results.

a) diet: Walker, Hoeck and Perez (1978) examined the microwear patterns of two sympatic species of hyrax - a browser and a seasonal grazer. It was found that the wear facets on the enamel displayed fine parallel striations less than 1 $\mu$ wide on the molars of both species, but the scratch density on the teeth of the grazer varied according to seasonality. They proposed therefore that information regarding the diet of extinct species, including hominids, may be obtained from examination of the dental microwear. Studies of the East African fossils seems to show great potential. Walker (1981) argued that the occlusal surfaces of the robust australopithecines (*A. boisei*) showed a pattern of microwear indicative of fruit-eaters (probably fairly hard seasonal fruit), while *Homo erectus* had patterns of microwear associated with a more omnivorous and eclectic diet. In another study, Grine (1981) examined the microwear of the Sotuh African australopithecines. He was able to show that the robust australopithecines had a different pattern of wear from that seen in more gracile forms, and argued that this indicated that the former had a diet that involved more crushing and puncture crushing. All the Southern African australopithecines, though, were said to be herbivorous on the basis of their microwear.

Covert and Kay (1981) adopted an experimental approach to microwear. They fed captive opossums on foods aimed to simulate insectivorous and herbivorous diets. In addition, some animals were fed on a soft diet as a control, and one animal was fed with a diet that included a fine-ground pumice component. Analysis of wear facets showed that little difference could be seen between the patterns on the control specimens and those animals with extra dietary components, except for the animal with pumice additives, which showed distinctive scratches akin to those on the teeth of hyraxes caused by silicates in grasses. These results led Covert and Kay to propose that microwear is by no means conclusive in establishing different dietary patterns between populations eating insectivorous and herbivorous diets. They note, however, that the method can provide information on whether the animal included a dietary component with exogenous grit or silicate-containing palnts.

These results led to much controversy, (Gordon and Walker, 1983) and Gordon (1982) examined the microwear of chimpanzees to ascertain intraspecific variability of the patterns and to test the methodology. This study highlighted the fact that microwear is the product of <u>both</u> diet and masticatory movement, and was thus difficult to interpret. Further important variables included the position of the tooth or the facet in the mouth and the age of the specimen examined.

b) <u>mastication</u>: analysis of microwear and jaw mechanics was conducted by Ryan (1979 a and b) by producing masticatory movement artificially to assess types and patterns of wear. Ryan's model suggested that pitting, or widening, at the lingual end of a microscratch indicates lingually directed movements, and buccal broadening indicated buccal movement.

If it should be proved that chewing patterns can be reliably assessed from microwear analysis, the evolution of masticatory processes could be reconstructed. This may be used to contribute to the understanding of phylogenetic and taxonomic relationships between hominids and other primates.

The current debate in microwear analysis focuses on several points of interest. Firstly, the question of variability and its causes must be determined. Secondly, the role of functional morphology in determining microwear must be more closely examined. Finally, there is the question of whether the scratches on the teeth are truly representative of the diet of an individual during its entire lifetime, or whether it indicates only what was eaten immediately prior to death. Microwear is a comparatively new area of research. At this stage these studies have yet to achieve their full potential, and have still to be extended to assess the great variability in more recent human populations.

<u>Macrowear</u> can be used by the anthropologist to give an indication of age, diet, patterns of mastication, and occasionally para-functional habits of an individual. The factors which either cause or influence toothwear are various. Masticatory function may vary between the sexes (in terms of the amounts of load and force exerted, and the size of the teeth), age groups (masticatory vigour may be lost during senescence or with increasing periodontal and dental disease), and between groups and populations. The

degree of hardness or fibrosity of the diet will cause differences in wear patterns. However, as with microwear, it is difficult to ascribe a wear pattern to a single aetiological factor. Rare examples would be the unique grooves and slopes which have been observed on the teeth of some populations, caused by a specific phenomenon such as labrets in the Canadian Inuit or making thread from seal sinews among the East Greenland Inuit (Pedersen 1955). However, in terms of major anthropological issues, such as the proportion of meat in the diet, it would seem that wear is not a particularly sensitive variable. Differences between types of vegetable diet, which can vary enormously in their fibrosity and hardness, are more likely to be reflected in macrowear than animal/vegetable proportions.

Other factors which may influence the degree and rate of toothwear include the chemistry of the food and the biochemistry of the oral cavity. Ill health leading to digestive problems or recurrent vomiting may also cause extreme forms of wear (Smith and Knight, 1984). Chemical conditions may affect the resistance of teeth to abrasion or caries by altering the hardness or biochemical properties of the dental tissues. Genetic and environmental influences may contribute to this, as well as certain cultural practices (i.e. oral hygiene or artificial wear).

At this stage it may only be concluded that dental wear is produced by a combination of factors, including masticatory and dietary functions, genetic characteristics, the biochemistry of the dental tissue, the age, sex, and general health of the individual, and cultural practices. The importance of any of these factors may vary from population to population. For example, cultural practices and fibrous diets may be more important in causing toothwear in a group eating traditional foods, but dental health and bruxism may alter masticatory habits sufficiently to show abnormal wear patterns in more modern populations. However, until the proportion of variability caused by these different factors can be determined, toothwear will provide only general information in dental anthropology.

One important and longstanding use of toothwear in anthropology has been as an indicator of age in skeletal and fossil populations (Brothwell 1965). In conjunction with tooth eruption sequences, wear can provide reasonably accurate results, although dietary factors may make these relative within populations, rather than absolute and suitable for inter-population comparisons. Accuracy, howver, declines with increasing age and degree of wear. An analysis of the percentage of occlusal tooth surface covered by wear facets in a group of known-age British patients showed that accuracy of prediction decreased with increasing age, and that the 7s (M2s) provided the best estimate of the age of an adult.

<u>Biochemical analysis</u>: given its importance for understanding dental health it is not surprising that oral biologists have for a long time taken an interest in the biochemistry of teeth. This interest is now being extended to anthropology. The suggestion is that the chemical composition of teeth can provide information about an individual's life history, such as the diet. Teeth, during their formation and growth, take up minerals, and relative proportions of minerals are indicative of the environment in which individuals live. Fluorine has received the most attention in this context on account of its importance in dental health. Archaeologists have also taken considerable interest in strontium levels, as this has often been thought to reflect the nature of the diet, particularly the level of meat consumption. While many of the simplistic assumptions underlying this

research have been questioned, there is no doubt that the analysis of the chemical composition of teeth represents an important field of research in dental anthropology. Teeth, rather than bone, may be particularly useful here as they are less susceptible to pre-mortem, post-mortem and post-depositional changes in chemical composition.

## Dental Anthropology

While both traditional and new techniques are critical for the development of research in dental anthropology, ultimately future directions depend upon the nature of the problems in which anthropologists and oral biologists are interested. Anthropology is characterised by a particular perspective: it is broadly comparative, attempting to place human attributes into a wider, inter-specific context. Consequently, it is essentially a branch of evolutionary biology. The questions anthropologists ask relate to the function of particular features of humans and hominids, or, in other words, their selective advantage and survival value. With this basic interest anthropologists have tended to focus on large scale patterns of variation, and have sought explanations of this variation in terms of environmental factors and genetic considerations.

More immmediate clinical problems have inspired research in oral biology. Questions have been equally concerned with function, but in a more proximate context. Attention has thus focussed on the mechanisms underlying tooth formation, growth, development and use. From this field has come the understanding of the way in which the human masticatory system works.

The fusion of these two perspectives - proximate function and mechanisms and ultimate evolutionary and biological context - should be the basis for inter-disciplinary co-operation. Anthropologists have much to learn from oral biology about the complexity of the teeth which form such an important element of the skeletal and fossil record, while they in turn can perhaps contribute a longer term and broader perspective to our knowledge of human dental health. It is the aim of this volume to draw together some of these areas of common interest under the title Teeth and Anthropology.

## References

Biegert, J. (1981) Folia Primitalogica vol 35. Karger, Basel.

Boesen, P., Eriksen, J.H. and Helm, S. (1976) Timing of permanent tooth emergence in two Greenland Eskimo populations. Community Dental Oral Epidemiology 4: 244-247.

Boyde, A. (1976) Amelogenesis and the structure of enamel. In: Cohen, B. and Kramer, I.R.H. (eds.) Scientific Foundations of Dentistry: 335-352. William Heinemann Medical Books, London.

Boyde, A. and Martin, L. (1984) Primate enamel microstructure. In: Chivers, D., Wood, B.A. and Bilsborough, A. (eds.) Food Acquisition and Processing in Primates: 341-367. Plenum Press, New York.

Brace, C.L. (1962) Cultural factors in the evolution of the human dentition. In: Montagu, M.F.A. (ed.) Culture and the Evolution of Man. Oxford University Press, London.

Bromage, T.G. and Dean, M.C. (1985) Re-evaluation of the age at death of immature fossil hominids. Nature 317: 525-526.

Brothwell, D.R. (1965) Digging up Bones British Museum (Natural History), London.

Carbonell, V.N. (1963) Variations in the frequency of shovel shaped incisors in different populations. In: Brothwell, D.R. (ed.) Dental Anthropology: 211-35 Pergamon, London.

Covert, H.H. and Kay, R.F. (1981) Dental microwear and diet: implications for determining the feeding behaviours of extinct primates, with a comment on the dietary pattern of Sivapithecus. American Journal of Physical Anthropology 55: 331-336.

Cruwys, E. and Foley, R. (1986) Tooth size, dental arch dimension and crowding in populations from Newcastle and Bradford. Journal of Dental Research 65(4): 520.

Dahlberg, A.A. (1963) Analysis of the American Indian dentition. In: Brothwell, D.R. (ed.) Dental Anthropology: 149-78. Pergamon, London.

Darwin, C. (1871) Descent of Man Murray, London.

Gantt, D., Pillbeam, D. and Steward, D. (1977) Hominoid enamel prism patterns. Science 198:1155-1157.

Garn, S.M., Lewis, A.B. and Kerewsky, R.S. (1965) X-linked inheritance of tooth size. Journal of Dental Research 44: 439-441.

Garn, S.M., Lewis, A.B. and Kerewsky, R.S. (1966) Tooth size and body size in families. Archives of Oral Biology 12: 575-81.

Gordon, K.D. (1982) A study of microwear on chimpanzee molars: implications for dental microwear analysis. American Journal of Physical Anthropology 59: 195-215.

Gordon, D.K. and Walker, A.C. (1983) Playing 'possum: a microwear experiment. American Journal of Physical Anthropology 60: 109-112.

Grine, F.E. (1981) Trophic differences between 'gracile' and 'robust' australopithecines: a scanning electron microscope analysis of occlusal events. South African Journal of Sceince 77: 203-30.

Hrdlicka, A.A. (1920) Shovel shaped teeth. American Journal of Physical Anthropology 3: 429-65.

Hylander, W.L. (1977) The adaptive significance of Eskimo craniofacial morphology. In: Dahlberg and Graber (eds.) Orofacial Growth and Development. Mouton Press, The Hague.

Kay, R.F. (1981) The nut crackers - a new theory of the adaptations of Ramapithecinae. American Journal of Physical Anthropology 55: 141-151.

Koski, K. and Hautala, E. (1952) On the frequency of shovel shaped incisors in the Finns. American Journal of Physical Anthropology 10: 127.

Klevezal, G.A. and Kleinenberg, S.E. (1967) Age determinations of mammals by layered structure in teeth and bones. Translation by Israel Program for Scientific Translations Jerusalem 1969.

Lasker, G. (1950) Genetic analysis of racial traits of the teeth. Cold Spring Harbour Symposia on Quantitative Biology 15: 191.

Laws, R.M. (1952) A new method for age determination in mammals. Nature 169: 972-73.

Martin, L. (1985) Significance of enamel thickness in hominoid evolution. Nature 314: 260-263.

Moorrees, C. (1957) The Aleut Dentition. Harvard University Press. Cambridge, Mass.

Morris, P. (1978) The use of teeth for estimating the age of wild animals. In: Butler, P.M. and Joysey, K.A. (eds.) Development, Function and Evolution of Teeth. Academic Press, London.

Pedersen, P.O. (1949) The East Greenland dentition. Meddeleserom Grønland 142(3): 1-244.

Pedersen, P.O. (1955) Eine besondere Form der Abnutzung von Eskimozähnen aus Alaska. Deutsche Zahnärztliche Zeitschrift 10(1): 41-46.

Pilbeam, D. (1979) Recent finds and interpretations of Miocene hominoids. Annual Review of Anthropology 8: 333-52.

Ryan, A.S. (1979a) A preliminary scanning electron microscope examination of wear striation direction on primate teeth. Journal of Dental Research 58: 525-530.

Ryan, A.S. (1979b) Wear striation direction in primate teeth: a scanning electron microscope examination. American Journal of Physical Anthropology 50: 155-168.

Smith, B.G.N. and Knight, J.K. (1984) A compariosn of patterns of toothwear with aetiological factors. British Dental Journal 157(16): 16-19.

Vrba, E.S. and Grine, F.E. (1978a) Australopithecine enamel prism patterns. Science 202: 890-892.

Vrba, E.S. and Grine, F.E. (1978b) Analysis of South African australopithecine patterns. Proceedings of the Electron Microscopy Society of Southern Africa 8: 125-26.

Walker, A.C. (1981) Diet and teeth. Philosophical Transactions of the Royal Society of London (Series B) 292:57-64.

Walker, A.C., Hoeck, H.N. and Perez, L. (1978) Microwear of mammalian teeth as an indicator of diet. Science 201: 908-11.

Wolpoff, M.H. (1971) Metric trends in hominid dental evolution. Studies in Anthropology: Case Western Reserve University. Cleveland.

Wolpoff, M.H. (1978) Analogies and interpretations in palaeoanthropology. In: Jolly, C.J. (ed.) Early Hominids of Africa.

Wood, B.A. and Abbott, S.A. (1983) An analysis of the dental morphology of Plio-Pleistocene hominids. Journal of Anatomy 136: 198-219.

Y'edenak (1978) Culture, diet and dental reduction in mesolithic forager-fishers of Yugoslavia. Current Anthropology 93: 616-118.

# PART I

# THE BIOLOGY OF TEETH

Chapter 2

# TOOTH GROWTH AND STRUCTURE IN LIVING AND FOSSIL HOMINOIDS.

A.D. Beynon,

Department of Oral Biology
Dental School
Newcastle upon Tyne.

## INTRODUCTION

All dental tissues, including enamel, dentine and cementum, grow in a regular incremental manner, which can provide much information on tooth growth, and by inference, on growth of the animal in question. A major advantage of dental tissus is that they are not usually remodelled (except deciduous teeth) during life, unlike bone. Fully mineralised enamel, following enamel maturation (see below), is very highly mineralised at approximately 97% by weight and greater than 85% by volume, rendering it virtually fossilised from its date of completion. Dentine and cementum are dental examples of calcified connective tissues and are mineralised at about 70% and 50% by weight respectively. Dentine is penetrated by vast numbers of dentinal tubules ranging from 15,000/mm$^2$ in outer dentine to 65,000/mm$^2$ in inner dentine, which renders this tissue highy permeable, although with increasing age there is deposition of hypermineralised peritubular dentine within the original tubular space, thereby diminishing the permeability and even blocking it in certain instances. At the same time the deposition of this hypermineralised tissue increases the mineral level by weight of dentine. Cementum is comparable to bundle bone (bone of attachment), and is mineralised at similar levels. Cementum is usually thin on the coronal of the root and does not contain cells, whereas cementum in the apical part of the root is thick and contains cementocytes. Acellular cementum is relatively impermeable, although cellular cementum is permeable through the communicating channels linking cementocyte lacunae. Details of histology and patterns of growth of dental tissues are described in Bhaskar (1985).

## A. ENAMEL

In enamel there are two separate manifestations of incremental growth with differing periodicities. Enamel is laid down in successive waves, eccentrically outwards on the crown of the tooth. Disturbances or re-adjustments within cells forming enamel cause an interuption in enamel formation, which corresponds to the surface of the enamel formed at the time of the interuption (see Figs. 2.1a, b, c). These lines are called striae of Retzius and they are broadly analogous to growth rings in trees, with the two exceptions:-

(i) they grow outwards on only one half of the tooth surface (on the other surface dentine is forming in a comparable manner)

(ii) enamel formation begins at the cusp tip and layers are laid down successively from the enamel-dentine junction outwards, i.e. layers 1-1'

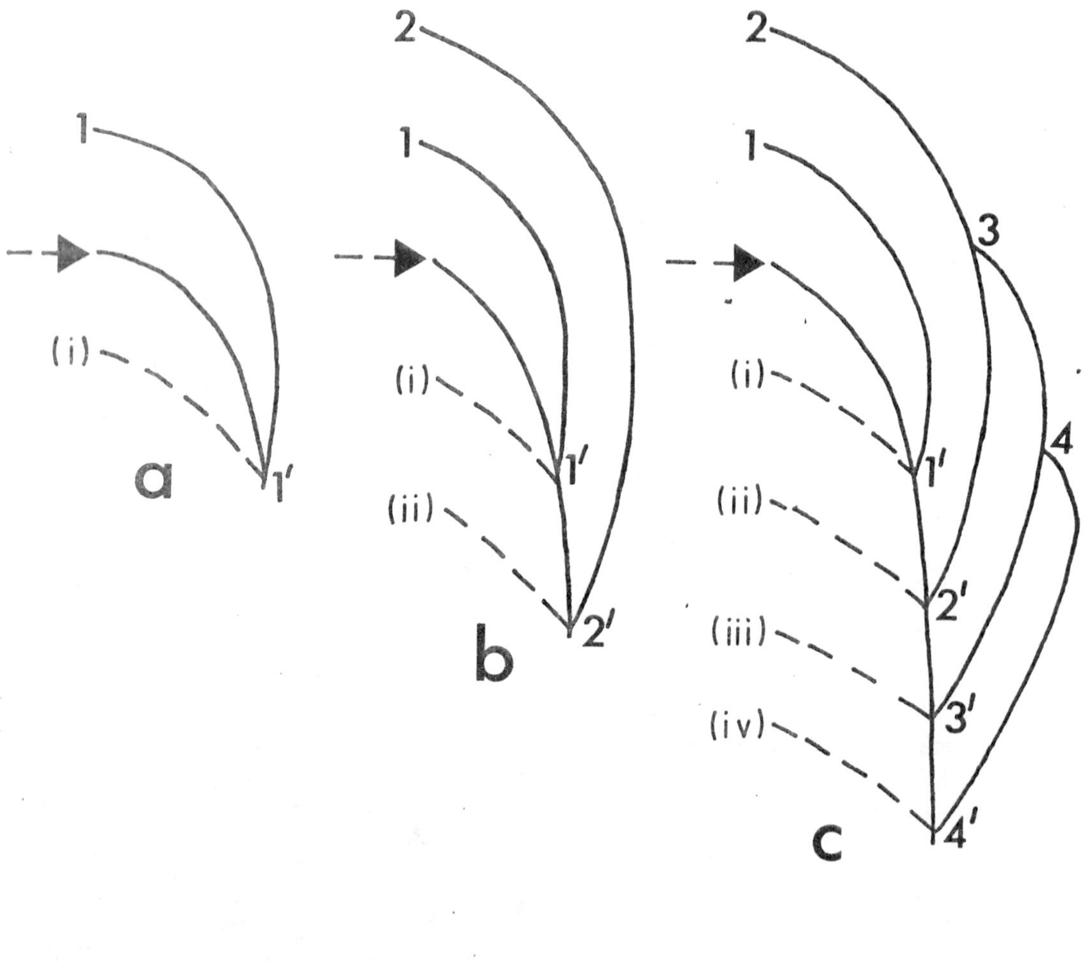


Figure 2.1. Shows successive increments of enamel (and dentine). Arrows denote enamel-dentine junction, at same level across three figs. Layers 1-1', 2-2' etc. represent successive enamel increments, 'buried' lines correspond to striae. Layers (i), (ii) etc. represent dentine increments, 'buried' lines corresponding to lines of Owen.

and 2-2' in Figure 2.1a and b, until the full thickness of enamel is formed at that site.

Subsequently, further increments which are necessary both to increase the width of the enamel on the lateral margins of the crown, and also to extend the height of the crown, are deposited eccentrically in the manner illustrated in Fig. 2.1c. The earliest growth lines in the occulusal enamel are buried (i.e. 1-1', Fig. 2.), whereas growth lines reach the surfaces of the enamel on the sides of the tooth (Fig. 1c, Fig. 2.2), producing alternating depressions. These correspond to the ends of striae, separated by elevations called perikymata (Risnes, 1984) which appear as transverse bands (open arrow Fig. 2.2) on the surface of recently erupted teeth.

The basic structural unit of enamel is the prism, which runs from the enamel-dentine junction in a near perpendicular direction to the enamel surface, transverse to the striae of Retzius. Enamel prisms show a short period cross-striation repeat interval of 4-8um in primate enamel, which is believed to reflect daily increments of enamel growth (Boyde, 1976). Shellis (1984) has described a method of measuring crown extension rates, derived from slopes of striae, in modern deciduous and permanent teeth. He showed that the enamel extension rate varied with distance from the cusp along the enamel-dentine junction in permanent teeth, with an earlier rate being higher on tall cusps. In deciduous teeth the rate appears to be fairly constant, although the extension rate is approximately five times greater in deciduous than in permanent teeth. He concludes that the rate of extension may have an effect upon the ameloblast secretory area and influence prism size.

There is evidence in the literature that the spacing between cross striations and striae of Retzius is relatively constant (Gustafson & Gustafson, 1967; Poole, 1967) showing a consistent pattern of between 5 & 10 cross striations between adjacent striae of Retzius. This averages 7-8, suggesting that striae are formed with a periodicity of 7-8 days, a theory confirmed by Newman & Poole (1974). This independence of the two incremental patterns of formation of enamel are diagrammatically illustrated in Figure 2.2, in which rates of daily increments (cross striations) of enamel formation are the same in Figs. 2.2a and 2.2b, but the rates of crown extension are faster in Fig. 2.2b, in which the slope of striae at the enamel dentine junction is shallower than in Fig. 2.2a. The diagrams shows that the time it takes to complete the crown in a tooth forming with a slow extension rate (Fig. 2.2a) will be longer than in teeth with a fast extension rate (Fig. 2.2b), although the daily incremental rate and enamel thickness may be the same. Beynon & Wood (1985; Beynon & Wood in press) have presented evidence in East African fossil hominids that the rate of crown coverage is faster in Australopithecus boisei than in early Homo.

A further expression of this pattern of enamel growth is the manifestation of growth lines on the surface of enamel in the form of perikymata. Perikymata are visible in recently erupted (unworn) human permanent and fossil hominid incisors, although they are absent in human deciduous teeth and in pongid incisors. Bromage & Dean (1985) have recently shown that it is possible by counting the number of perikymata, giving allowance for incisal 'buried' increments, to arrive at an estimate of the crown completion time assuming an average 7 days interval between striae of Retzius. Their results suggest that crown formation times of incisors in East African and South African hominids, including specimens

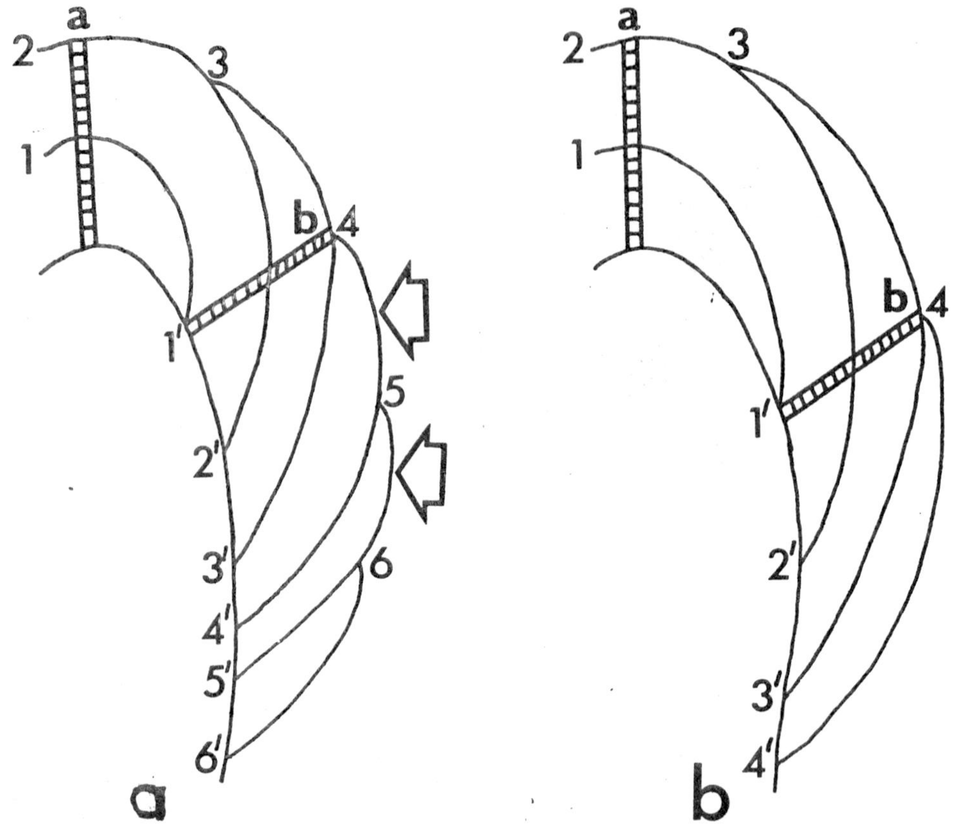


Figure 2.2. Diagram illustrating effect of slow (2a) and fast (2b) crown extension rates. Daily prism secretory rates are similar (cross hatched lines a & b represent prisms with 7 day periodicity, crossing striae), and final enamel thickness is the same. Open arrows indicate perikymata.

attributed to early Homo, are appreciably shorter than in modern man, resembling modern great apes more closely. Preliminary studies on East African hominids confirm this finding (Beynon, in preparation). These findings are of interest since they suggest that the characteristic prolongation of the growth period known in modern humans had not yet begun.

Enamel forms in two distinct stages, the first stage being the production of enamel matrix which is mineralised at around 30% by volume, which is succeeded by a prolonged maturation period when the mineral levels are increased to their final level of 97% by weight. Disturbances may occur during enamel formation which, if they affect the early matrix production stge, will cause a deficiency in the amount of enamel formed, giving rise to hypoplastic enamel, which typically encircles the tooth crown and will be present on all teeth that are forming at the time of the disturbance. Hypoplastic enamel is usually deficient in quantity, but may be fully mineralised. Illnesses which give rise to fevers, including viral infections, commonly give rise to enamel defects of this kind (chronological hypoplasia), which will be present at different levels on the teeth forming at different stages during the time of the injury. Disturbances in diet, vitamin intake and hormone balance may also influence tooth development (review Jenkins, 1978). Such defects in archaeological material would be relatively permeable and would bind 'foreign' ions and extrinsic staining. Examples of chronological hypoplasia in early Homo material, which are more consistent with modern pongid rather than modern Homo dental chronology, have been noted in East African hominids (Beynon, in preparation).

Enamel thickness It has been recognised for many years that hominoid enamel is thick, although the evidence for this until recently has been based on qualitative assessment of wear patterns (i.e. Simons & Pilbeam, 1972). The significance of thick enamel has been discussed extensively in relation to hominoid evolution (Key, 1981). Martin (1983, 1985) has provided quantitative information on enamel thickness in Miocene hominoids, including Sivapithecus, Ramapithecus, and modern pongid and human material. The only previous author to provide quantitative evidence in fossil hominids was Robinson (1956) who measured enamel thickness in only 6 molars of Paranthropus. Our studies (Beynon & Wood, 1985; Beynon & Wood, 1986, in press) on fractured surfaces in East African Homo and robust Australopithecines show that robust Australopithecines have thicker enamel than early Homo and this difference remains significant after correction for body size.

Enamel Prism Shape Early reports by Gantt et al (1977) reported that enamel prism shape was circular or hexagonal (pattern I), although this was disputed by Vrba & Grine (1978). These findings have been reviewed by Boyde & Martin (1984a) in an exhaustive study on primate enamel microstructure, who showed that prism shape in hominoids is predominantly arcade shaped (pattern 3). Pattern 3 enamel has been described in Paranthropus boisei (Boyde & Martin, 1984b) and in A. boisei and early Homo (Beynon, in preparation).

Enamel Prism Decussation Enamel prisms do not follow a straight course from the enamel-dentine junction to the periphery but follow a sinusoidal course as they pass out through the enamel. Kawai (1955) surveyed decussation patterns in primate enamel and Shellis & Poole (1977) discussed the possible significance of decussation in primate enamel. They commented that there was relatively little enamel decussation in gorilla enamel, although this has been subsequently disputed by Boyde & Martin (1984a). Beynon & Wood have presented observations on enamel prism decussation in East African hominids (1985; in press) in Australopithecus boisei and early Homo. Enamel prism decussation appeared to be very limited in robust australopithecine enamel.

## B. DENTINE

Dentine is formed incrementally inwards from the enamel-dentine junction towards the pulp, with longer period incremental lines of Owen (which probably correspond to striae of Retzius), and shorter period incremental lines of von Ebner (which may correspond to cross striations in enamel). Kawasaki et al (1977) described patterns of incremental growth in dentine and orientation of Owen lines in modern human teeth. Dean & Wood (1981) showed a very shallow slope of contour lines of Owen in pongid teeth, which is similar to the pattern observed in deciduous teeth, in which the roots form quickly. Dean (1985) has presented evidence that early Homo (KNM-ER 820) had a foreshortened period of root growth compared with modern man.

## C. CEMENTUM

Growth lines in human and hominoid cementum have been studied relatively little, although annual cemental annulations have been described in primates (references Stott et al, 1982). These authors have reported that annual growth rings can be identified in modern human teeth.

I have found it very difficult to identify chronological incremental lines in cementum, even when using calcified tissue markers including tetracycline. Lines are present, but are inconsistent, and may be very closely spaced in acellular cementum, which is the least unfavourable measuring site. Cementum deposition is a functional adaptation for the re-attachment of periodontal fibres following tooth movement, and continues throughout life. Following the inital rapid phase of active tooth movement, the tooth continues to migrate occlusally in the juvenile animal until jaw growth is complete, and continues to move in the adult to compensate for occlusal and interstitial wear; this process is likely to vary markedly between individuals and populations, being influenced by numerous factors including strength of bite, masticatory cycles and habits, and diet consistency and abrasivity.

## REFERENCES

Beynon, A.D. & Wood, B.A. (1985). The enamel of the posterior dentition of East African fossil hominids. J. Anat. 140: 534-536.

Beynon, A.D. & Wood, B.A. (in press). Variation in enamel thickness and structure in East African hominids. Am. J. Phys. Anthropol.

Bhaskar, S.N. (1985). Orbans Oral Histology & Embryology, 10th Ed. Mosby, St. Louis.

Boyde, A. (1976). Amelogenesis and the structure of enamel. In 'Scientific Foundations of Dentistry'. Ed. B. Cohen & L.R.H. Dramer, Heinemann, London : pp. 335-352.

Boyde, A. & Martin, L. (1984a). The microstructure of primate dental enamel. In: 'Food Acquisition and Processing in Primates'. Edited by J. Chivers, B.A. Wood & A.B. Bilsborough, Plenum, New York: pp. 341-367.

Boyde, A. & Martin, L. (1984b). A non-destructive survey of prism packing patterns in primate enamels. In: 'Tooth Enamel IV'. Edited by R.W. Fearnhead & S. Suga. Elsevier, Amsterdam: pp. 417-421.

Bromage, T.G. & Dean, M.C. (1985). Re-evaluation of the age at death of immature fossil hominids. Nature 317: 525-527.

Dean, M.C. (1985). Variation in the developing root core angle of the permanent mandibular teeth of modern man and certain fossil hominids. Am .J. Phys. Anthropol. 68: 233-238.

Dean, M.C. & Wood, B.A. (1981). Developing pongid dentition and its use for ageing individual crania in comparative cross-sectional growth studies. Folia Primatol, 36: 111-127.

Gantt, D.G., Pilbeam, D. & Steward, G.P. (1977). Hominoid enamel prism patterns. Science 198: 1155-1157.

Gustafson, G. & Gustafson, A.G. (1967). Microanatomy and histochemistry of enamel. In: 'Structural and Chemical Organisation of Teeth II'. Edited by A.E.W. Miles. Academic Press, London: pp. 75-134.

Jenkins, G.N. (1978). The Physiology & Biochemistry of the Mouth. Blackwell, Oxford.

Kawai, N. (1955). Comparative anatomy of the Bands of Schreger Okajimas Folia Anat. Japan. 27: 115-131.

Kawasaki, K, Tanaka, S. & Ishikawa, T. (1977). On the incremental lines of human dentine as revealed by tetracycline labelling. J. Anat. 123: 426-436.

Kay, R.F. (1981). The nut-crackers - a new theory of the adaptions of the Ramapithecinae. Am. J. Phys. Anthropol. 55: 141-151.

Martin, L.B. (1983). The relationships of the later Miocene Hominoidea. Ph.D. Thesis, University of London.

Martin, L.B. (1985). Significance of enamel thickness in hominoid evolution. Nature 314: 260-263.

Newman, H.N. & Poole (1974). Observations with scanning and transmission electron microscopy on the structure of human enamel surface. Archs. Oral Biol. 19: 1135-1143.

Poole, D.F.G. (1967). Phylogeny of tooth tissue: enameloid and enamel in recent vertebrates, with a note on the history of cementum. In: 'Structural & Chemical Organisation of Teeth I. Edited by A.E.W. Miles. Academic Press, London: pp. 111-149.

Risnes, S. (1984). Rationale for consistency in the use of enamel surface terms: perikymata and imbrications. Scand. J. Dent. Res. 92: 1-5.

Robinson, J.T. (1956). The dentition of the Australopithecinae. Trans. Mus. Mem. No. 9.

Shellis, R.P. (1984). Variations in growth of the enamel crown in human teeth and a possible relationship between growth and enamel structure. Archs. Oral Biol. 29: 697-705.

Shellis, R.P. & Poole, D.F.G. (1977). The calcified dental tissues of Primates. In: 'Evolutionary changes to the Primate Skull and Dentition'. Edited by L.L.B. Lavelle, R.P. Shellis & D.F.G. Poole. Thomas, Illinios: pp. 197-279.

Simons, E.L. & Pilbeam, D.R. (1972). Hominid paleoprimatology. In: 'The Functional and Evolutionary Biology of Primates'. Edited by R. Tuttle. Aldine, Chicago: pp. 36-62.

Stott, G.G., Sis, R.F. & Levy, B.M. (1982). Cemental annulation as an age criterion in forensic dentistry. J. Dent. Res. 61: 814-817.

Vrba, E.S. & Grine, F.E. (1978). Australopithecine enamel prism patterns. Science 202: 890-892.

## Chapter 3

## DENTAL ENAMEL - A LIVING FOSSIL.

C. Robinson, J. Kirkham, J.A. Weatherell & M. Strong

MRC Dental Tissues Research Group
Department Oral Biology
School of Dentistry
University of Leeds

### INTRODUCTION

Biological tissues which have provided the greatest amount of archaeological information about man and other mammals are invariably those which have the greatest potential for surivival *post mortem*. Almost inevitably therefore attention has been focussed on the skeleton. Skeletal material itself however is variable in its capacity for archaeological survival. Compact cortical bone for example survives much more frequently than spicules of trabecular bone, dentine survives better than cortical bone and enamel more effectively than either.

This survival depends on the ability of the tissue to withstand chemical and physical change. Broadly this ability rests with the tissue's propensity to resist degradation by, for example, acids and bases in the burial environment and penetration of extraneous material into the tissue.

In this respect all calcified tissues derived from man are very poor since the calcium phosphate phase they contain, hydroxyapatite, is well known for its capacity to take up and accumulate other ions into its crystal lattice. The most obvious of these is fluoride, but aluminium, lead, tin, sulphate and a whole range of other ions can accumulate within the hydroxyapatite lattice (Losee *et al*., 1974, Weatherell and Robinson, 1982).

With this in mind, tissues which exhibit low porosity and high physical density will obviously be least susceptible to alteration by their surrounding *post mortem* matrix. Dental enamel is by far the hardest, most dense and most highly calcified of the mammalian tissues (Fig. 3.1) and because of this has the greatest potential to provide historical data about the period of tissue formation and its subsequent functional period in the oral cavity. Such data, however, requires a sound understanding of the chemistry of enamel formation and its subsequent behaviour in the oral environment.

The intention behind this presentation is to outline the chemistry of enamel formation and describe the composition of the final mature tissue and its behaviour in the oral environment.

### Developing enamel

Enamel development occurs via a series of visibly and chemically distinct stages (Robinson *et al*., 1978). These are summarised in Fig. 3.2.

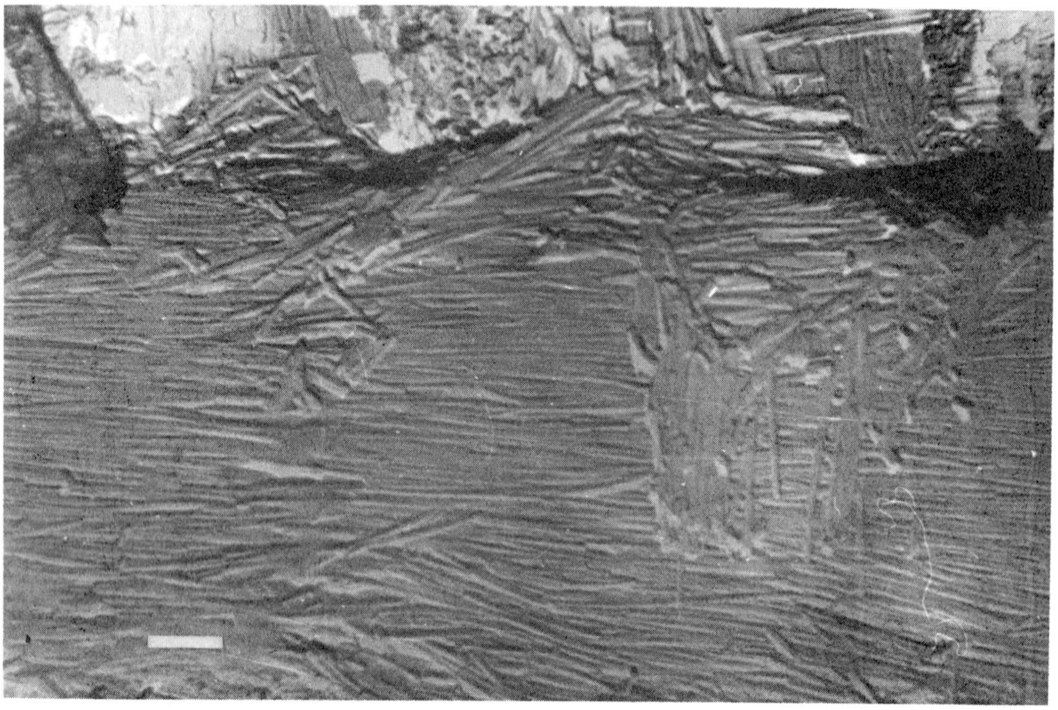

Figure 3.1. T.E.M. appearance of freeze-fractured rat incisor enamel taken from the maturation stage (stage 3). The crystallites are closely packed, with no apparent intercrystalline material.
White bar = 24000A.

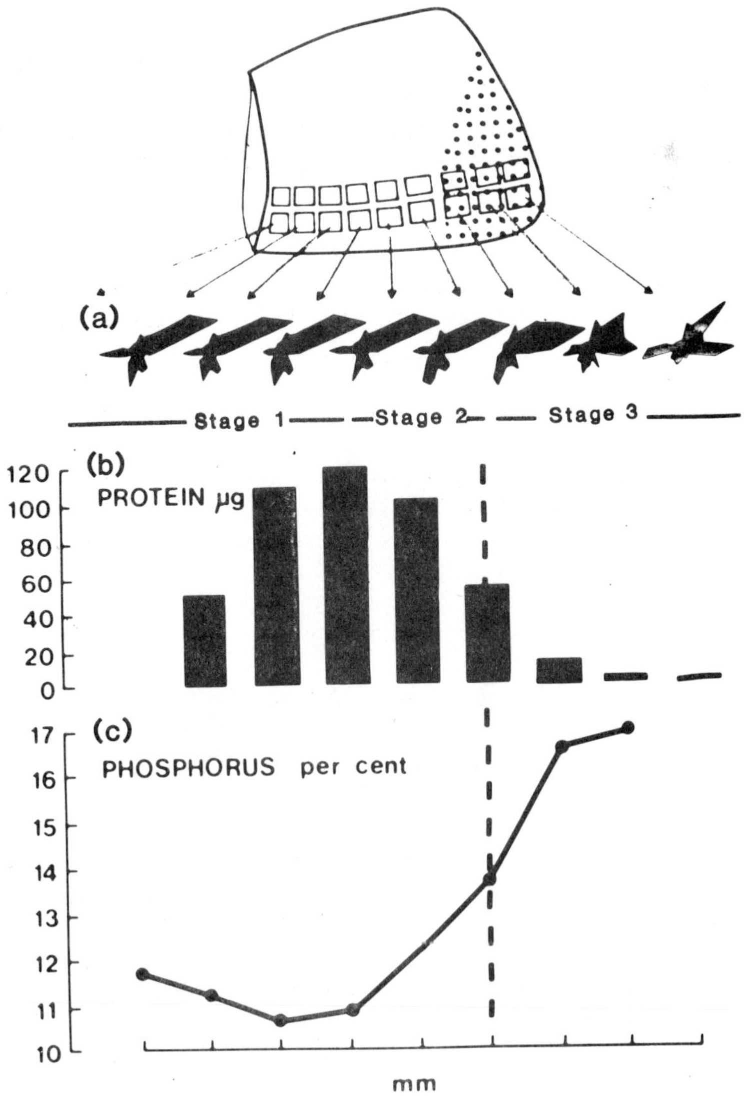


Figure 3.2. Changes in enamel chemistry at each developmental stage of a developing deciduous bovine tooth.

(a) Changes in amino acid composition (shown as rose diagrams, Robinson et al., 1975) of enamel matrix proteins at each stage of development.

(b) Changes in protein content of enamel from each developmental stage. Protein content can be seen to increase initially with enamel thickness during secretion then fall to very low levels in the maturation stage (stage 3).

(c) Changes in mineral content, expressed as %P, of enamel from each stage of developent.

Phosphorus concentrations can be seen to increase in the maturation stage (stage 3).

Robinson and Kirkham (1985). Proc. Royal Soc. Health (In press).

1. Secretion

A complex protein framework (Fincham, 1971, Seyer and Glimcher, 1977, Robinson et al., 1977a, 1982a) is laid down which dictates the micro-architecture of the tissue and organises the deposition and growth of the inorganic phase i.e. the crystals of hydroxyapatite.

2. Transition

Secretion of protein ceases and replacement of matrix protein by tissue fluid becomes apparent. (Hiller et al., 1975, Robinson et al., 1977b, 1978, 1982a).

3. Maturation

Almost all of the protein matrix is lost (Deakins, 1942, Burgess and Maclaren, 1965, Robinson et al., 1978, 1980) and more calcium and phosphate enters the porous tissue to replace fluid (Hiller et al., 1975, Robinson et al., 1980).

4. Mature tissue

The porosity generated by loss of organic matrix is finally occluded by growth of hydroxyapatite crystals to occupy almost the entire tissue volume (Hiller et al., 1975, Robinson et al., 1984).

The largely proteinaceous nature of stages 1 and 2, while crucially important from a biological viewpoint, makes them unlikely to survive for any length of time post mortem due to chemical and biological degradation.

Maturing enamel (stage 3) on the other hand, although porous, is quite well mineralised (Hiller et al., 1975) and could therefore persist long after the protein has disappeared.

Maturing enamel is also known to accumulate extraneous materials, such as magnesium (McCann and Bullock, 1957, Robinson et al., 1984) and fluoride (Weatherell et al., 1975), during tooth development in vivo and could conceivably provide data about physiological or even dietary conditons during life. The fact that it is porous, however, would render it susceptible to post portem alterations related to the burial environment. Unless well protected in the bony crypt of the jaw, interpretation of chemical information would be extremely difficult.

In addition, the relative position and size of these developmental zones could provide some indication of the age of the individual at death.

## Enamel in the mature human tooth

Dental enamel is the most highly mineralised (80% by volume calcium phosphate) (Hiller et al., 1975), the hardest (3 on the Moh scale) and most dense ( $\sim$ 3gm/cc) (Weatherell et al., 1967) of the calcified tissues. Little penetration of the intact tissue occurs in vivo, most reactions being confined to the tissue surface.

However, the composition of the tissue is not uniform. There are

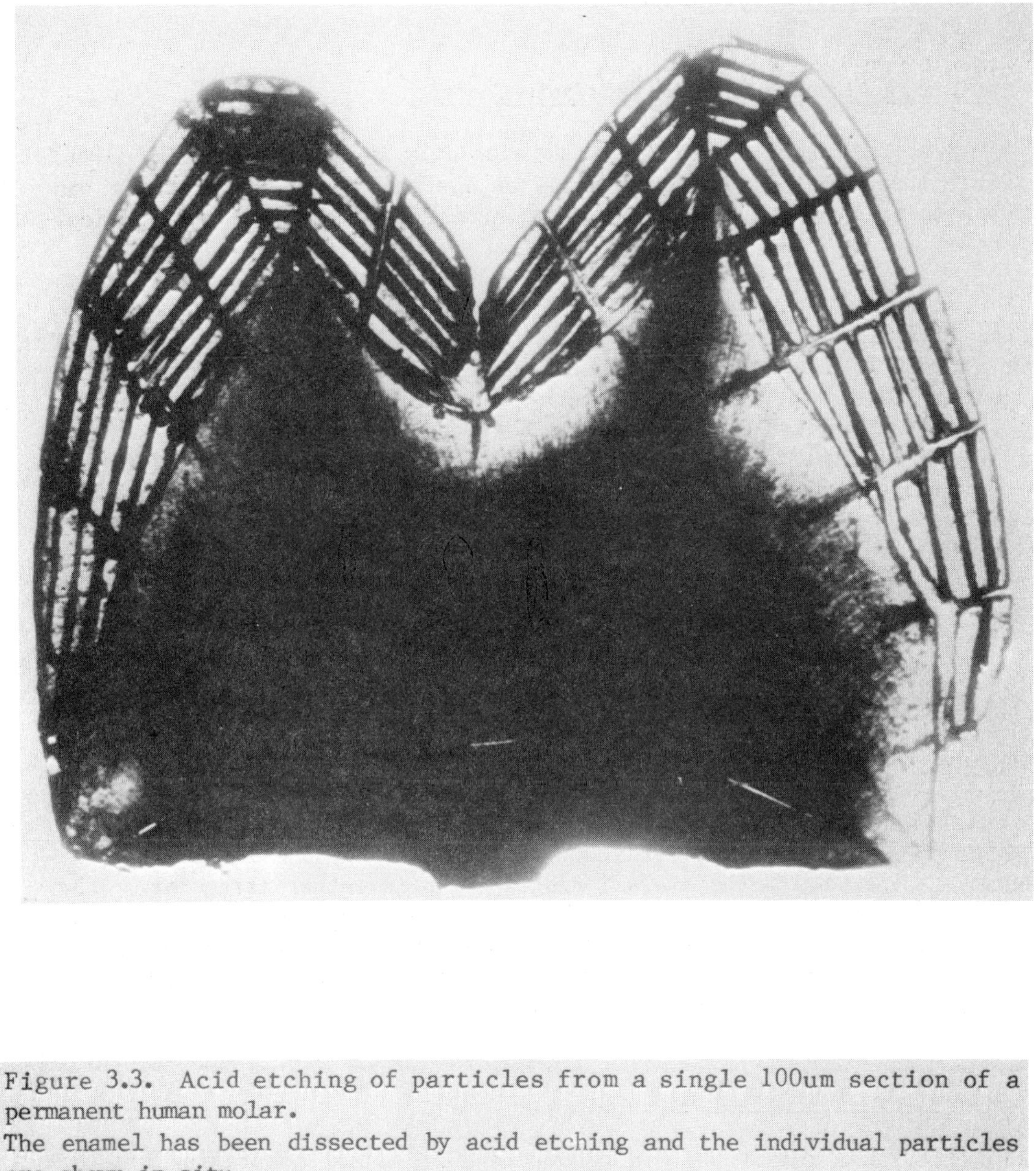

Figure 3.3. Acid etching of particles from a single 100um section of a permanent human molar.
The enamel has been dissected by acid etching and the individual particles are shown *in situ*.
Weatherell *et al*., (1967). Caries Res. 1: 42-51.

distinct patterns in the content and distribution of both mineral and organic phases as well as the physical properties of the tissue (Weatherell et al., 1974). Fundamental knowledge of this nature is an essential prerequisite to provide a baseline for understanding any alterations which might result in post mortem changes.

1) Mineral Density and Calcium Phosphate Content

Using an acid etching procedure developed by Weatherell et al., (1966) to sample the enamel at different sites on a single tooth (Fig. 3.3) it has been possible to create contour maps of enamel chemistry and its physical properties.

The density of the tissue decreases from the tooth surface towards the dentine fairly regularly (Angmar et al., 1963; Weatherell et al., 1966), as shown in Fig. 3.4. There are often, however, pockets of low density near the dentine and beneath the tooth cusps. Calcium (Fig. 3.5) and phosphorus (Fig. 3.6) distribution also decreases towards the dentine but in a much less regular fashion (Robinson et al., 1982b). Once again pockets of low mineral content occur beneath the fissures and immediately beneath the enamel cusps. The irregularity of calcium and phosphorus distribution, when compared with density, probably reflects the fact that density, unlike calcium and phosphorus is a compound parameter of mineral, space, water and protein.

2) Protein content and distribution

Mature enamel contains only very small ( $\sim$ 1%) amounts of protein (Burgess and Maclaren, 1965, Weatherell et al., 1968a). Much of this is highly insoluble and is distributed close to the dentine, although pockets of higher concentration are often found in the region of the enamel fissures as shown in Fig. 3.7. The overall distribution is rather irregular. The high insolubility of this organic material (Robinson et al., 1975) and its presence in such a dense, impenetrable tissue raises the possibility of isolating unchanged organic material fron tissues of considerable archaeological age (Doberenz et al., 1969).

3) Carbonate content and distribution

Carbonate is a relatively minor component of enamel comprising 1-4% by weight. The concentration rises from the tooth surface towards the dentine in a fairly regular way (Little and Brudevold, 1958, Weatherell et al., 1968b, Fig. 3.8). The reason for this pattern of distribution is unclear but Weatherell and Robinson, (1973) suggested that it is a reflection of $pCO_2$ in the environment of the enamel-forming cells during tissue development. Carbonate confers considerable acid-lability on the enamel (Sobel, 1960), and enamels with high carbonate content would not be expected to survive under conditions of low pH. Interior enamel is, in this regard, much more acid soluble than the outer, carbonate poor, denser and more highly mineralised tissue.

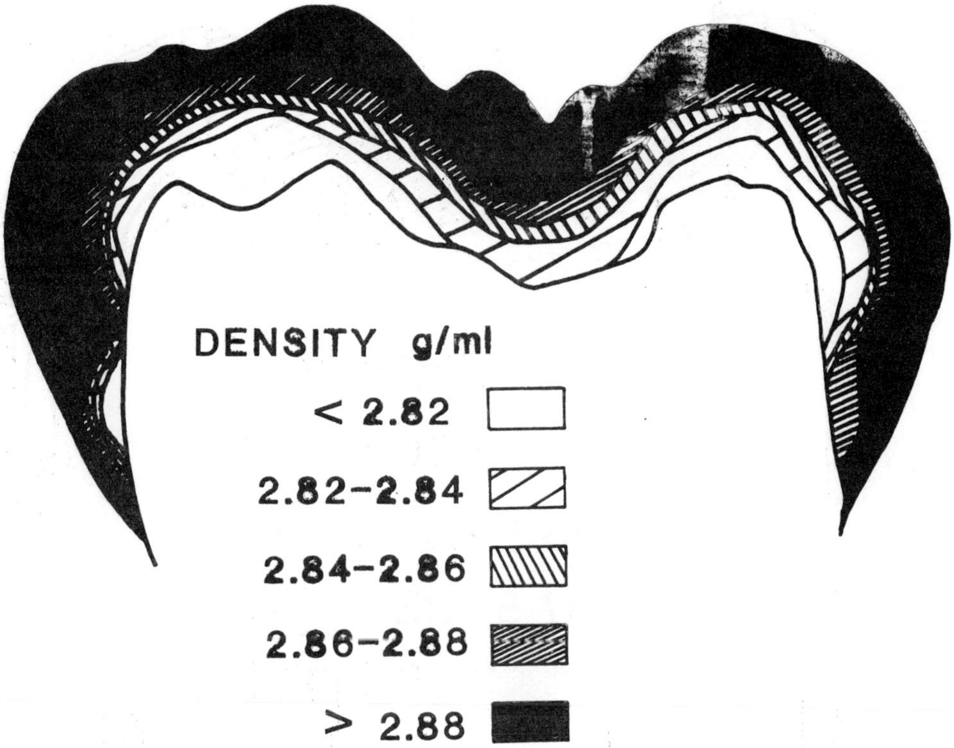


Figure 3.4. Variations in Density in a single section of permanent human molar enamel.
Regions of highest density can be seen at the enamel surface decreasing towards the inner enamel at the junction within the dentine.

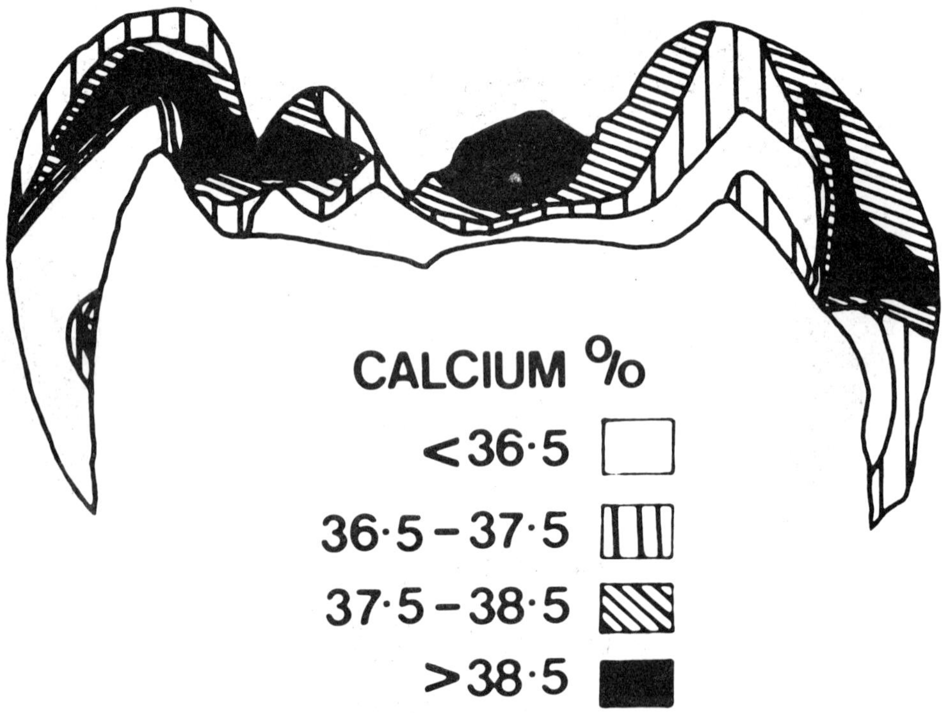


Figure 3.5. Distribution of Calcium in a single section of permanent human molar enamel.
Calcium concentration can be seen generally to increase from the interior of the enamel at the junction with the dentine to the outer enamel at the tooth surface.

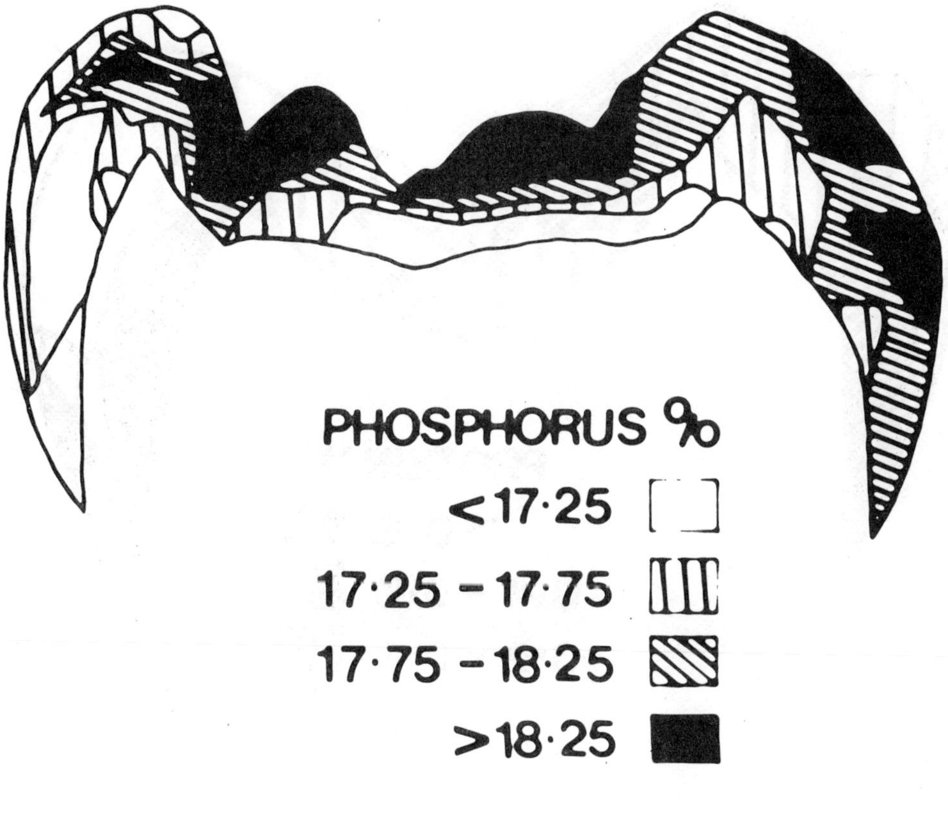


Figure 3.6. Distribution of Phosphorus in a single section of human molar enamel.
The distribution pattern can be seen to be very similar to that of calcium, with highest concentrations of phosphorus tending to be located in the outer enamel at the tooth surface.

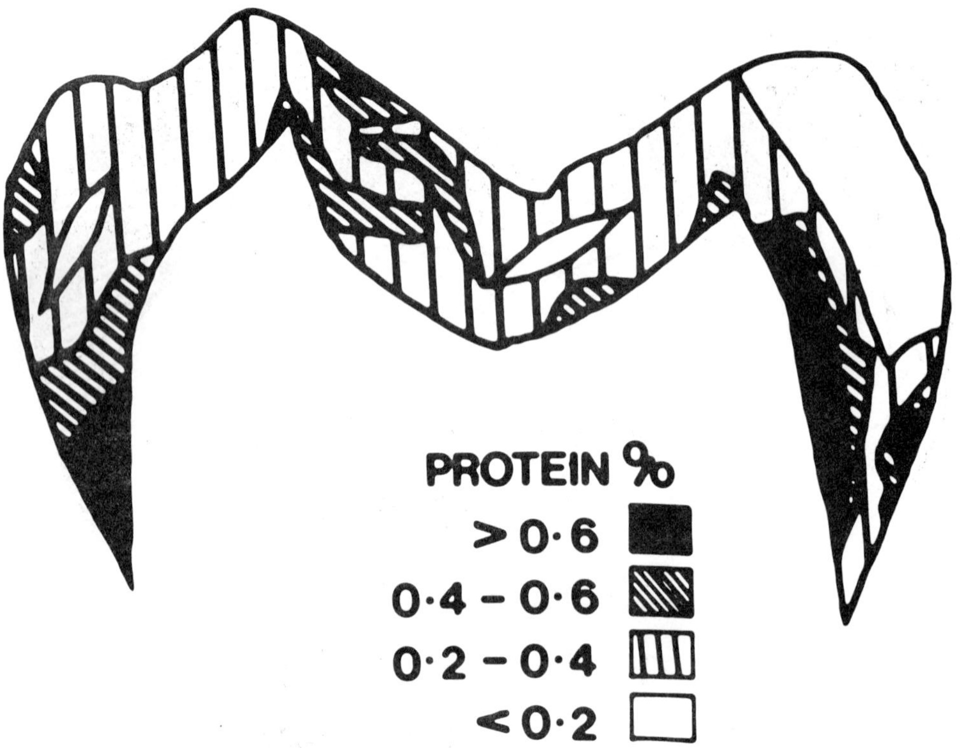


Figure 3.7. Distribution of Protein in a single section of human molar enamel.
Relatively high concentrations of protein can be seen in inner enamel, towards the cervical margin and in the fissure region.
Robinson et al., (1981). In: Demineralisation and Remineralisation of the Teeth. Ed. Leach, S.A. and Edgar, W.M. IRL Press, pp. 209–223.

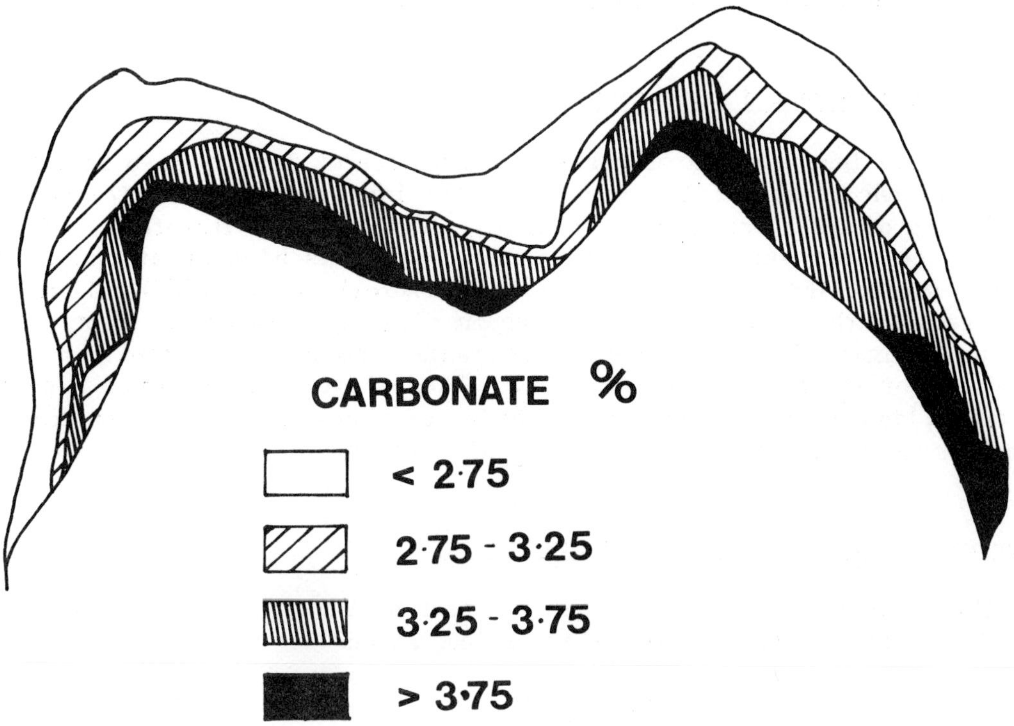


Figure 3.8. Distribution of Carbonate in a single section of human molar enamel.
Carbonate concentrations can be seen to decrease from the interior of the enamel at the junction with the dentine to the outer enamel at the tooth surface.
Robinson et al., (1981). In: Demineralisation and Remineralisation of the Teeth. Ed. Leach, S.A. and Edgar, W.M. IRL Press, pp. 209-223.

4) Magnesium content and distribution

There is much less magnesium in enamel compared with carbonate i.e. 0.1-0.4% (Robinson et al., 1981). Although the distribution pattern is similar in that magnesium concentrations rise towards the interior of the tissue it is a little more irregular than carbonate showing distinct pockets of relatively high magnesium concentrations near the dentine, in the cuspal regions and in the fissure enamel (see Fig. 3.9). In this respect magnesium resembles protein distribution (Fig. 3.7) and it is tempting to speculate that it may in some way be associated with residual organic matrix in the less dense regions of enamel. A high magnesium content is also associated with an increase in enamel solubility (Bachra et al., 1965).

5) Fluoride content distribution

Fluoride in enamel is of particular importance, largely as a result of the fact that it is avidly taken up by the hydroxyapatite lattice and in doing so produces a more stable material. Its uptake is therefore confined largely to tooth surfaces. Its concentration is highest at the outer enamel surface (Brudevold et al., 1956, Weatherell et al., 1972) falling to a plateau in the interior, to rise again slightly towards the dentine as shown in Figure 3.10. Concentrations range from a few hundred ppm to a thousand or so at the outer surface. These levels can be much higher, however, depending on the concentration of fluoride in the diet during development (Fig. 3.11) (Weatherell et al., 1973).

## Changes in erupted enamel in the oral cavity

The most visible alterations which occur during life are physical wear and destruction of the enamel due to carious attack.

1. Wear

Considerable tooth wear can occur such that interior enamel and even dentine may be exposed to the oral environment.

Chemical analysis of the outer surface of such severely worn teeth revealed basic chemical patterns characteristic of inner tissue (Fig. 3.12) i.e. low mineral content and high levels of carbonate and magnesium (Weatherell et al., 1971). This indicates that no alteration of the intrinsic patterns built into the tissue during tooth development takes place due to the oral environment. Analysis of the extreme outer surface with regard to fluoride has indicated that even moderate to slight wear will remove the fluoride-rich outer surface (Fig. 3.13). This can occur due to contact with the soft tissues of the buccal mucosa as well as occlusal surfaces with tooth/tooth contact (Weatherell et. al., 1973). Accumulation of fluoride during the life of the tooth may occur in certain locations i.e. between teeth and near the gum margin. These protected sites, as well as not being subject to wear also harbour bacteria which are known to facilitate fluoride uptake into the surface which they have colonised.

2. Dental Caries

Destruction of the enamel, and eventually the underlying dentine, by

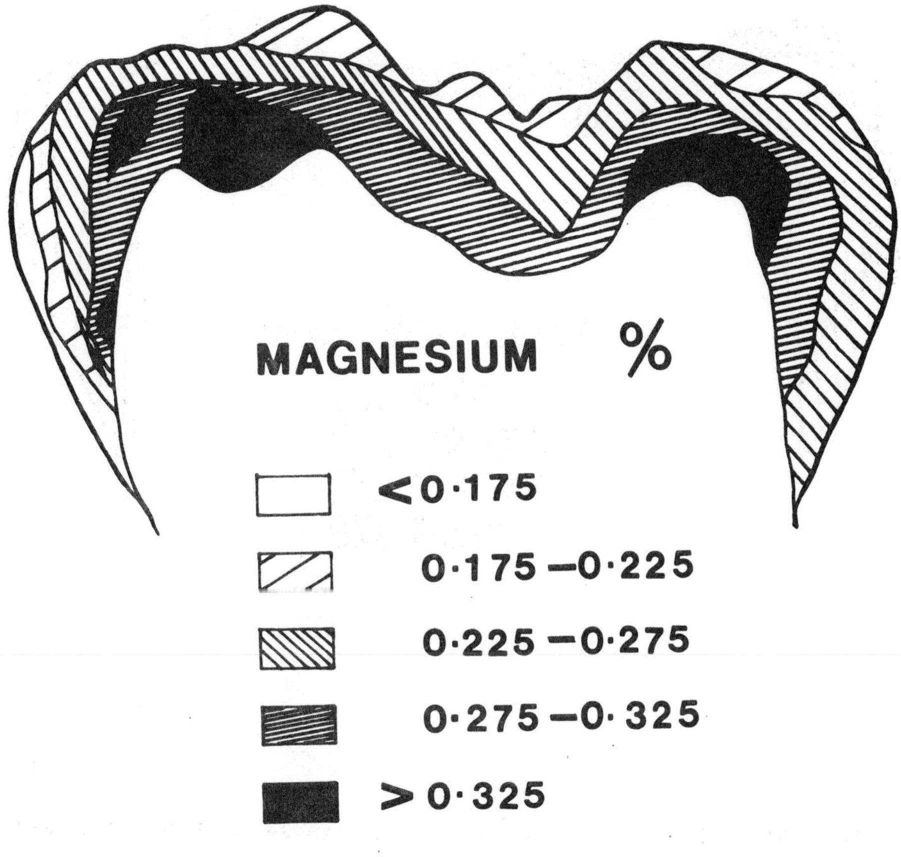


Figure 3.9. Distribution of Magnesium in a single section of human molar enamel.
Magnesium concentrations can be seen to decrease from the interior of the enamel at the junction with the dentine to the outer enamel at the tooth surface.

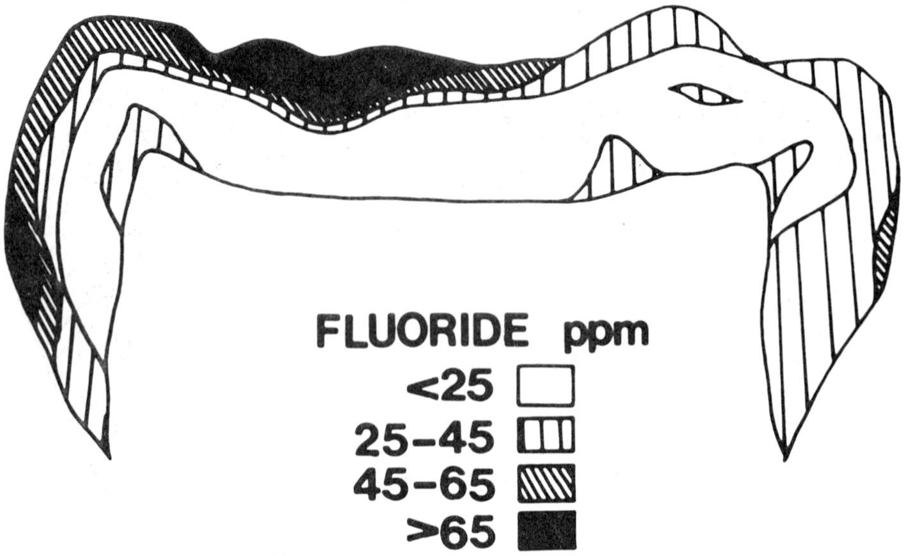


Figure 3.10. Distribution of Fluoride in a single section of human molar enamel.
Fluoride concentrations can be seen to be highest at the enamel surface falling to a plateau in the interior and rising slightly again at the junction with the dentine.
Weatherell, J.A. (1975), The British Medical Bulletin, 31, (2): 117.

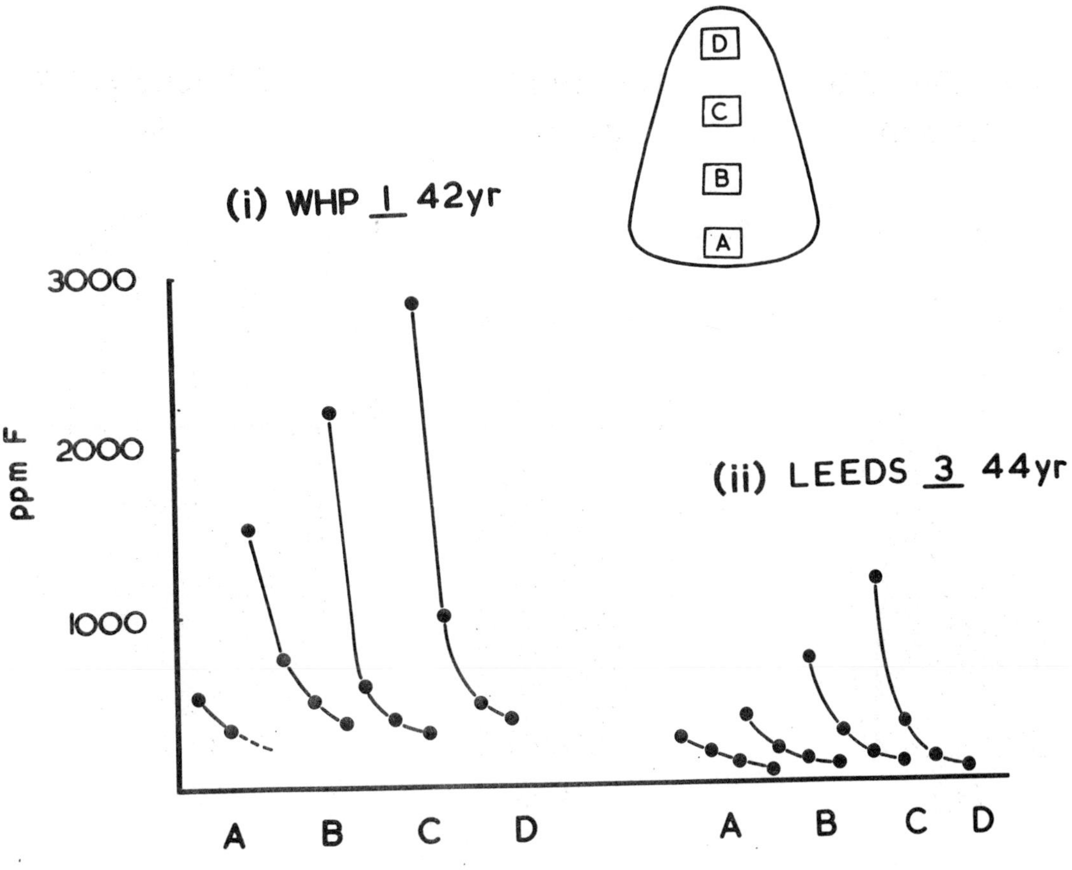


Figure 3.11. Effect of diet on enamel fluoride concentrations.
Fluoride distribution from surface to interior in enamel from different sites of human mandibular incisors from a resident of West Hartlepool (fluoride content of drinking water 1.9 ppm) compared with a resident of Leeds (fluroide content of drinking water 0.1 ppm).

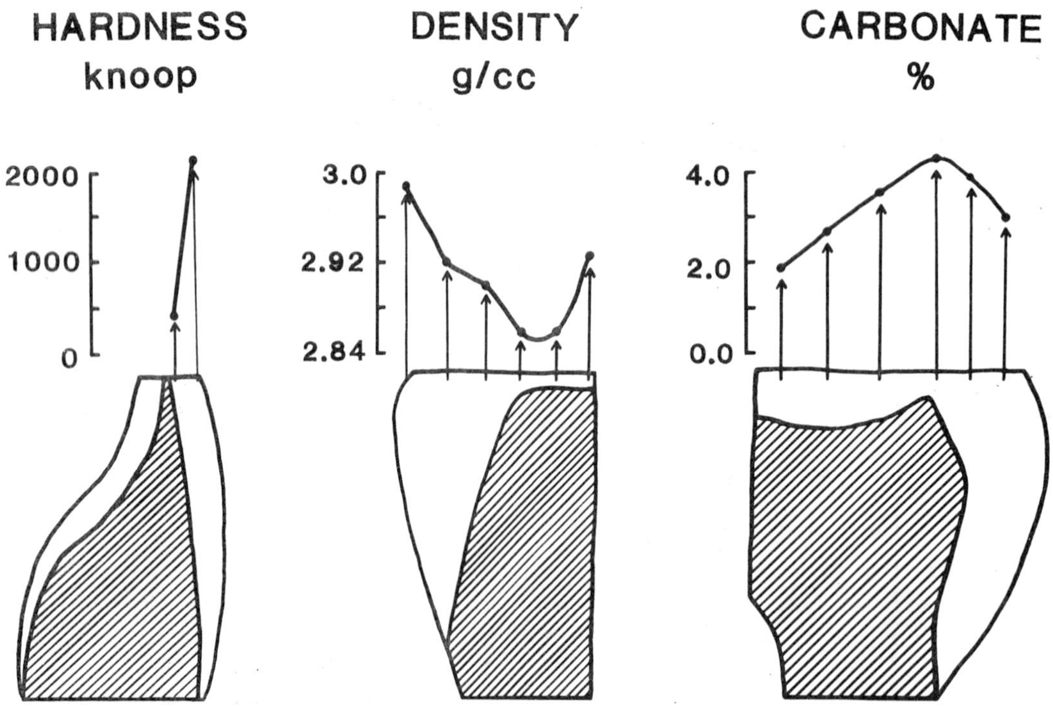


(a) (b) (c)

Figure 3.12. (a) Hardness (b) Density and (c) Carbonate content of interior enamel exposed by wear to the oral environment. No leaching out of carbonate or increase in hardness or density due to mineral uptake from the saliva is apparent.

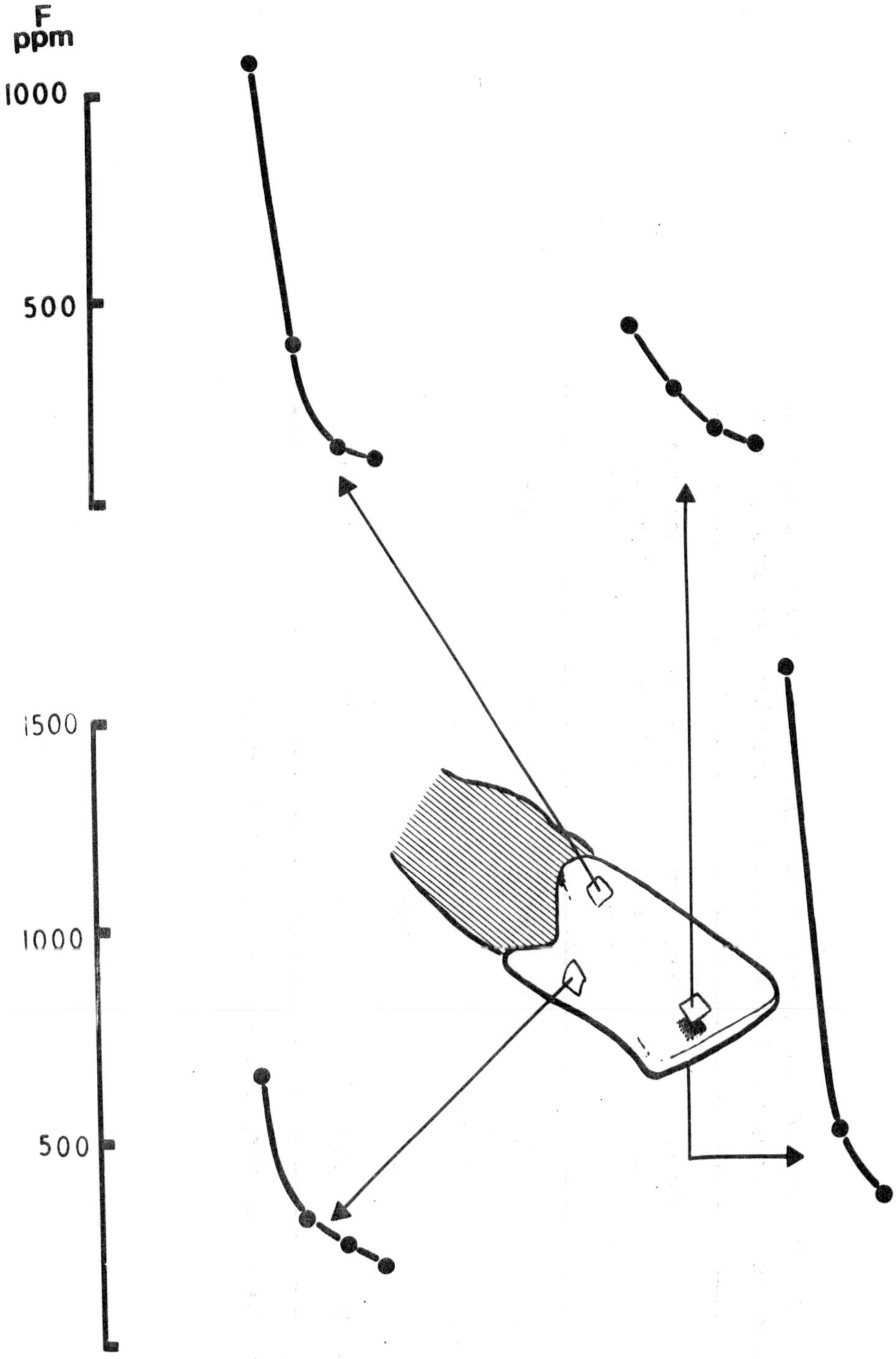


Figure 3.13. Fluoride distribution from surface to interior in enamel from different sites of a human mandibular incisor. The concentrations of fluoride can be seen to be low in those regions exposed to wear, and high in protected sites e.g. near the gum margin, where accumulations of bacterial plaque may facilitate fluoride uptake.
Weatherell et al., (1974). J. dent. Res. 53: 180-192.

Table 3.1 Calculated composition of material removed from each zone of a carious lesion compared with sound enamel. (from Robinson et-al., 1981).

| | Sound Enamel | Lost from translucent zone | Lost from dark zone | Lost from Body of Lesion |
|---|---|---|---|---|
| *Calcium | 37% | 30% | 35% | 37% |
| *Phosphorus | 18.55 | 15% | 16.6% | 18.5% |
| Carbonate | 2-4% | 28% | 3% | 1.0% |
| Magnesium | 0.2-0.4% | 2% | 3% | 0.16% |

* Calculated assuming Ca:P similar to hydroxyapatite.

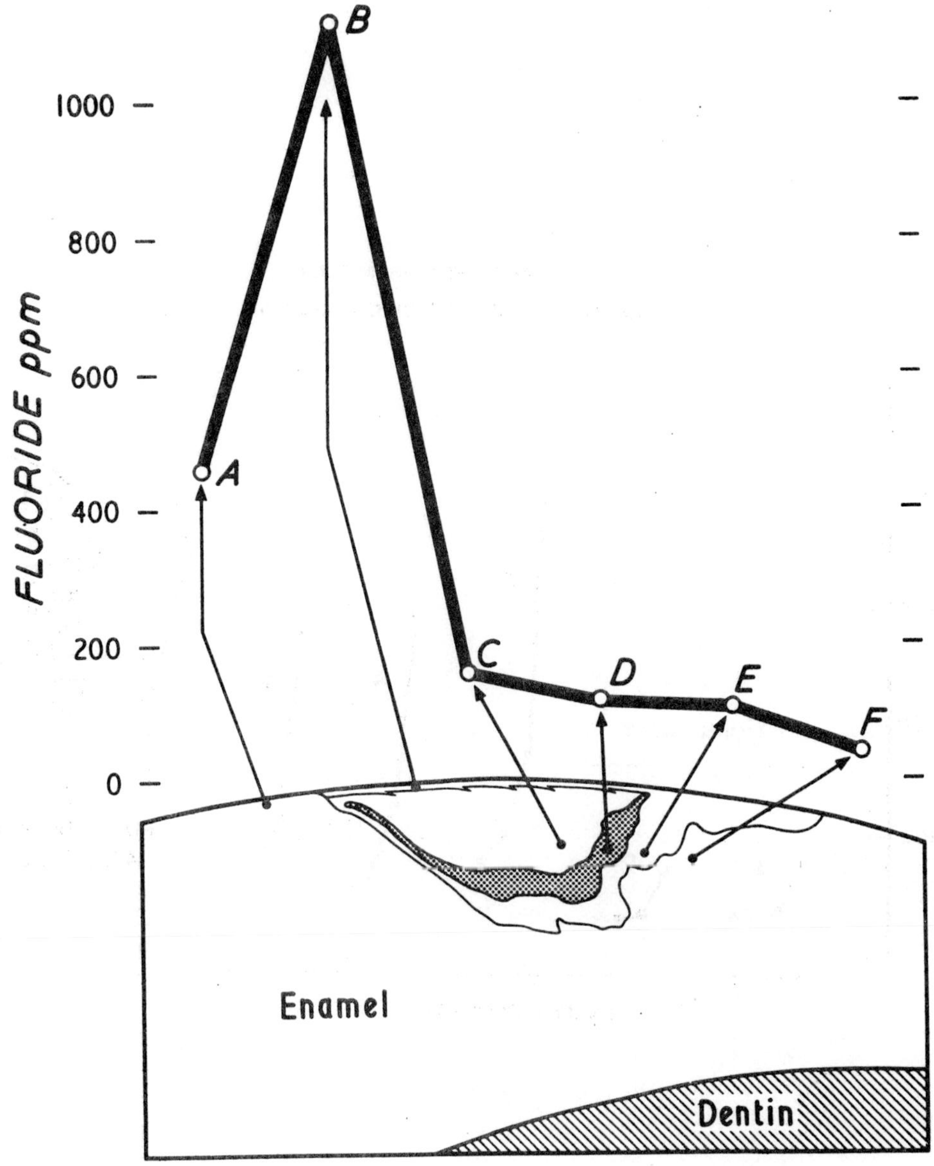


Figure 3.14. Distribution of Fluoride within a carious lesion. Fluoride can be seen to accumulate within the lesion reaching higher concentrations than those seen in the adjacent, sound enamel.

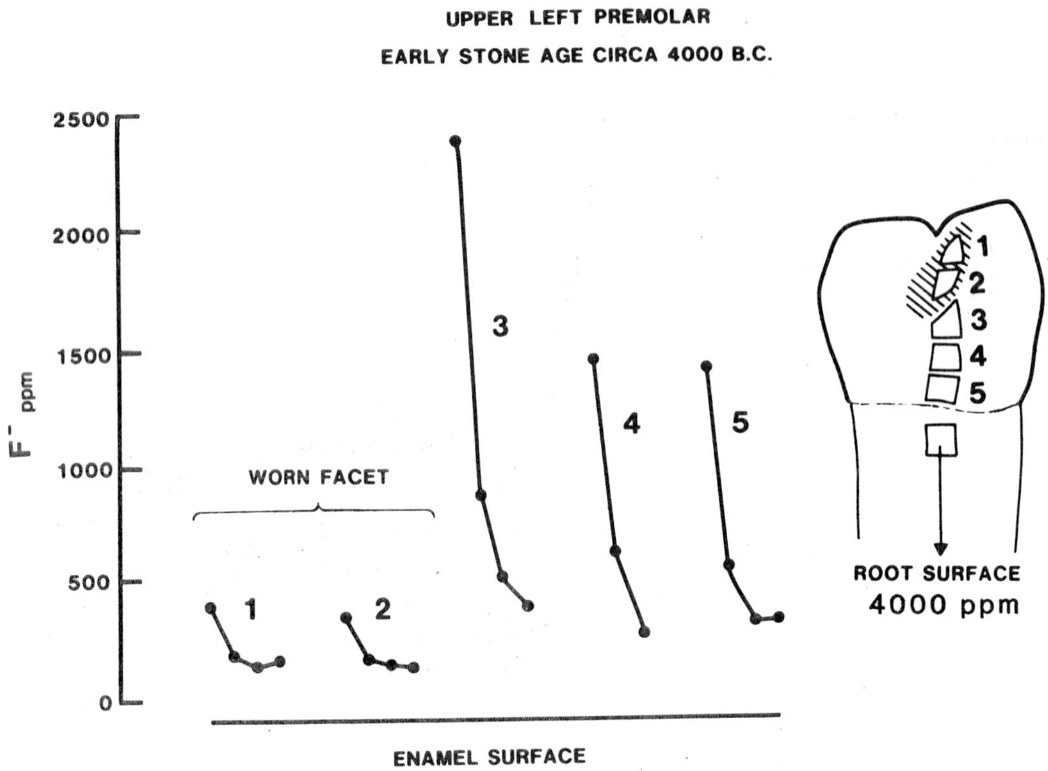


Figure 3.15. Concentrations of Fluoride from surface to interior of enamel from different sites of a human premolar tooth circa. 4,000 BC.
The pattern of fluoride distribution can be seen to correspond with that of contemporary teeth, the worn facet showing characteristic fluoride loss.

bacterially produced acid is the condition known as dental caries. The chemical and histological changes which occur during the caries process are now well known. Initially, small amounts of mineral are removed creating a porosity which results ultimately in mechanical tissue destruction (Hallsworth et al., 1972). Initially, selective removal of magnesium and carbonate rich material occurs (Coolidge and Jacobs, 1957, Johansen, 1963, Hallsworth et al., 1973) such that carious enamel can be identified chemically by its lowered concentration of magnesium and carbonate (Table 3.1). Fluoride on the other hand accumulates in the lesion at all stages of its development, acquiring concentrations over and above those of the adjacent enamel as seen in Fig. 3.14 (Weatherell et. al., 1971).

## Discussion

### Analysis of archaeological material

In order to interpret analytical findings derived from archaeological tissue, in this case dental enamel, it is crucially important to possess a comprehensive knowledge of enamel chemistry, both healthy and diseased, from non-archaeological material.

This presentation has attempted to outline the background of data now available concerning enamel chemistry together with some of the techniques required for sampling and analysis. Since little work of this sort has been carried out using archaeological specimens we have included some data concerning fluoride concentrations in a premolar tooth surface *circa* 4000 BC (Strong et al., 1985). The results are shown in Fig. 3.15.

The worn facet has lost much of its fluoride as in contemporary teeth, whilst adjacent enamel, which would have been protected by an adjacent crown shows values and a distribution again similar to unworn contemporary teeth.

Analysis of the root surface produced a fluoride value of 4000 ppm. This is higher than usual for normal root surfaces and suggests that some fluoride had been absorbed by the dentine *post mortem*. In contrast to this, values for the enamel were not unusually high and supported the view that enamel chemistry can remain unchanged for considerable periods *post mortem*.

While a great deal more of this kind of work needs to be done, this example together with the data presented earlier does indicate that dental enamel, if carefully examined and analysed, offers, if not an ideal tissue, perhaps the best available for studies of archaeological material.

## ACKNOWLEDGEMENT

The authors would like to acknowledge the Medical Research Council of Great Britain for their considerable financial support of projects which resulted in a great deal of the information in this paper.

Figs. 3.2, 3.3, 3.7, 3.8, 3.10, 3.11, 3.12 and 3.13 are reproduced by kind permission of the publishers.

REFERENCES.

Angmar, B., Carlstrom, D. and Glas. J.E. (1963). Studies on the ultrastructure of dental enamel. IV. The mineralization of normal human enamel. J. Ultras. Res. 8: 12-23.

Bachra, B.N., Trautz, O.R. and Simon, S.L. (1965). Precipitation of calcium carbonates and phosphate. III. The effect of magnesium and fluoride ions on the spontaneous precipitation of calcium carbonates and phosphates. Archs. Oral Biol. 10: 731-738.

Brudevold, F., Gardner, D.E. and Smith, F.A. (1956). The distribution of fluoride in human enamel. J. Dent. Res. 35: 420-429.

Burgess, R.C. and Maclaren, C. (1965). Proteins in developing bovine enamel. In: Tooth Enamel edited by R.W. Fearnhead and M.V. Stack. John Wright & Sons, Bristol: 74-82.

Coolidge, T.B. and Jacobs, M.H. (1957). Enamel carbonate in caries. J. dent. Res. 36: 765-768.

Deakins, M. (1942). Changes in the ash, water and organic content of pig enamel during calcification. J. Dent. Res. 21: 429-435.

Doberenz, A.R., Miller, M.F. and Wykoff, R.W.G. (1969). An analysis of fossil enamel protein. Calcif. Tiss. Res. 3: 93-95.

Fincham, A.G. (1971). Experiments of the DEAE-cellulose chromatography of bovine foetal enamel matrix and the isolation of a low molecular weight fraction. In: Tooth Enamel edited by R.W. Fearnhead and M.V. Stack. John Wright & Sons, Bristol: 79-87.

Hallsworth, A.S., Robinson, C. and Weatherell, J.A. (1972). Mineral and magnesium distribution within the approximal carious lesion of dental enamel. Caries Res. 6: 156-168.

Hallsworth, A.S., Weatherell, J.A. and Robinson, C. (1973). Loss of carbonate during the first stages of enamel caries. Caries Res. 7: 345-348.

Hiller, C.R., Robinson, C. and Weatherell, J.A. (1975). Variations in the composition of developing rat incisor enamel. Calcif. Tiss. Res. 18: 1-12.

Johansen, E. (1963). Ultrastructural and chemical observations on dental caries. In: Mechanisms of Hard Tissue Destruction. edited by R.F. Sognnaes. Washington: 187-211.

Little, M.F. and Brudevold, F. (1958). A study of inorganic carbon dioxide in intact human enamel. J. Dent. Res. 37: 991-1000.

Losee, F.L., Curzon, M.E.J. and Little, M.F. (1974). Trace element concentrations in human enamel. Archs. Oral Biol. 19: 467-470.

McCann, H.G. and Bullock, F.A. (1957). The effect of fluoride ingestion on the composition and solubility of mineralized tissues of the rat. J. Dent Res. 36: 391-398.

Robinson, C., Lowe, N.R. and Weatherell, J.A. (1975). Amino acid composition, distribution and origin of "tuft" protein in human and bovine dental enamel. Archs. Oral Biol. 20: 29-42.

Robinson, C., Lowe, N.R. and Weatherell, J.A. (1977a). Changes in the amino acid composition of developing rat incisor enamel. Calcif. Tiss. Res. 23: 19-31.

Robinson, C., Fuchs, P. and Weatherell, J.A. (1977b). The fate of matrix proteins during the development of dental enamel. Calcif. Tiss. Res. 23: 185-190.

Robinson, C., Fuchs, P., Deutsch, D. and Weatherell, J.A. (1978). Four chemically distinct stages in developing enamel from bovine incisor teeth. Caries Res. 12: 1-11.

Robinson, C., Weatherell, J.A., El Attar, I. and Deutsch, D. (1980). The pattern of mineral uptake in developing bovine incisors. Caries Res. 14: 389-393.

Robinson, C., Weatherell, J.A. and Hallsworth, A.S. (1981). Distribution of magnesium in mature human enamel. Caries Res. 15: 70-77.

Robinson, C., Weatherell, J.A. and Hallsworth, A.S. (1982b). Alterations in the composition of permanent human enamel during carious attack. In: Demineralisation and Remineralisation of the Teeth edited by S.A. Leach and W.M. Edgar. IRL Press: 209-223.

Robinson, C., Kirkham, J., Briggs, H.D. and Atkinson, P.J. (1982a). Enamel proteins from secretion to maturation. J. Dent Res. 61: 1490-1495.

Robinson, C., Hallsworth, A.S. and Kirkham, J. (1984). Distribution and uptake of magnesium by developing deciduous bovine incisor enamel. Archs. Oral Biol. 29: 479-482.

Seyer, J.M. and Glimcher, M.J. (1977). Evidence for the presence of numerous protein components in immature bovine dental enamel. Calcif. Tiss. Res. 24: 253-257.

Sobel, A.E. (1960). Interrelationship of tooth composition, body fluids, diet and caries susceptibility. Ann. N.Y. Acad. Science. 85: 96-109.

Strong, M., Athanassouli, T. Kröncke, A. and Weatherell, J.A. (1985). Fluoride absorption by sound enamel. J. Dent. Res. 64: 675 (Abstract).

Weatherell, J.A., Weidmann, S.M. and Hamm, S.M. (1966). Sampling of enamel particles by means of strong acids for density measurements. Archs. Oral Biol. 11: 107-111.

Weatherell, J.A., Weidmann, S.M. and Hamm, S.M. (1967). Density patterns in enamel. Caries Res. 1: 42-51.

Weatherell, J.A., Robinson, C. and Hiller, C.R. (1968b). Distribution of carbonate in thin sections of dental enamel. Caries Res. 2: 1-9.

Weatherell, J.A., Weidmann, S.M. and Eyre, D.R. (1968a). Histological appearance and chemical composition of enamel protein from mature human molars. Caries Res. 2: 281-293.

Weatherell, J.A., Robinson, C. and Hallsworth, A.S. (1971). Micro-analytical studies on single sections of enamel. In: Tooth Enamel II edited by M.V. Stack and R.W. Fearnhead. Wright, Bristol: 31-38.

Weatherell, J.A., Robinson, C. and Hallsworth, A.S. (1972). Changes in the fluoride concentration of the labial enamel surface with age. Caries Res. 6: 312-324.

Weatherell, J.A., Hallsworth, A.S. and Robinson, C. (1973). Effect of tooth wear in the distribution of fluoride in the enamel surface of human teeth. Archs. Oral Biol. 18: 1175-1189.

Weatherell, J.A. and Robinson, C. (1973). The inorganic composition of teeth. In: Biological Mineralisation edited by J. Zipkin. John Wiley, New York: 43-74.

Weatherell, J.A., Robinson, C. and Hallsworth, A.S. (1974). Variations in the chemical composition of human enamel. J. Dent. Res. 53: 180-192.

Weatherell, J.A., Deutsch, D., Robinson, C. and Hallsworth, A.S. (1975). Fluoride concentrations in developing enamel. Nature 256: 230-232.

Weatherell, J.A. and Robinson, C. (1982). Action of trace elements in the mineralisation of hard tissues. Proc. Finn. Dent. Socy. 78: 81-92.

Chapter 4

# DENTAL CALCULUS: ITS RELEVANCE TO ANCIENT DIET AND ORAL ECOLOGY.

Keith Dobney and Don Brothwell
Institute of Archaeology
University of London

## INTRODUCTION

The enamel surface of the tooth provides a locus for direct interaction with imbalances in the oral environment and it is at this point that the health status of the tooth is decided. Normally a dynamic equilibrium exists between the calcifying forces that contribute to the integrity of the tooth and the decalcifying forces which disrupt it (Navia 1972: p. 298).

This paper is concerned with those secondary calcifying forces which result in the deposition of dental calculus, the most common ectopic calcified deposit in man (Lustmann et al 1976: p. 47). Its origins lie in the yellowish layer of soft organic matter known as plaque which collects on the surface of the enamel in a relatively short period of time. Colonisation of the enamel by numerous types of micro-organisms occurs and incorporated within this matrix may be epithelial cells, leucocytes and, importantly for this study, remnant food debris. When relatively mature this deposit can mineralise, depending on the flora composition and trophic environment, to form a durable calcified matrix.

Based on its position on the tooth surface there are two recognised categories differentiated only by position, colour and degree of calcification: supragingival calculus situated above the gingival margin and more common, and subgingival calculus usually found isolated in gingival pockets. In humans this calcified matrix consists mainly of inorganic apatitic calcium phosphates, including hydroxyapatite, brushite and whitlockite, proportions of which vary with species, age and geographic location (Unmack and Rowles 1963). Approximately 20% of this matrix consists of an organic fraction similar in its constituents to dental plaque.

Its formation appears to be associated with variable aspects of our oral biology rather than simply with diet, although laboratory animals, such as rats and ferrets, have been shown to produce plaque and calculus more effectively when subjected to certain dietary regimes (King and Glover 1945; Fitzgerald and McDaniel 1960; Baer et al 1961).

## The archaeology of calculus

Dental calculus occurs in relative abundance archaeologically, being found on a wide variety of fossil and sub-fossil human and other mammals material as is shown in Fig. 4.1-4.3 (Baker and Brothwell 1980; Levitan 1984; Rielly in press). Because of its mineral composition it survives well in all but acid burial environments, varying in consistency from very friable to solid and compact. In its more friable condition it can easily be lost during excavation and post-excavation work by over-zealous cleaning.

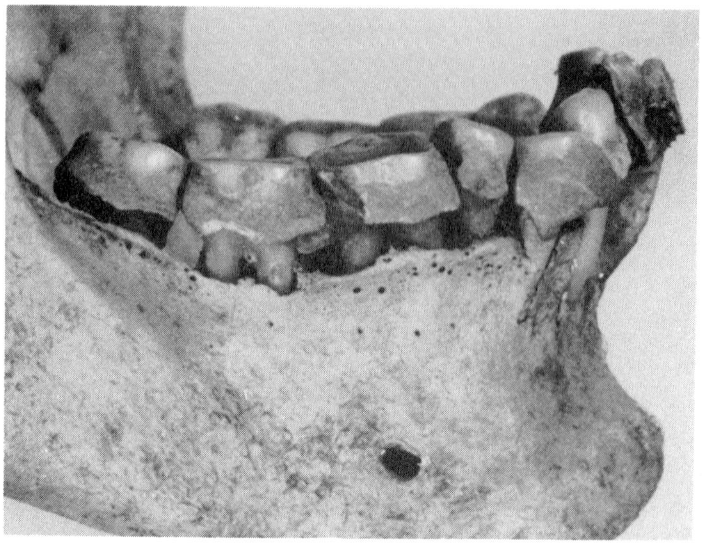

Figure 4.1. Gross calculus deposits on Norse human dentition, Newark Bay.

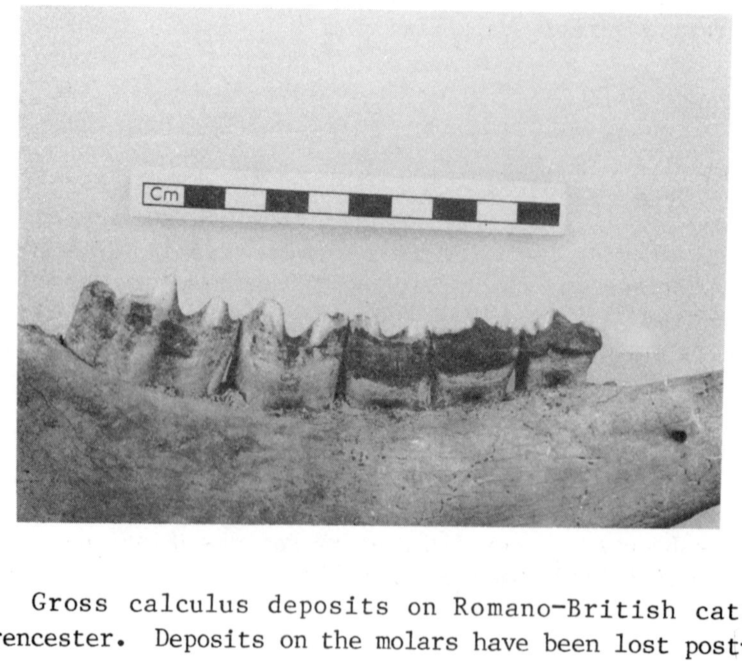


Figure 4.2. Gross calculus deposits on Romano-British cattle teeth, Ditches, Cirencester. Deposits on the molars have been lost post-mortem.

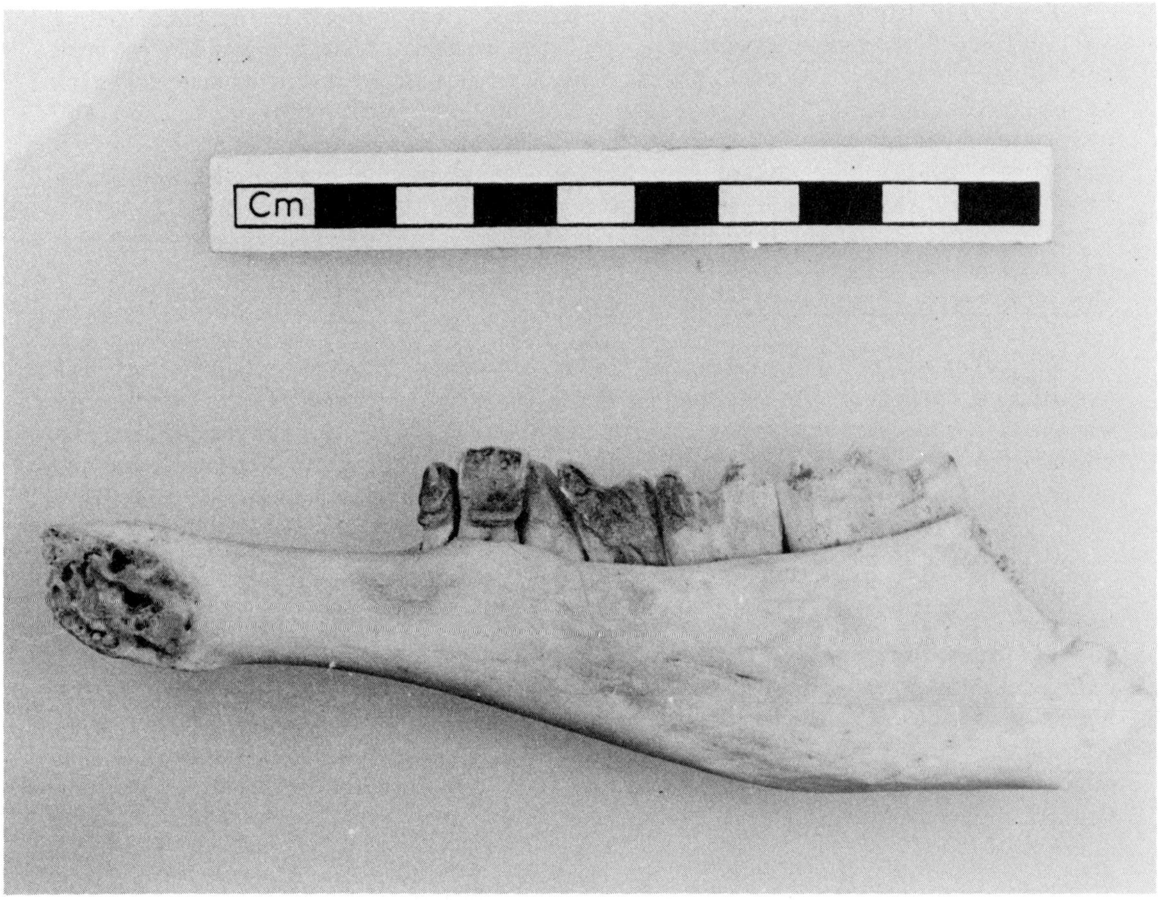


Figure 4.3. Severe calculus deposits on 8th-10th century sheep teeth from Naples. Note the association with abnormal positioning of the teeth, attrition and abscess development.

Storage and curation of material will also be a major factor determining its survival for future study.

Human examples showing its survival rate include a number of burials from early mediaeval Jewbury and Anglo-Saxon Raunds. From the Jewbury cemetery, of a total of approximately 300 individuals, 201 showed signs of at least slight deposits, i.e. 60% of the sample. From Raunds 93 of a total of 141 individuals studies showed signs of calculus formation, i.e. over 65%.

Similarly high proportions were observed in a number of archaeological collections of domestic livestock. A large number of cattle mandibles from the Romano-British site of Ditches, Cirencester showed quite severe deposits of calculus (Rielly, in press), as did a large collection of Iron Age ovi/caprid mandibles housed at the British Museum (Natural History). Calculus deposits were also prevalent on many of the ovi/caprid mandibles from Danebury and the near eastern site of Tel Nebi Mend.

## The importance of archaeological calculus

An interest in archaeological calculus arose, not only because of its prevalence on teeth, but because it forms part of a range of oral pathology which deserves far more detailed study. Until recently concentration appears to have been on secular changes in caries frequency, tooth loss and apical infection to the neglect of calculus formation and composition.

Our initial aim was to investigate the organic constituents of calculus in order to locate microscopic fragments of food debris which may have become trapped within the calcified matrix. If these did survive in an identifiable form then calculus could make significant contributions to our understanding of past human and other mammalian diet. This direct association of diet with the individual occurs rarely in archaeological contexts, usually in the form of coprolites associated with burials or the gut contents of individuals from unusual burial environments, e.g. the Danish bog bodies.

## Methodology

At a methodological level there are many problems ranging from the basic recording of its position and extent on the tooth surface to the destructive and non-destructive analysis of the material itself.

Scoring and recording of calculus: studies of the occurrence of dental calculus are at an early stage (Baker and Brothwell 1980; Levitan 1984; Rielly in press) Fig. 4.4, 4.5a and b, and 4.6).

Since a number of methods of examination used in this study are destructive, a basic recording system was devised, based loosely on modern dental methods, which would not be too time-consuming but which would evaluate the extent and amount of dental calculus in detail (Dobney and Brothwell, in preparation).

Initially we were surprised to find no modern dental recording system detailed enough for our purpose. Most only recorded presence/absence or

4.4

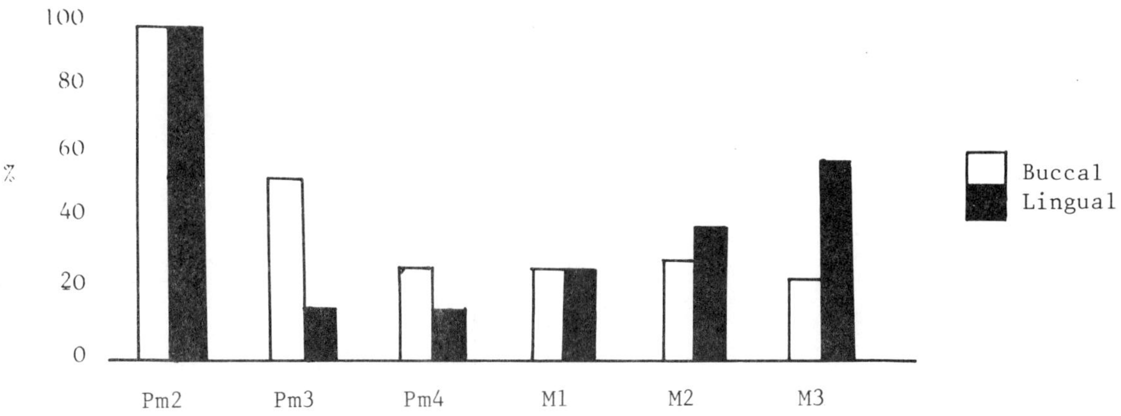


4.5a

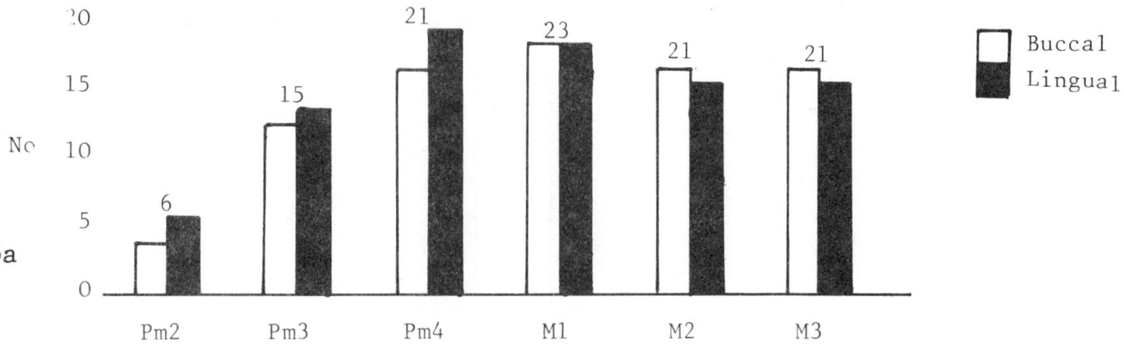


4.5b

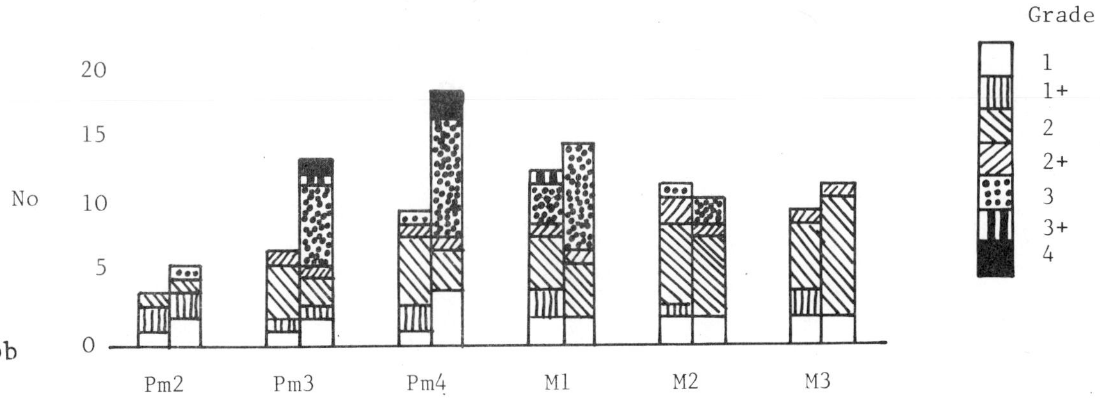


Figure 4.4. Occurrence of dental calculus in sheep mandibles from Middleton Stoney (After Levitan, 1984).

Figure 4.5a. Occurrence of dental calculus in cattle mandibles. Total calculus records from Ditches (After Rielly in press).

Figure 4.5b. Cattle mandibles from Ditches where grade of calculus could be seen or estimated. (After Rielly, in press).

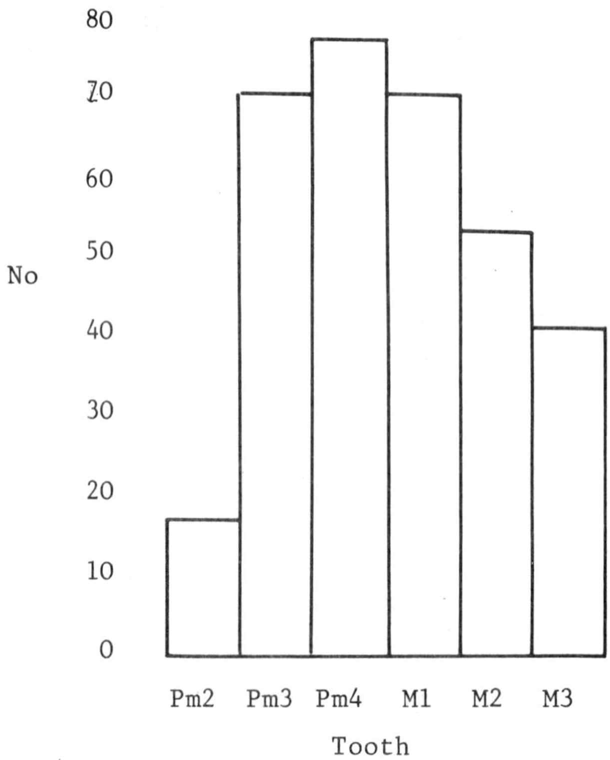


Figure 4.6. Calculus frequencies on sheep molars and premolars. Wicken Bonhunt Saxon samples. (After Baker and Brothwell, 1980).

its severity over the buccal, lingual and occlusal surface of the tooth, giving no indication of position or thickness. Our system divides the tooth surface into a number of morphological zones according to tooth structure and the observed way calculus is deposited for that particular species (Fig. 4.6 and 4.7). Thus a detailed assessment of the position of calculus deposits is possible. As well as recording the position, each zone is allocated a numerical grade, i.e. 0, 1, 2, 3 or 4 (0 = normal, 1 = slight, 2 = mild, 3 = severe, 4 = gross) (Mellanby 1934) to give an idea of the severity/thickness of the calculus covering (Figs. 8b and 9b). In addition to this detailed recording, an overall grade for each mandible was established for simple and rapid evaluation of the severity of calculus throughout the sample (Figs. 4.8, and 4.9b). Dry-weight was also considered as a means of assessing calculus loads of individuals. Fig. 4.10 shows the distribution of total calculus weights from early mediaeval Jewbury.

As well as detailed recording, a photographic archive was established for each mandible/maxilla where calculus had been removed for further analysis.

Specimen preparation and cleaning

Closer examination of calculus necessitates careful cleaning to avoid contamination from the adhering soil matrix. Obviously, when dealing with micro-scopic fragments any extraneous material could confuse and greatly distort any conclusions regarding diet. It is important to show that organic and inorganic debris associated with the ingestion of food is definitely trapped within and therefore contemporaneous with the calculus.

Since chemical cleaning may have detrimental effects on microscopic organic particles a physical method of cleaning was devised. Air abrasive cleaning, using particles of sodium bicarbonate less than 125 m as a gentle abrasive, was employed. This not only successfully removes any debris from the surface or trapped within surface hollows, but also has the advantage of being soluble, thus in no way inhibiting further analysis.

Location of food debris: one of our initial concerns was to establish whether archaeological calculus did contain within its matrix fragments of identifiable food debris remaining in the mouth after mastication. If this is the case archaeologically then it seems likely to contrast with the rather fine deposits, free from larger food particles, which still plague many people today.

A number of techniques were employed to attempt to establish beyond doubt that debris was trapped within archaeological calculus:-

i) Archaeological calculus specimens from various species were immersed for up to two hours in a standard dental decalcifying agent. During this period every attempt was made to ensure that the fragment remained intact. The fully decalcified specimen was then stained, immersed in alcohol and transferred to a medium power binocular microscope for viewing. Microscopic inclusions were stained red and could be seen within the semi-opaque matrix. However, at such low magnification actual identification proved impossible.

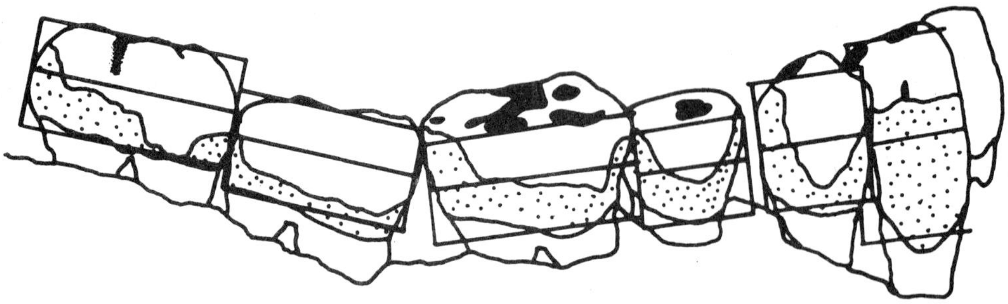


Figure 4.7a. Diagram of human dentition showing mild calculus deposits. The various boxes demonstrate the use of zones for recording calculus covering.

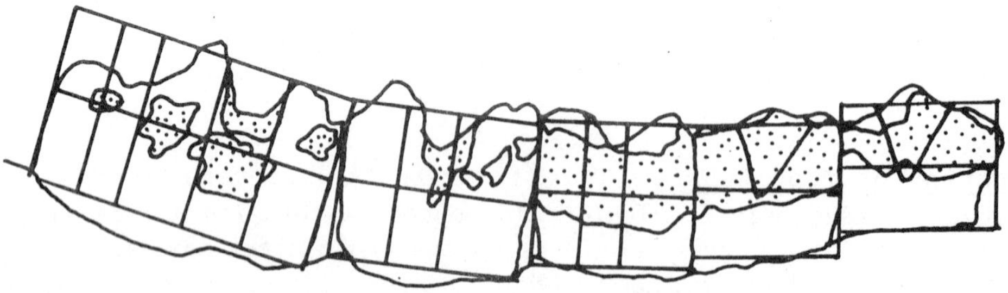


Figure 4.7b. Diagram of *Bos* dentition showing gross calculus deposits.

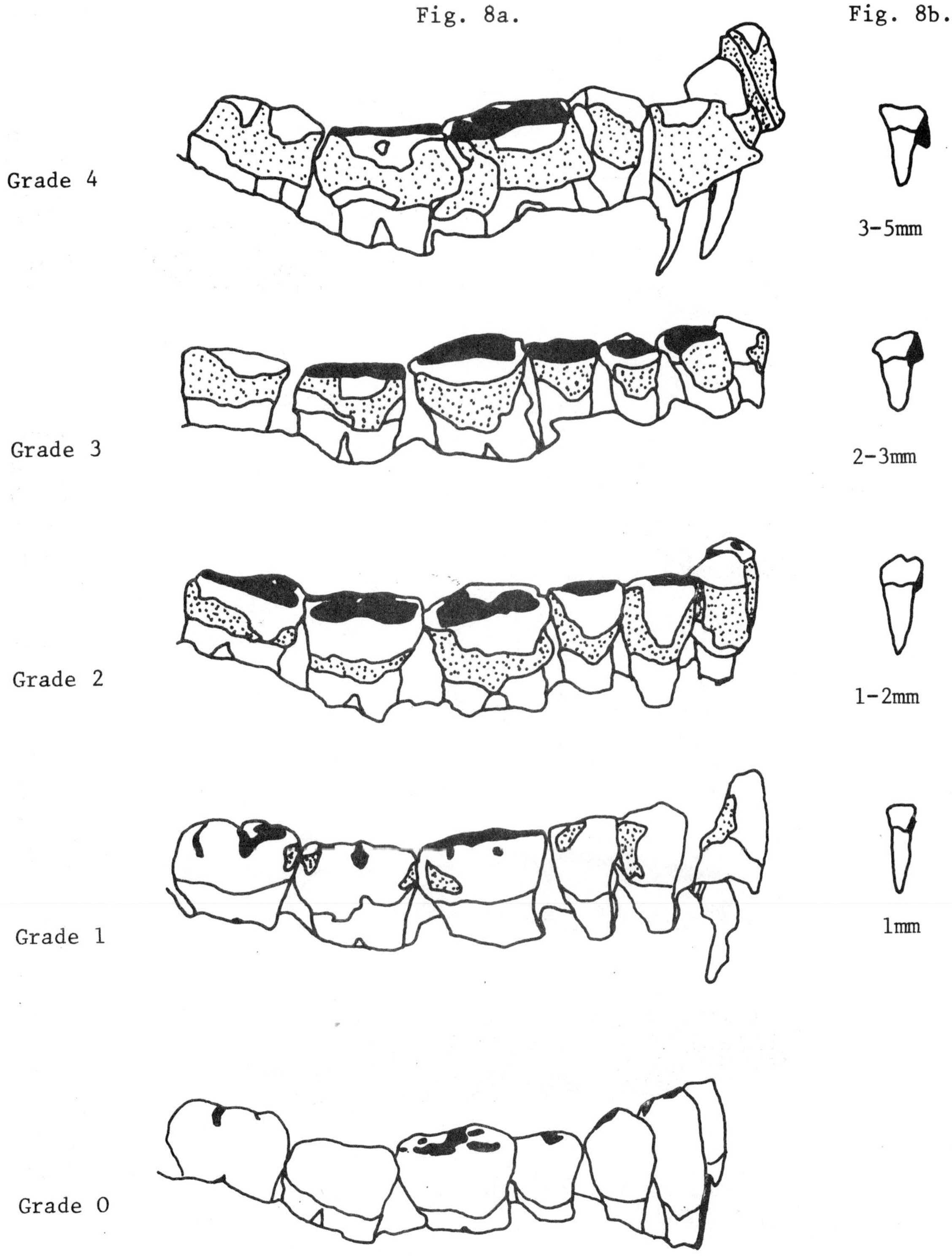


Figure 4.8a. Ranges of calculus development, grade 0-4 (normal-gross) on archaeological human teeth.

Figure 4.8b. Actual thickness measurements corresponding to the various grades defined.

Fig. 4.9a

4.9b

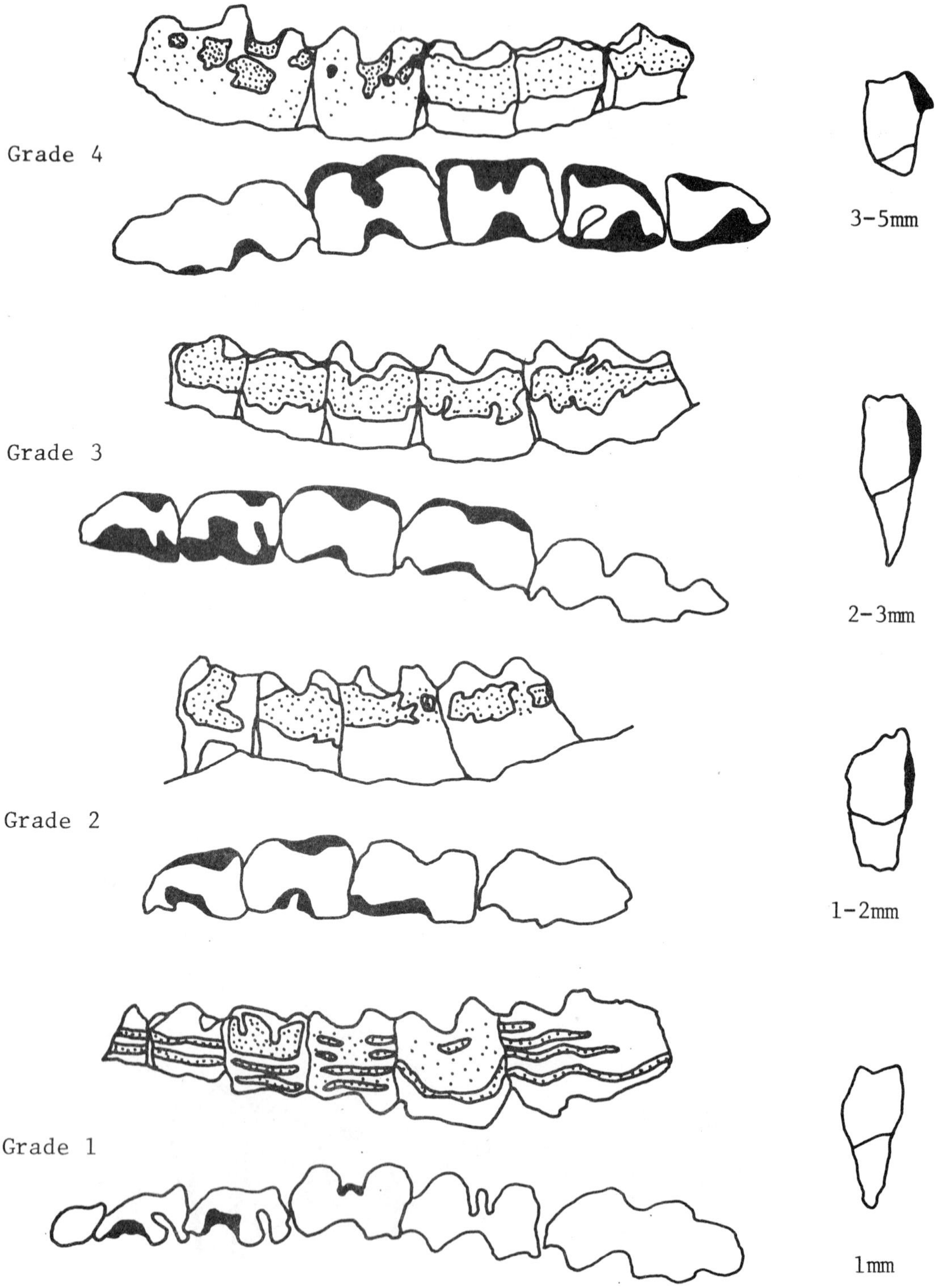


Figure 4.9a. Ranges of calculus development graded 1-4 (slight-gross) on archaeological cow teeth. Occlusal views give additional evidence of severity and thickness.

Figure 4.9b. Range of thickness measurements corresponding to the various grades defined.

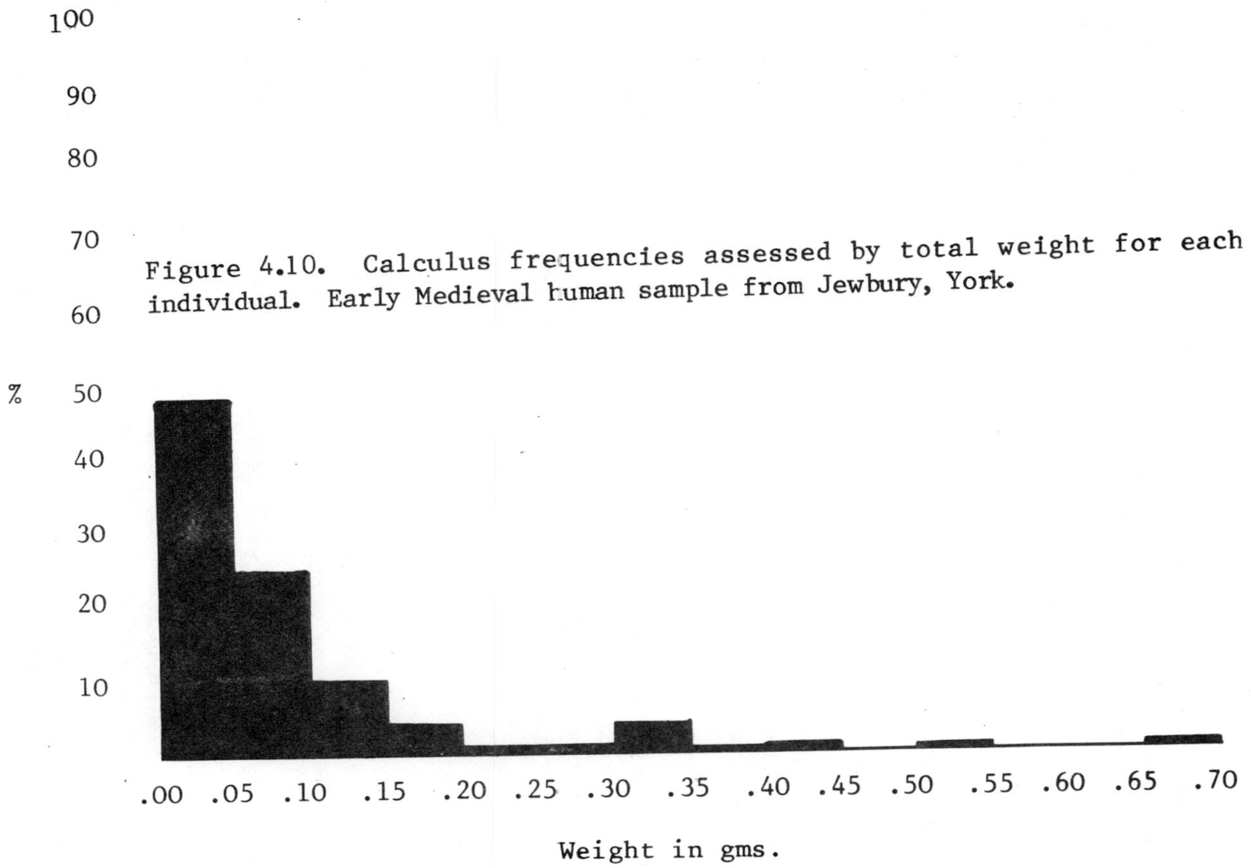


Figure 4.10. Calculus frequencies assessed by total weight for each individual. Early Medieval human sample from Jewbury, York.

ii) The scanning electron microscope (SEM), capable of much greater magnification, was also used in this respect. Since the SEM can give excellent detail of surface structure coupled with an increased depth of field, fresh fracture surfaces were viewed for evidence of food inclusions. Only a small proportion of those viewed showed this directly since the probability of a fracture occurring directly where an inclusion is situated remains fairly remote. Neverthless inclusions were found in one or two specimens conclusively trapped within the matrix (Fig.s 4.11a and 4.11b).

iii) Attempts were made to view the interior of the calculus with the SEM by physical and chemical removal of small amounts of its exterior. This was achieved by prolonged use of the air abrasive unit and by etching the surfaces with dilute hydrochloric acid. However, these methods proved inconclusive and in fact were probably responsible for the removal of whatever organic debris was originally present.

iv) Since the above are destructive processes we are considering ways of scanning non-destructively for those specimens which may be most productive of food debris. One possibility is to use the Tandem scanning reflected light microscope housed at University College, London. This remarkable piece of equipment allows visual penetration of the surface of a specimen depending on its reflective properties (Boyde et al 1983). Initial results on modern calculus seem promising although more work is needed on archaeological specimens.

An alternative as far as gross calculus deposits are concerned is the use of radiographic techniques. Distinctive zoning has been noted by others in modern calculus (Spouge 1973: p. 76) and by ourselves in archaeological specimens (Fig. 4.12). With the use of softer X-rays other heterogeneities within the calculus may be highlighted.

Decalcification and location of food debris

To discover the potential range of debris that may survive archaeologically we looked at calculus from a number of species from a number of sites of differing periods and environments.

Method: after basic recording, each calculus fragment was cleaned, using the method previously described, and subsequently weighed. Each was then immersed in 5 mls of Villanueves decalcifying solution, a dental decalcifying agent, for approximately 2-2½ hours, depending on the size of the fragment. Distilled water was then added and the specimen centrifuged for three minutes. The supernatant was then decanted and distilled water with two drops of saffranine stain were added to the residue. The specimen was again centrifuged for a further three minutes and the supernatant decanted.

Semi-permanent mounts of each were then made on glass slides which were subsequently viewed using normal transmission light microscopy. Each slide was scanned systematically, as is normally undertaken when counting pollen grains, with the position and provisional identification/observations of each recognisable inclusion being recorded.

A photographic record is kept of each representative fragment of a larger group or of unusual isolated fragments showing reasonable anatomical

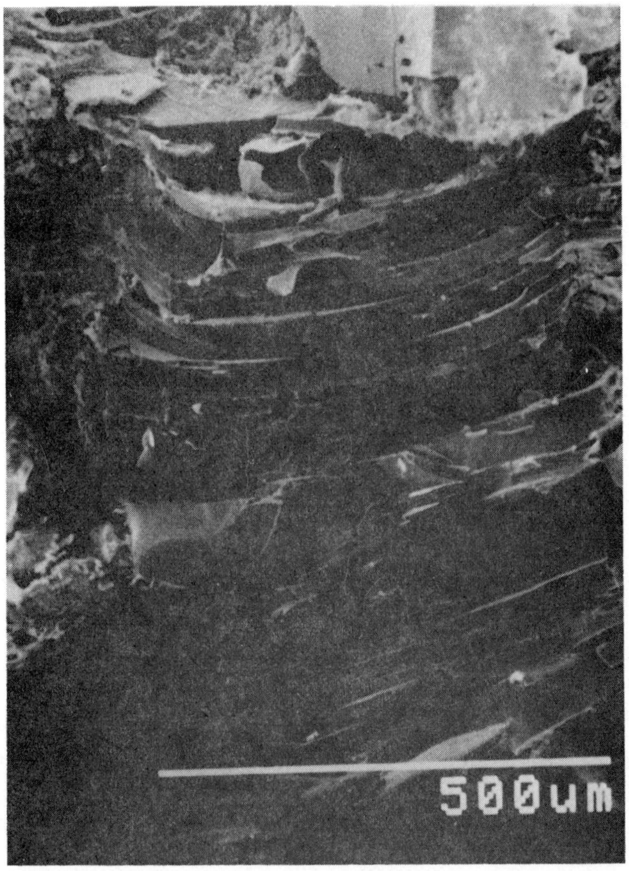


Figure 4.11a. Scanning electron micrograph of a fresh fracture surface showing what appears to be an opal phytolith trapped in the matrix. Early Medieval human calculus, Jewbury York. Mag. X500.

Figure 4.11b. Scanning electron micrograph of archaeological cattle fracture surfaces showing two spherical objects trapped in the matrix. Mag. X80.

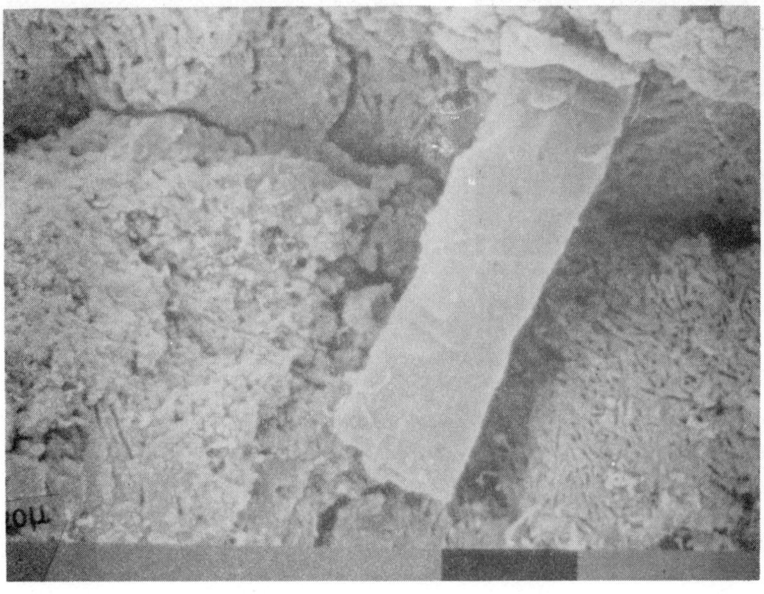

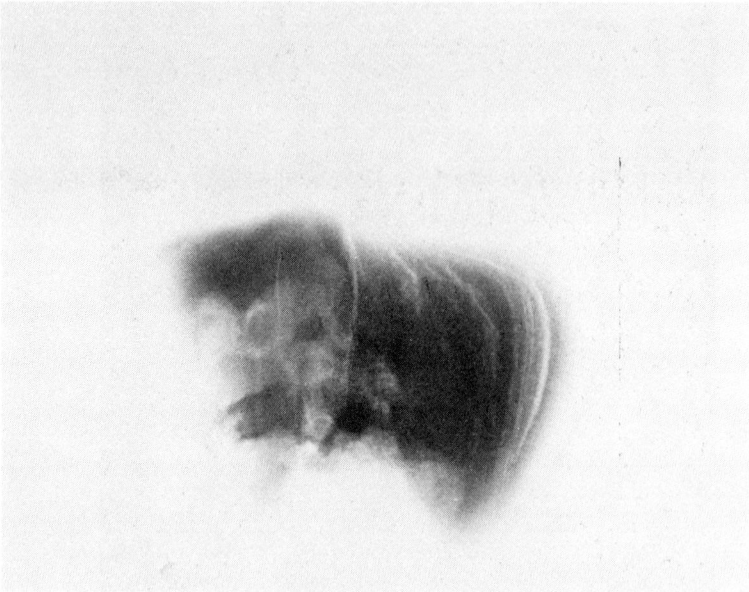

Figure 4.12. Radiograph of gross calculus deposits from a human molar. Note distinct layering within the dense matrix. Jewbury, York.

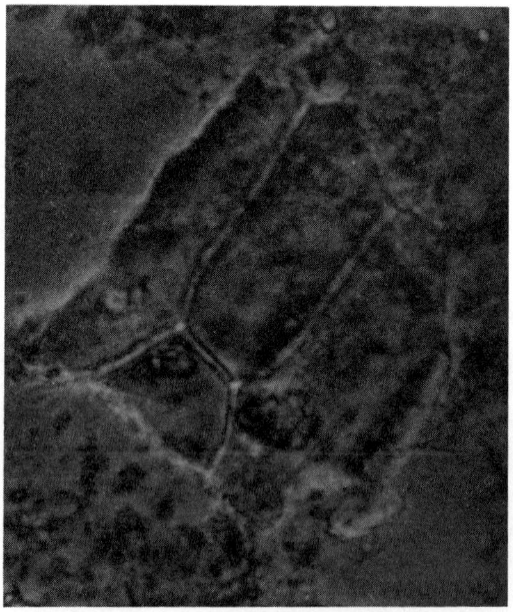

Figure 4.13a. Cereal testa fragment. Sheep calculus from Iron Age Danebury. Mag. X250.

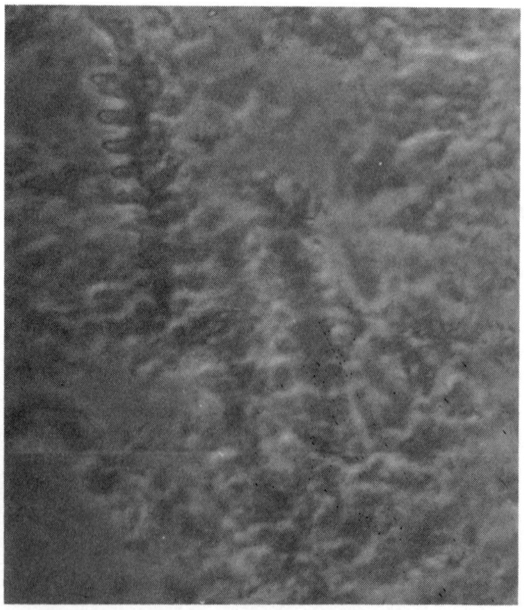

Figure 4.13b. Chaff epidermis fragment from prehistoric human calculus, Dalkey Island. Mag. X250.

detail. Contact prints of each as well as detailed line drawings were mounted on index cards along with additional information regarding the fragment itself and the individual from which it derived. These cards proved extremely useful when seeking further help with the various levels of identification.

Identification of food debris: once the debris has been isolated and initial recording achieved, the very basic problem of identification arises. At present there are very few comprehensive atlases of food particles that can be adequately related to this type of material. Some of the archaeological fragments can be readily identified and these include fragments of cereal testa, opal phytoliths, pollen grains, charcoal, animal hairs and accidental insect inclusion (Figs. 4.13a-h). Many more however, remain as yet unidentified and thus demand careful checking with modern tissue specimens (Figs. 4.13i-j).

It is perhaps fortunate that some palaeobotanists, already aware of the problems of identifying the various categories of archaeobotanical material, have begun to tackle similar problems. Precedents have been set by workers such as Hans Helbaek in the 1950s when working on the gut contents of several of the more notable Danish bog bodies, i.e.. the Tollund and Grauballe men (Helbaek 1950; 1958). More recently Korber-Gröhne has used the SEM to attempt to resolve cellular detail from various species of grasses, in particular the cereals (Korber-Gröhne 1980 and 1981).

Similar work to both Helbaek's and Korber-Gröhne's is at present being carried out in our own department at the Institute of Archaeology, London. One of these projects involves detailed study of the stomach and upper-intestinal contents of the now-famous Lindow man. In this study very similar problems arise regarding the identification of small comminuted fragments and co-operation with the preparation of comparative material has helped resolve a number of points regarding the identification of cereal fragments derived from prehistoric human calculus.

Case Study

An example of the diversity of fragments which may be recovered from one small fragment of calculus is given below. A piece of supra-gingival calculus weighing 0.042 gms was decalcified and mounted as already outlined. The material was obtained from a prehistoric Irish individual from Dalkey Island. In this case provisionally identifiable organic and inorganic fragments were abundant and the frequencies of each major category are shown in Table 4.1.

Fragments which could be readily identified included a number of tiny pieces of cereal chaff epidermis probably from the genus *Hordeum* (Barley) Fig. 4.14a. These consisted of characteristic elongate, coarse wavy cells which interlocked with one another. Located on this tissue are a number of stomata. Although some fragments are somewhat decayed both of these features are as clearly visible on the archaeological material as they are on the modern comparative tissue preparation (Fig. 4.14b).

A number of categories of opal phytoliths were also present from the Dalkey calculus. Seventeen coarse wavy phytoliths, almost certainly deriving from the characteristic *Hordeum* cells already mentioned, were found

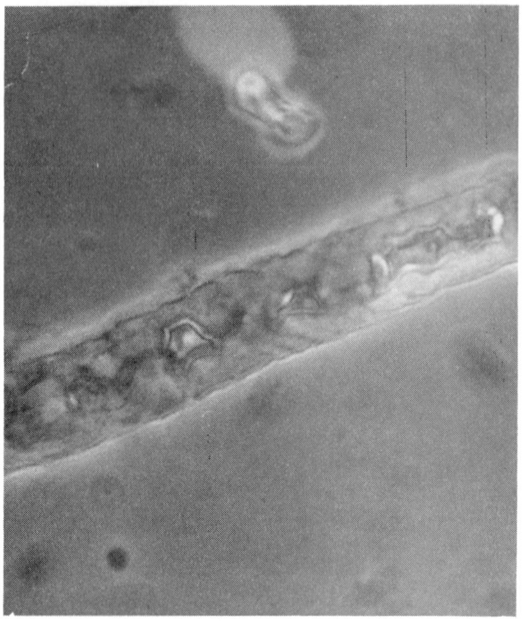

Figure 4.13c. Straight rod shaped phytolith from sheep calculus Tel Nebi Mend. Mag. X250.

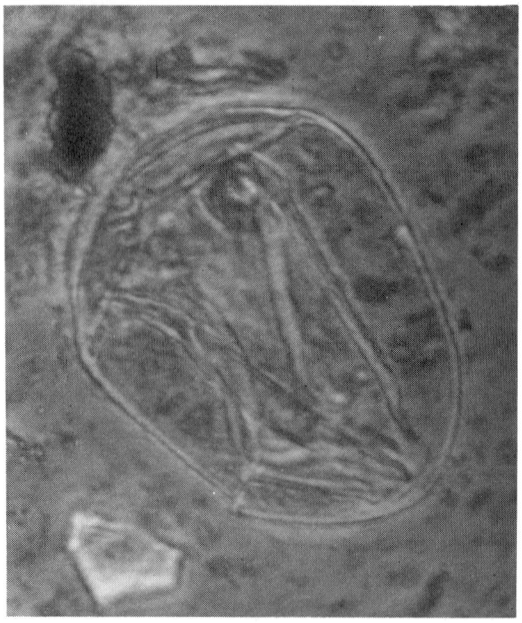

Figure 4.13d. Large Graminae pollen grain, probably cereal, from human calculus, early Medieval, Jewbury, York, Mag. X400.

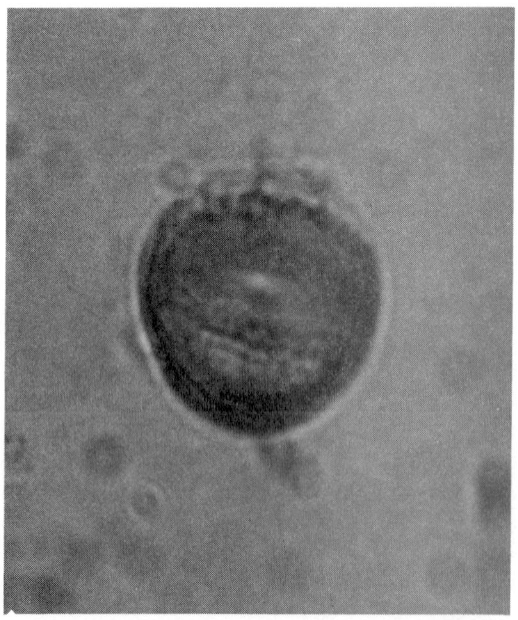

Figure 4.13e. Eroded Artemisium pollen grain. Sheep calculus from Tel Nebi Mend. Mag. X400.

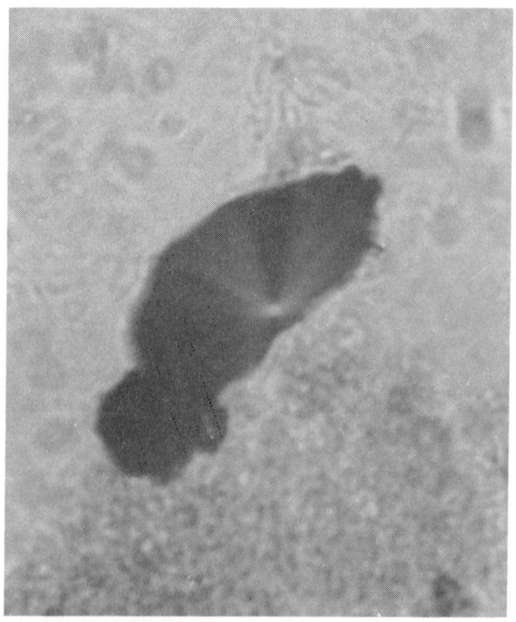

Figure 4.13f. Small carcoal fleck from human calculus, early Medieval Jewbury, York. Mag. X400.

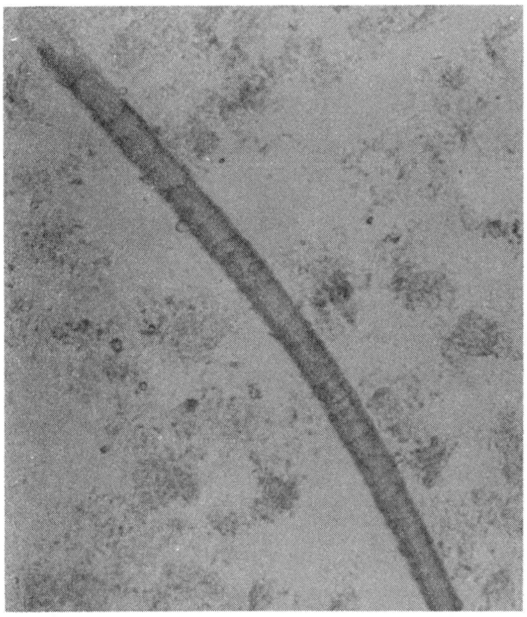

Figure 4.13g. Animal hair. Human calculus from prehistoric Dalkey Island. Mag. X100.

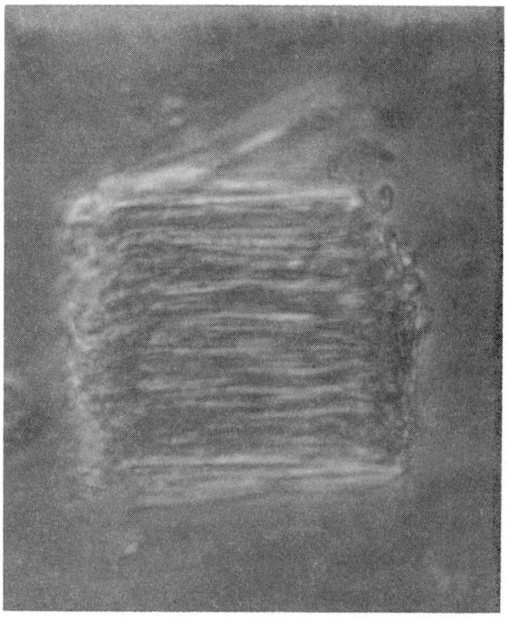

Figure 4.13h. Spiral strengthening vessels of plant origin. Human calculus from early Medieval Jewbury. Mag. X250.

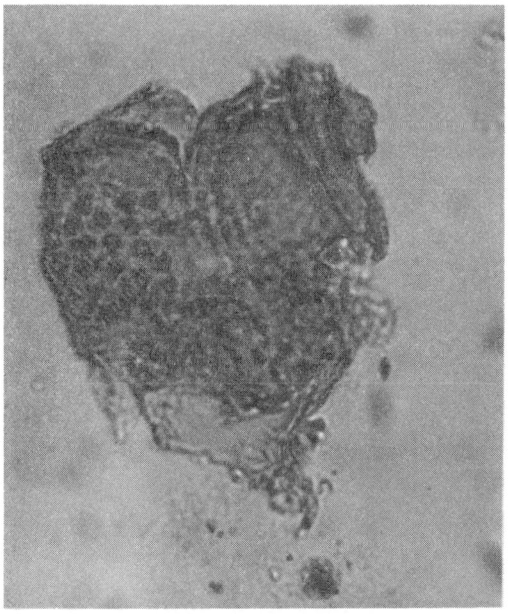

Figure 4.13i. Unidentified fragment, possibly insect in origin, from sheep calculus, Tel Nabi Mend. Mag. X250.

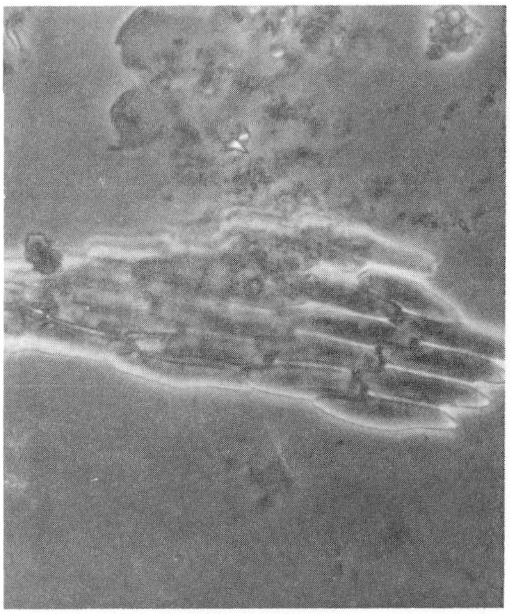

Figure 4.13j. Unidentified fragment, resembling pith cells from Iron Age Sutton Walls. Mag. X250.

| IDENTIFIABLE FRAGMENTS | | | | | | | | | UNIDENTIFIABLE FRAGMENTS | | |
|---|---|---|---|---|---|---|---|---|---|---|---|
| CEREAL TISSUE | | | PHYTOLITHS | | POLLEN AND FUNGAL SPORES | | PSEUDO-PARASITE | CHARRED | | | |
| *Hordeum* chaff epidermis | *Triticum* spermoderm | *Triticum* spermoderm? | Coarse wavy | Straight rod | Pollen | Fungal spores | *Psorospermium haeckelii* | Charcoal | Thin tissue fragments | Interwoven fragments | Remaining fragments |
| 10 | 2 | 76 | 17 | 26 | 3 | 2 | 3 | 49 | 76 | 36 | 75 |

Table 4.1. Total numbers of identifiable and unidentifiable fragments of food debris isolated from human prehistoric calculus, Dalkey Island.

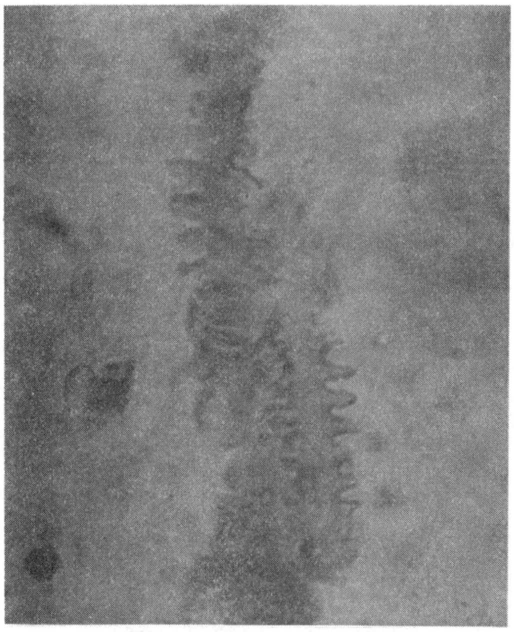

Figure 4.14a. Hordeum sp. (Barley) chaff epidermis fragment. One of 20 such fragments from a prehistoric Dalkey Island specimen. Note distinctive wavy cells and stomatum. Mag. X250.

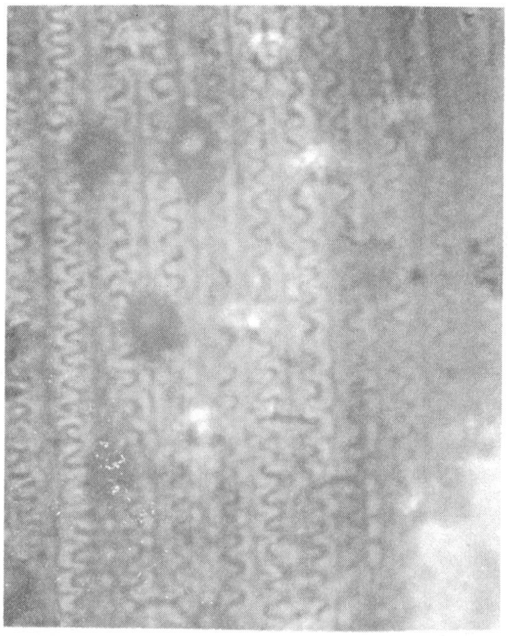

Figure 4.14b. Modern tissue preparation of Hordeum chaff epidermis. Note similarities to fig. 4.14a. Mag. X250.

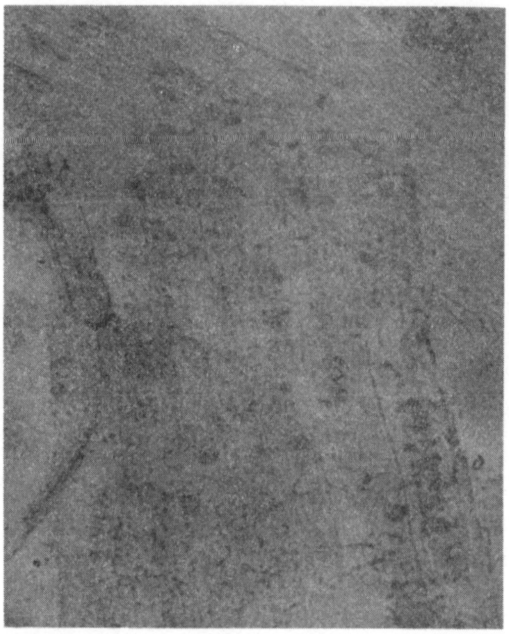

Figure 4.14c. Triticum sp. (Wheat) spermoderm fragment from Dalkey Island preparation. Note strand-like structures noticeable in the bottom left hand corner. Mag. X400.

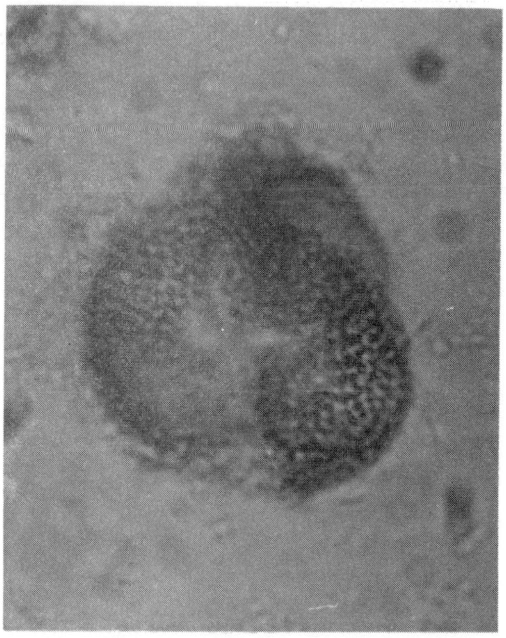

Figure 4.14d. Cruciferae pollen grain of Sinapsis type, noticeably eroded but still retaining good anatomical detail. Mag. X400.

scattered randomly over the slide. Less characteristic straight plain rods (Twiss et al 1969) occurred in more abundance. These are perhaps the least diagnostic category, being found in all major categories of Gramineae (Rovner 1971).

By far the most abundant fragment type recovered from this specimen was at first not readily identifiable. It consisted of a long, flattened 'thread-like' object with little visible structure except barely visible cell walls. Seventy-six were present in this sample, occurring isolated or in pairs. However, in the course of scanning the slide two large tissue fragments were located. These consisted of a number of individual strands criss-crossing one another in two distinct layers (Fig. 4.14c). Closer inspection and comparisons with modern tissue preparations revealed that these were probably fragments of Triticum (wheat) spermoderm.

More readily identifiable are pollen grains and a total of three grains were recovered. Only two were preserved well enough for positive identification to be made and although few in number they provided an interesting insight into possible diet. These were identified as Crusiferae grains of Sinapsis type (Moore and Webb 1978) (Fig. 4.14d). These derive from the charlocks, rapes or mustards which may have been a component of the diet. These are considered to prefer disturbed open habitats and thus, if contemporary with the calculus, are consistent with a prehistoric context.

The discovery of what appeared at first to be insect or parasite ova produced possibly the most interesting inference of diet from this human individual. These were elongate with thin cell walls, a lumen devoid of any internal structures and small apertures at each tapering end (Fig. 4.14e). Initially specific identification was not possible; however, with the aid of the photographic record and associated drawings a tentative identification has been made. They are very similar, although flattened and slightly distorted to an organism found only in the tissues of crayfish (Jones pers comm). This organism, Psorospermium haecklii, sometimes known as a 'beaver body' have been found in the stools of persons who have recently ingested crayfish but their origin and significance are still a mystery (Spencer and Monroe 1975). Only the direct ingestion of crayfish would result in the liberation of these organisms into the mouth and subsequent incorporation in the calculus.

Many fragments which could not readily be identified were present in large numbers. Charcoal flecks were found throughout the specimen with a total of 49 being recognised (Fig. 4.13f). Tiny fragments of charcoal attached to food or part of a charred portion of food would not be an unusual thing to ingest. Being carbonised they would tend to survive well in the mild digestive environment of the mouth. Unfortunately these fragments are almost impossible to identify.

As can be seen from Table 4.1, a number of similar fragments, all unidentifiable, could be grouped into a number of categories. These included 24 fragments of what appeared to be thin tissue lacking any visible structure and 36 thick elongate fibre-like objects which seem to consist of a number of finer interwoven fibrils (Fig. 4.14f). The remaining 75 unidentifiable fragments consist of seemingly unrelated organic and inorganic objects with little or no anatomical detail present.

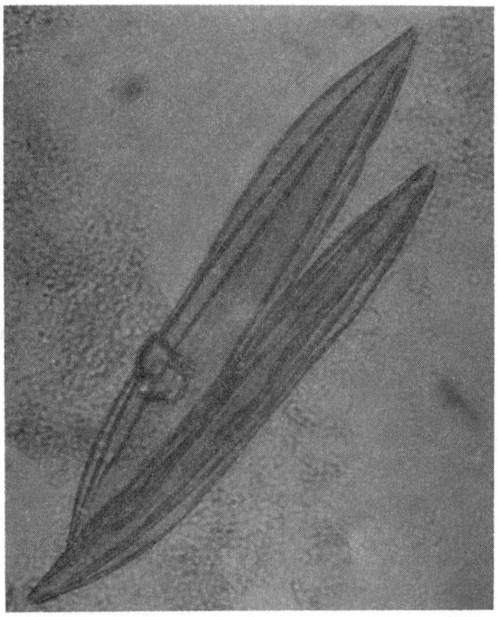

Figure 4.14e. Possible flattened spore of Psorospermium haecklii from the Dalkey Island specimen. Note small apertures at either end. Mag. X250.

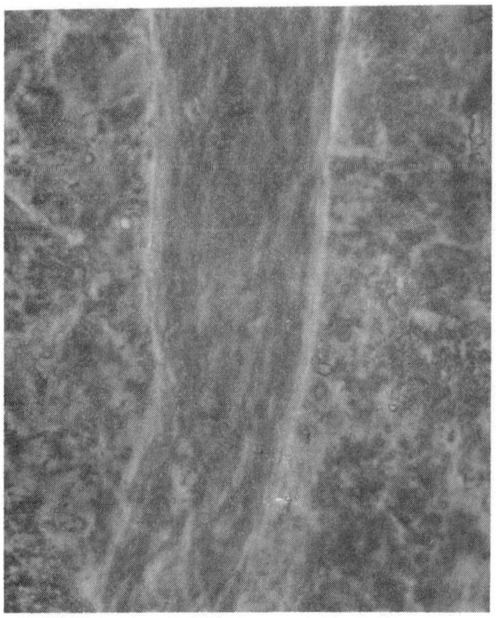

Figure 4.14f. Unidentifiable object showing interwoven appearance possibly deriving from animal tissue. Dalkey Island. Mag. X250.

## The microbiology of archaeological calculus

An exciting avenue of study was realised when relatively early in the research fragments of archaeological calculus were scanned with the SEM in order to isolate incorporated food debris.

At magnifications of greater than x 2000 it became obvious that large numbers of micro-organisms were present in a remarkable state of preservation from both human and other mammalian calculus. These were originally constituents of the dental plaque which, during the rapid calcification process, became petrified into the calculus matrix. It was obvious from these archaeological specimens that preservation was similar to that in modern calculus (Lustmann et al 1976).

The ancient micro-organisms are variable in form as they are during life, some resembling colonies of lactobacilli or cocci (Fig. 4.15a), other similar to filamentous mycetes (Figs. 4.15b) and oral treponemes (Fig. 4.15c), while others defy identification at present (Fig. 4.15d). Due to their abundance it may be possible to gain an impression of hominid oral ecology in the past. Has it always been the same or are there differences to be found through time or in relation to marked dietary contrasts?

More recent dental research has dealt extensively with dental plaque with rather less concentration on dental calculus (Gibbons and Van Houte 1973; McHugh 1970; Newman 1974, 11980; Poole and Newman 1971a and b and 1974; Shroeder 1970). Modern SEM analysis of calculus has concentrated on its deposition and formation (Friskopp and Hammerstrom 1980; Jones 1972a and b; Lustman et al 1976). The archaeological micro-organisms were originally viewed in hollows and voids at the enamel/calculus interface. Subsequent fracturing of a number of specimens, both human and other mammals, has shown that many more are located deep within the mature matrix.

There are formidable problems associated with the qualitative and quantitative evaluation of the surviving remnants of microflora. However, allowing for changes due to calcification, their size and shape can be analysed due to the numbers involved and their excellent preservation. Boyde and Williams (1971) have demonstrated subtle metrical differences between even closely related species from modern micro-organisms isolated from the mouth. Thus by grouping ancient microbes into varying size categories information regarding ancient human oral ecology can be compiled.

Due to the rapid calcification of dental plaque it is not surprising that remnant organic fragments of these micro-organisms remain petrified and preserved within their mineral shells. After decalcification a substantial amount of organic ground substance remains. When viewed at high magnification, i.e. x 500, this large mass consists mainly of a reticulate network of 'thread-like' objects. These would be consistent with the filamentous and rod-shaped micro-organisms which make up the bulk of modern dental plaque. This being the case, it would seem that a number of biochemical techniques may be employed as a possible means of confirming taxonomically distinctive groups of micro-organisms.

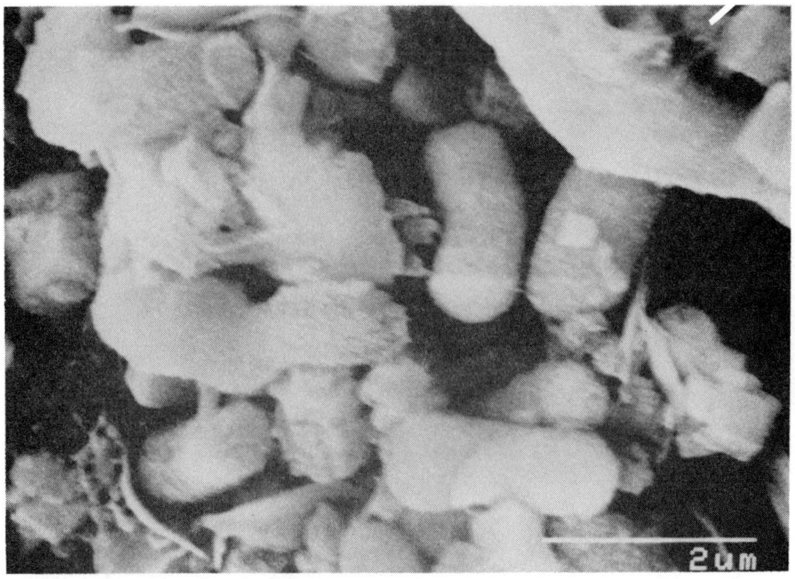


Figure 4.15a. Scanning electron micrograph of calcified rod shaped micro-organisms. Dalkey Island. Mag. X20K.

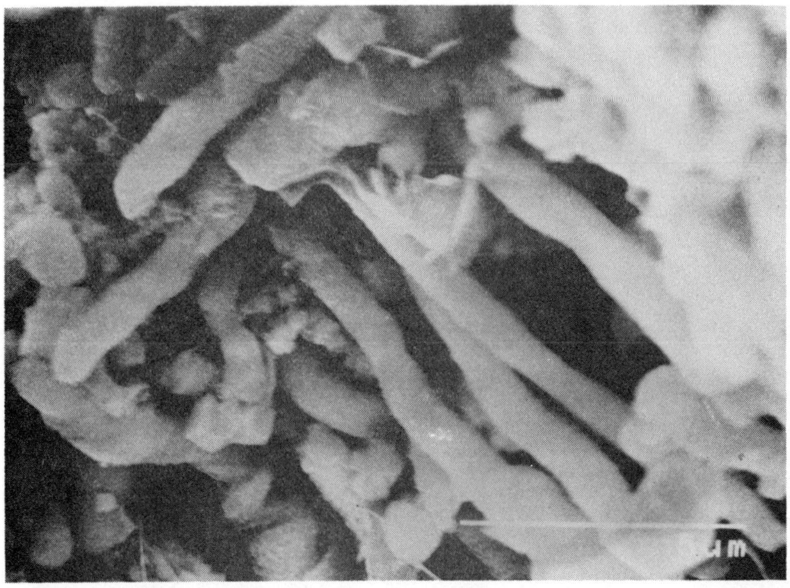

Figure 4.15b. Scanning electron micrograph of filamentous type micro-organisms from the same Dalkey Island calculus fragment. Mag. X15K.

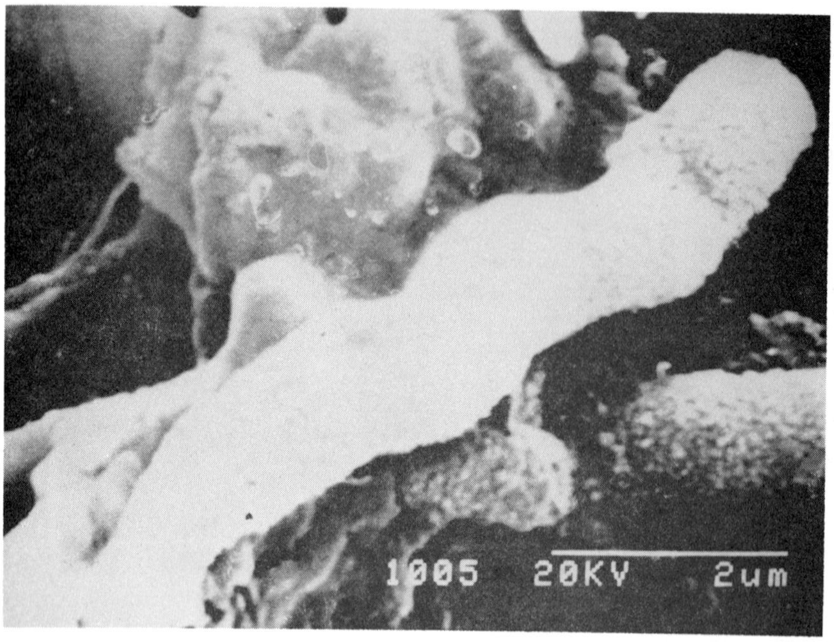


Figure 4.15c. Scanning electron micrograph of a single calcified oral treponeme. Early Medieval human calculus, Jewbury, York. Mag. X20K.

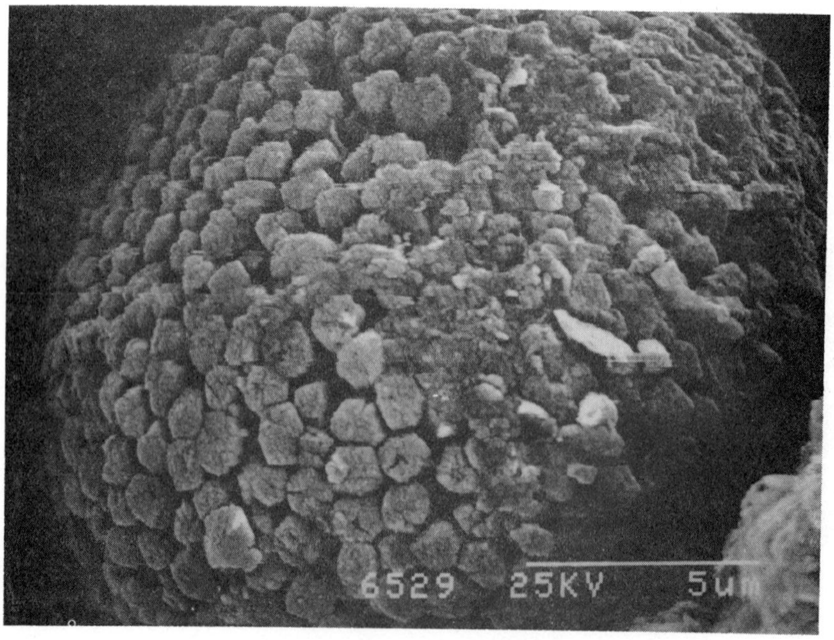


Figure 4.15d. Unidentified 'golf-ball' like object, possibly a colony of micro-organisms. Early Medieval human calculus, Jewbury, York. Mag. X10K.

## Conclusions

It is obvious that the information to be derived from the study of archaeological calculus promises to be varied. As has been shown from the Dalkey Island case study, dietary information can be specific and diverse even from a small amount of calculus. The amount of organic debris present in the calculus varies within and between individuals, as does preservation, but often anatomical detail is excellent.

The identification of the microscopic food inclusions is slow and highly specialised work, presenting problems not previously encountered in archaeological or indeed botanical fields. Similar problems arise when dealing with surviving calcified micro-organisms. However, the value of dental calculus in the reconstruction of past human diet and oral ecology is obvious. Further work is needed before the potential of this hitherto neglected source of archaeological information can be fully realised.


## ACKNOWLEDGEMENTS

The authors would like to thank the Science and Engineering Research Council for financing the research. Thanks are also due to Dr. R. Scaife, Dr. A. Jones, and T. Holden for their invaluable help with a number of problem identifications and references, B. Levitan and K. Rielly for generously allowing a number of tables to be incorporated into this paper, and Stephen Carter for useful comments on the final text.


## REFERENCES


Baer, P.N., Stephan, R.M. and White, C.L. (1961). Studies on experimental calculus formation in the rat. 1: effect of age, sex, strain, high carbohydrate, high protein diets. Journal of Periodontology 32: 190-96.

Baker, J. and Brothwell, D.R. (1980). Animal diseases in archaeology. 151-52. London: Academic Press.

Boyde, A. and Williams, A.D. (1971). Estimation of the volumes of bacterial cells by scanning electron microscopy. Archives of Oral Biology 16: 259-67.

Boyde, A., Petran, M. and Hadrovsky, M. (1983). Tandem scanning reflected light microscopy of internal features in whole bone and tooth samples. Journal of Microscopy 132: 1-7.

Dobney, K. and Brothwell, D.R. (in preparation). A method for evaluating the amount of dental calculus on teeth from archaeological sites.

Fitzgerald, R.J. and McDaniel, E.G. (1960). Dental calculus in the germ free rat. Archives of Oral Biology 2: 239.

Friskopp, J. and Hammarstrom, L. (1980). A comparative scanning electron microscopic study of supragingival and subgingival calculus. Journal of Periodontology 51: 553-62.

Gibbons, R.J. and Van Houte, J. (1973). On the formation of dental plaque. Journal of Periodontology 44: 347.

Helbaek, J. (1950). Tollunmandens sidste maltid. (The Tollund Man's last meal). Aarboger for Nordisk Oldkyndighed og Historie. 328-41.

Helbaek, J. (1958). Grauballemandens sidste maltid. (The Grauballe Man's last meal). Kuml. 111-16.

Jones, S.J. (1972a). Calculus on human teeth. Apex: 6.2.

Jones, S.J. (1972b). Morphology of calculus formation on the human tooth surface. Proceedings of the Royal Society of Medicine 65: 903-05.

King, J.D. and Glover, R.E. (1945). The relative effects of dietary constituents and other factors upon calculus and gingival disease in the ferret. Journal of Pathological Bacteriology 57: 353-62.

Körber-Grohne, U. (1980). Microstructure of the surfaces of carbonised and non-carbonised grains of cereals as observed in SEM and light microscopes as an aid in determining prehistoric finds. Journal of Archaeological Science 8: 1-9.

Körber-Grohne, U. (1981). Distinguishing prehistoric cereal grains of Triticum and Secale on the basis of their surface patterns using the scanning electron microscope. Journal of Archaeological Science 8: 197-204.

Levitan, B. (1984). The vertebrate remains in: Middleton Stoney: Excavation and survey in a north Oxfordshire parish 1970-1982. S. Rahtz and T. Rowley (eds.). Oxford: University Department of External Studies. 108-48.

Lustmann, J., Lewin-Epstein, J. and Shteyer, A. (1976). Scanning electron microscopy of dental calculus. Calcified tissue research 21: 47-55.

Mellanby, Lady M. (1934). Diet and the teeth: an experimental study. Part III. Special Report Series. Medical Research Council: London.

McHugh, P.D. (ed.). (1970). Dental plaque. London: Livingstone.

Moore, P.D. and Webb, J.A. (1978). An Illustrated Guide to Pollen Analysis. London: Hodder and Stoughton.

Navia, J.M. (1972). Prevention of dental caries: agents which increase tooth resistence to dental caries. International Dental Journal 22: 427-40.

Newman, H.N. (1974). Diet, attrition, plaque and dental disease. British Dental Journal 136: 491.

Newman, H.N. (1980). Dental Plaque: the Ecology of the Flora on Human Teeth. Illinois: Springfield.

Newman, H.N. and Poole, D. (1974). Structural and ecological aspects of dental plaque. In: F.A. Skinner and J.G. Carr (eds), The Normal Microbial Flora of Man. London: Academic Press.

Poole, D. and Newman, H.N. (1971a). Dental plaque and oral health. Nature 234: 329-31.

Poole, D. and Newman, H.N. (1971b). Topographical variations in dental plaque. Journal of Dental Research 50. 1175.

Rielly, K. (in press). The animal bones from Ditches, Cirencester.

Rovner, I. (1971). Potential of opal phytoliths for use in palaeoecological reconstruction. Quaternary Research 1: 343-59.

Schroeder, H.E. (1970). The structure and relationship of plaque to the hard and soft tissues: electron microscopic interpretation. International Dental Journal 20: 353.

Spencer, F.M. and Monroe, L.S. (1975). The Colour Atlas of Intestinal Parasites. Illinois: Springfield.

Spouge, J.D. (1973). Oral Pathology. St. Louise: C.V. Masby.

Twiss, P.C., Suess, E. and Smith, R.M. (1969). Morphological classification of grass phytoliths. Proceedings of Soil Science of America 33: 109-15.

Unmack, A. and Rowles, S.L. (1963). Constituents of dental calculus from sheep. Nature 197: 486-87.

## Chapter 5

# CEMENTUM DEPOSITION AMONG TROPCIAL AFRICAN UNGULATES: IMPLICATIONS FOR PALAEOECOLOGICAL STUDIES.

Robert Foley

Department of Physical Anthropology
University of Cambridge

## INTRODUCTION

Cementum, along with enamel and dentine, is one of the principal components of dental tissue (Figure 5.1). It is normally deposited throughout life. Consequently it has attracted the attention of biologists concerned with life history. Patterns of cementum distribution have been used by wildlife biologists, archaeologists and palaeontologists as a means of determining the age and season of death of an animal (Klevezal and Kleinenburg 1967; Morris 1972; Casteel 1976: Borque et al 1978; see Stallibras 1982 for a recent review). This method arises from the fact that among many species the rate and nature of deposition varies according to environmental conditions, and thus may appear as a series of lines or bands. These increments often represent seasonal or annual periods of growth, and may be counted for ageing purposes, or the final band used to determine the period of year in whch death took place.

The method has been used extensively for marine mammals, where cementum deposition may be very regular and the banding is remarkably clear (Laws 1952). Arctic and temperate terrestrial mammals have also proved to be susceptible to this form of analysis (Morris 1972; Stallibras 1982). In both cases it is the marked regularity of the seasonal conditions that results in clear banding.

Applications to tropical mammals, however, have been less successful, on account of the fact that seasonality is based on rainfall patterns (wet/dry seasons, rather than summer/winter; these are less regular and their effect on animals more variable) (Spinage 1973; Sinclair 1977). Consequently cementum deposition is frequently continuous and not marked by banding. Where banding does occur it is often irregular in width. This irregularity gives rise to problems in determining age, but it also offers various possibilities for palaeobiological research.

If, as is most likely, cementum deposition reflects environmental conditions, then the variability in band width should be a record of the variability in the environment. The pattern of cementum banding among tropical mammals should indicate conditions of rainfall and seasonality during the life of an individual. Measurements of the width of cementum layers should act as a means of monitoring life history. This hypothesis, which is explored in this paper, would take cementum analysis beyond an ageing technique and to a situation where it may be used to reconstruct environmental conditions.

Several problems in palaeoanthropology might be approached usefully from this direction. Very little is known about the seasonality of semi-arid

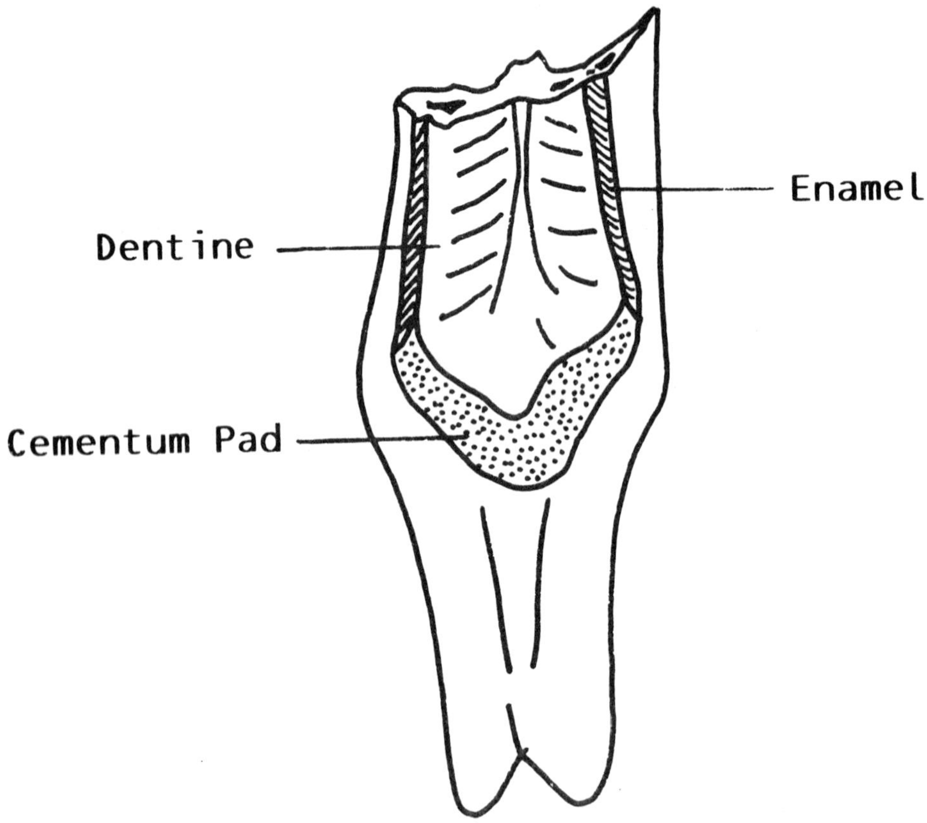


Figure 5.1 Section through the first permanent lower molar of a Cape Buffalo (Syncerus caffer), showing principal dental tissues and the cementum pad.

African environments in the Quaternary, and neither has it been possible to determine the seasonality of early hominid and prehistoric hunter-gatherer foraging behaviour. Analysis of the variability in deposition of cementum among tropical African mammals might be expected to yield some information on these points.

## Material and Methods

To test some of these ideas modern ungulate material was collected from East Africa. The National Parks of Tsavo East, Amboseli, Olorgesailie, Nairobi, and Nakuru were sampled for carcasses and skeletons that would form a control sample. Mandibles were collected, and where possible, a time of death was recorded. Some 120 complete and partial mandibles were collected. Species included Cape buffalo (*Syncerus caffer* Sparrman 1779), lesser kudu (*Tregelaphus imberbis* Blyth 1869), eland (*Taurotragus oryx* Pallas 1776), defassa waterbuck (*Kobus defassa* Ruppell 1835), wildebeest (*Connochaetes taurinus* Burchell 1823), kongoni (*Alcelaphus bucelaphus bucelaphus* Pallas 1776), Grant's gazelle (*Gazalla granti* Brooke 1872), Thomson's gazelle (*Gazalla thomsonii* Gunther 1884), impala (*Aepyceros melampus* Lichtenstein 1812), Burchell's zebra (*Equus burchelli* Gray 1824) and cow (*Bos taurus*).

Studies have shown that cementum banding is clearest in incisors and canines (Morris 1972), but as these are seldom preserved in fossil samples, premolars and molars were examined. These possess a pad of cementum between the roots of varying thickness. Various methods of sample preparation were employed, including decalcification and thin-sectioning, as well as embedding in plastic and thick-sectioning, etc., followed by microscopic examination. After experimentation the following method was used: the teeth were embedded in candle wax, cut in half bucally-lingually, and then a section removed from the exposed surface. This section was then ground down and dry mounted on a slide. The point of thickest cementum deposition was selected for the sectioning plane. The sectioning was carried out with a diamond-edged rotary saw driven at a very slow speed to prevent splintering of the sample, and enhance the polishing of the section surface. The teeth were then examined and photographed under a white light with a polarizing filter, using an Olympus Stereo Zoom Microscope, at magnifications of between x20 and x80.

On each tooth the metrical characteristics, particularly crown height, were recorded. Information on the thickness of the cementum, number of bands, width of each band and colouration were taken. As banding was often diffuse and so unclear, repeated observations were made.

## Results and Discussion

Only some preliminary results are presented here. These relate principally to the Cape buffalo, although some other species are referred to for comparative purposes.

1. Ageing. The well-established use of cementum lines for aging purposes can be seen to be of general utility for many of the specimens examined. (Figures 5.2 and 5.3). A correlation between crown height, the principal ageing technique for ungulates (Klein & Cruz-Ubibe 1984), and cementum line counts for M1 and P4 can be established, but there is considerable

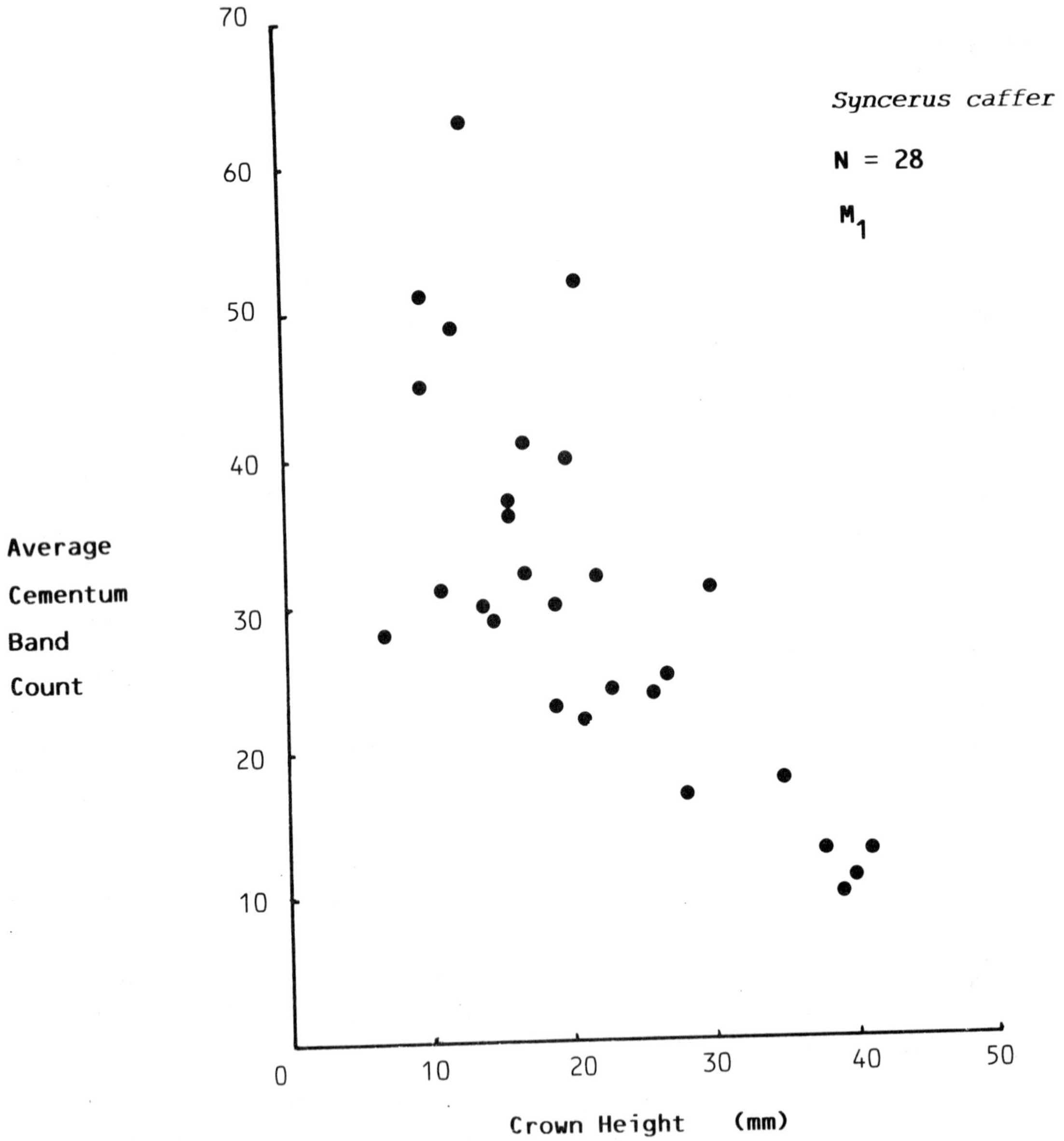


Figure 5.2. Relationship between crown height and cementum increment counts for a sample of Cape Buffalo permanent first molars.

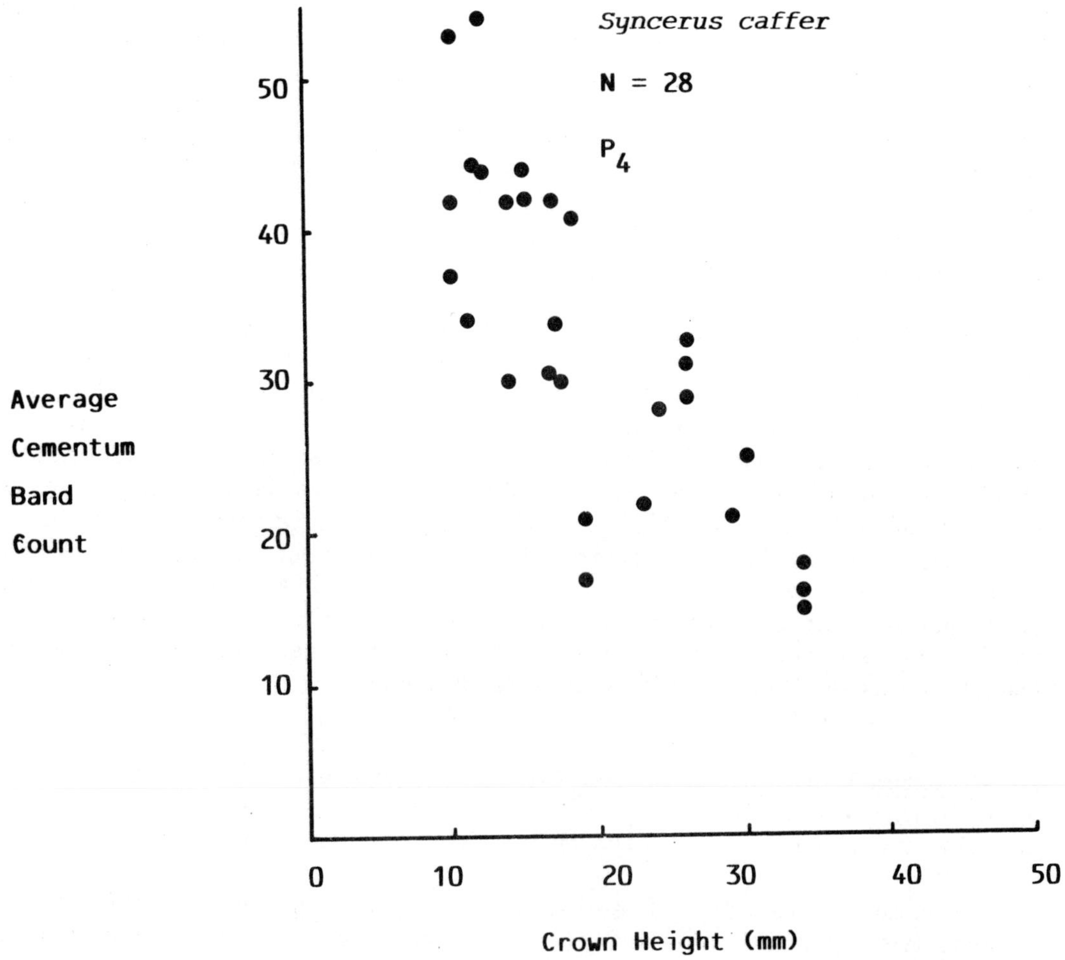


Figure 5.3. Relationship between crown height and cementum increments for a sample of Cape Buffalo P4s.

variability that remains unexplained. This may be illustrated by the fact that left and right M1s from the same animal may have different cementum bands counts (Table 5.1). If these left and right M1s are then plotted against crown height (Figure 5.4) it can be seen that while right teeth display very little patterning, those from the left side of the jaw show a much neater relationship. This suggests that there are biomechanical factors in the processes of mastication that affect crown height and/or the degree of cementum deposition. The implication of this is that the left and right sides of the jaw should be treated separately in analysis, and one side may be of more value than the other in ageing, either by crown height or by cementum deposition. This may raise great difficulties when dealing with isolated archaeological material as the separation of rights from lefts can be problematic. In both of these cases, though, it should be noted that with older animals the relationship between crown height and cementum lines becomes eratic. This is likely to be due to the resorption of dental tissue which is known to occur in old age.

As a technique for ageing, it may be suggested, as has been argued before, that analysis of cementum lines among tropical animals may provide a useful supplement to other techniques, but owing to irregular and diffuse deposition it is unlikely to be as reliable as among high latitude mammals. As alternative, potentially simpler, method, using maximum cementum thickness, also shows some relationship with crown height, although the scatter of points is fairly wide (Figure 5.5). Sample size for other species is very small, but Figure 5.6 shows that cementum increment growth varies from species to species. Although data is limited it might perhaps be suggested that the grazers and seasonally variable animals, particularly wildebeest, are more likely to have markedly banded cementum deposition, and therefore susceptible to this ageing technique.

2. Cementum Increment Thickness. The main purpose of this analysis, is to explore patterns of variability in the width of cementum deposition in animals, and the extent to which this reflects environmental conditions.

Incremental banding of cementum shows up under the microscope as alternative layers of dark and light tissue. The boundaries between these layers are sometimes diffuse, and sometimes clearcut. Most of the cementum consists of the lighter, less dense bands. Table 5.2 shows the mean thickness of dark and light bands for various specimens. With one exception the dark layers are always considerably narrower than the light. For *S. caffer* the mean ratio of dark to light is 0.57 +0.33 Other species doe not differ significantly from this value. The light bands, with less calcium and more cementocytes, are thought to represent periods of more rapid growth, and the dark bands attenuated growth. In other words, during growth periods thick layers of less densely packed tissue are deposited, but as growth slows down for various reasons the rate of cementum deposition also decreases. For herbivorous animals in the tropical savanna the dark lines may be assumed to be dry seasons, the light one wet seasons, although other factors, such as reproductive behaviour and age may also affect deposition. In an analysis of cementum increments among Serengeti buffalo, Sinclair (1977) related patterns of light and dark deposition to the bimodal rainfall distribution of the region, suggesting that two dark increments were deposited each year.

An examination of the cementum growth for various Tsavo East buffalo substantiates this general pattern. Figure 5.7 shows the thickness of each

| Specimen Number | Mean Number of Cementum Lines: Left | Right | Difference |
|---|---|---|---|
| TSE20 | 52 | 37 | 15 |
| TSE35 | 36 | 30 | 6 |
| TSE17 | 30 | 32 | 2 |
| TSE15 | 24 | 22 | 2 |
| TSE14 | 17 | 31 | 14 |
| TSE13 | 45 | 31 | 14 |
| TSE18 | 63 | 49 | 14 |
| TSE34 | 11 | 13 | 2 |
| TSE36 | 10 | 13 | 3 |

Table 5.1. Differences in the number of cementum lines in M1 (left and right) from Tsavo National Park (East).

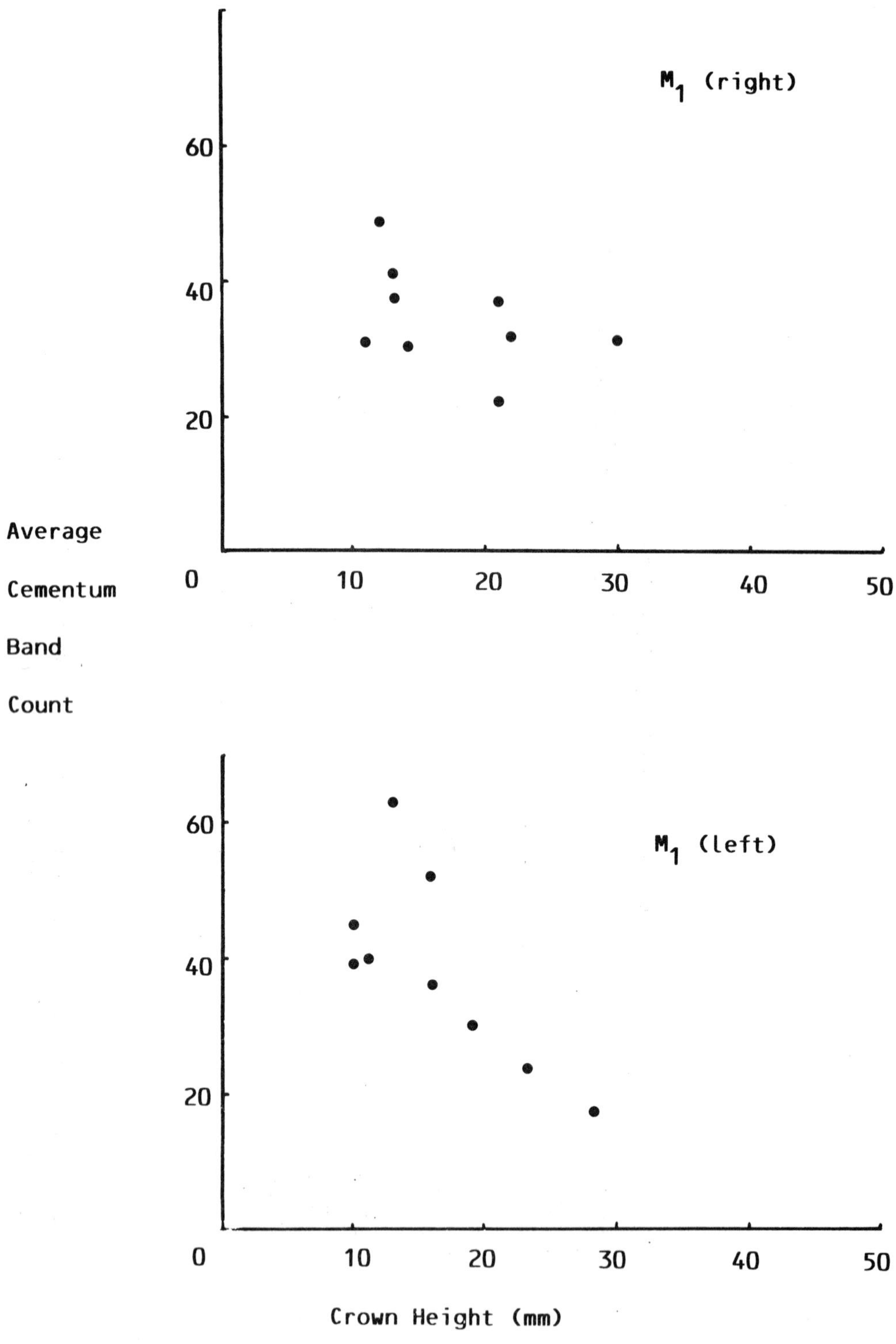


Figure 5.4. Relationship between crown height and cementum increment for a sample of Cape buffalo permanent first molars for matched left and right sides of the jaw.

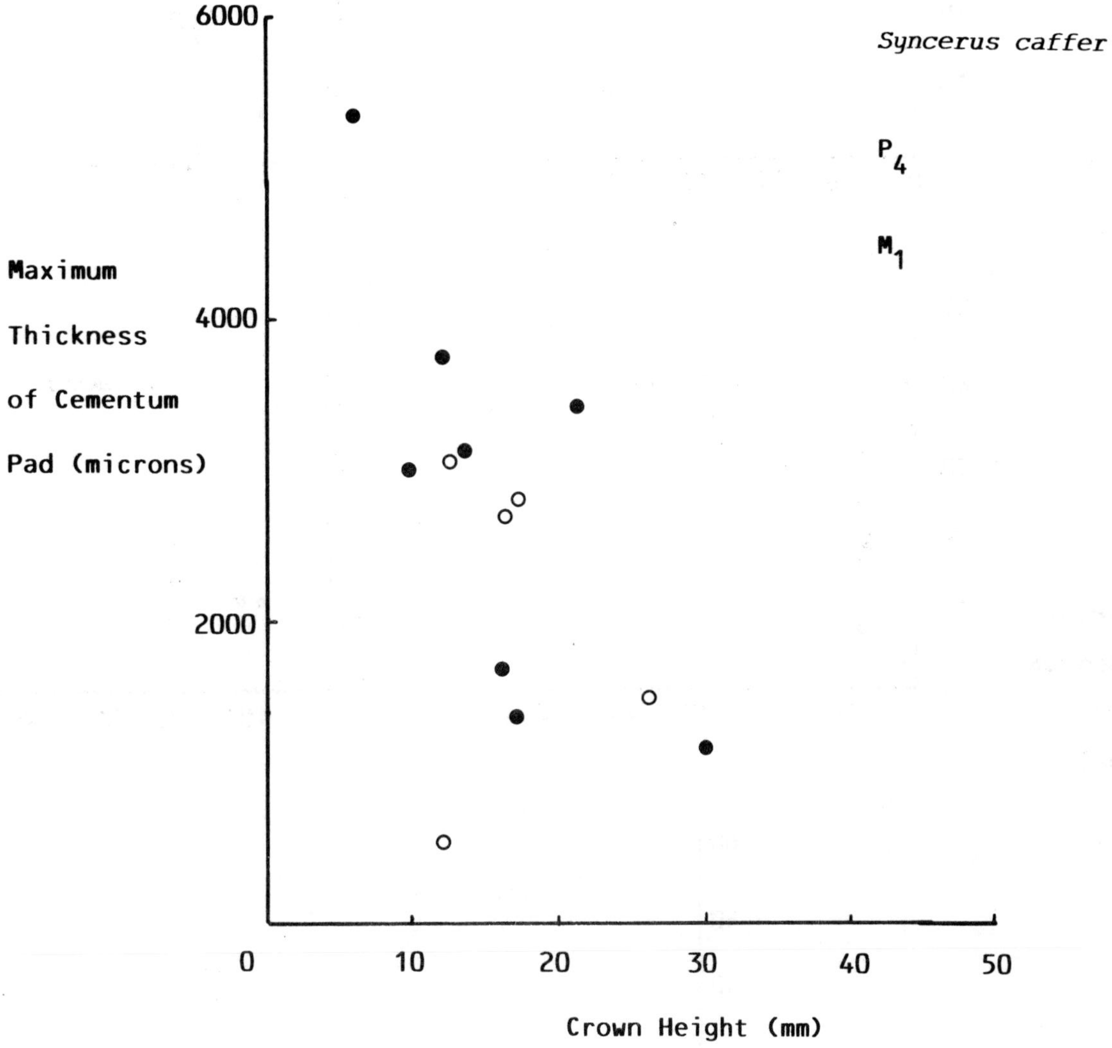


Figure 5.5. Relationship between crown height and maximum cementum thickness for Cape buffalo M1 and P4.

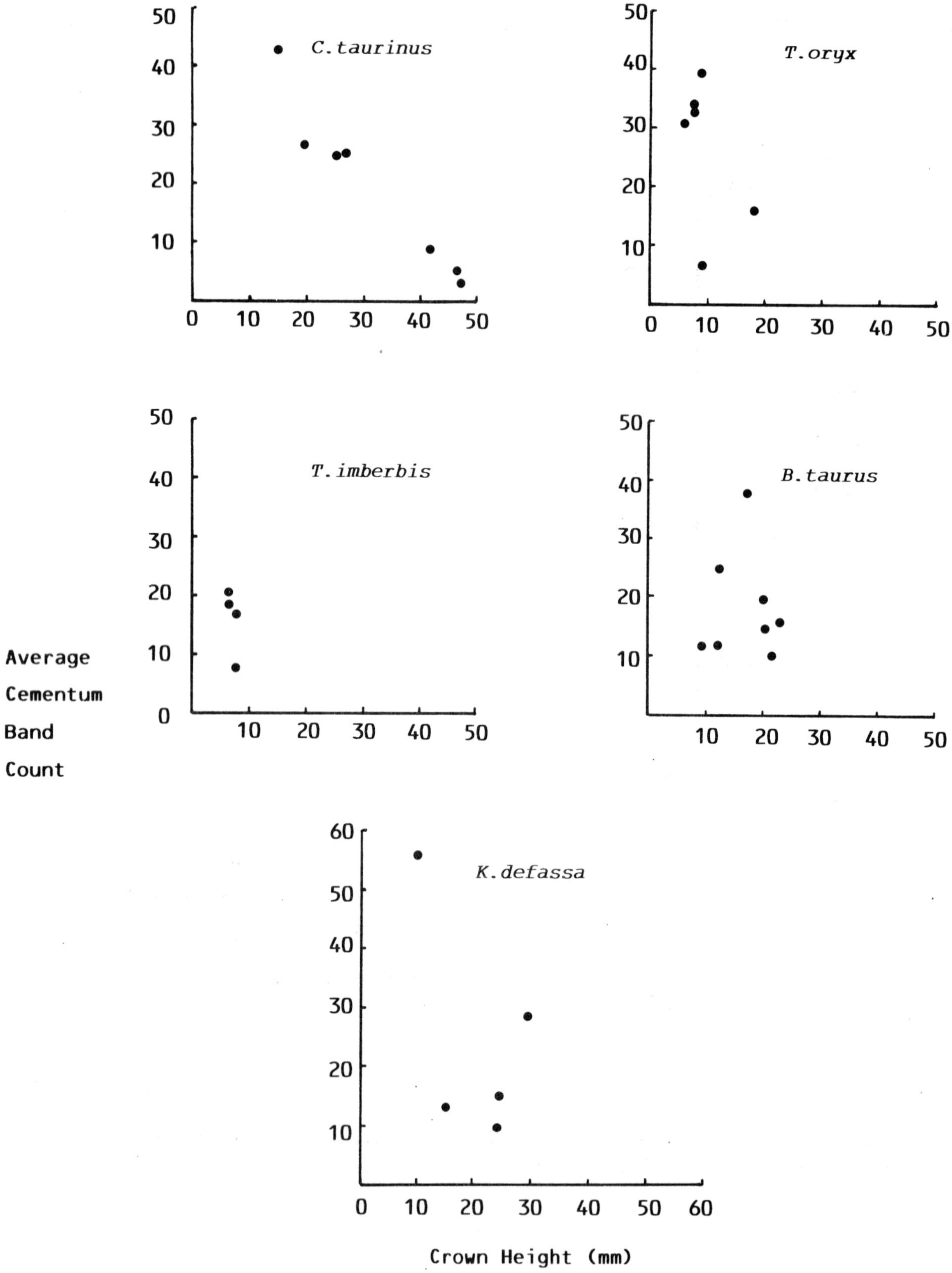


Figure 5.6. Relationship between crown height and cementum increment counts for M1 for various species.

| Specimen Number | | Dark | Light | Dark / Light |
|---|---|---|---|---|
| **Buffalo** | | | | |
| TSE14 | P4 | 126 | 319 | 0.39 |
| TSE16 | P4 | 135 | 1081 | 0.12 |
| TSE35 | P4 | 126 | 186 | 0.67 |
| TSE35 | P4 | 174 | 127 | 1.37 |
| TSE14 | M1 | 250 | 303 | 0.83 |
| TSE20 | M1 | 51 | 154 | 0.33 |
| TSE26 | M1 | 62 | 139 | 0.45 |
| TSE28 | M1 | 111 | 294 | 0.38 |
| TSE30 | M1 | 216 | 294 | 0.74 |
| TSE35 | M1 | 95 | 240 | 0.39 |
| **Domestic Cattle** | | | | |
| OLG02 | M1 | 131 | 131 | 1.0 |
| OLG02 | M1 | 43 | 135 | 0.32 |
| AMB17 | M1 | 96 | 379 | 0.25 |
| AMB39 | P4 | 36 | 149 | 0.24 |
| **Thomson's Gazelle** | | | | |
| NBI10 | M1 | 233.4 | 486.6 | 0.48 |
| **Waterbuck** | | | | |
| NBI08 | M1 | 72.4 | 73.75 | 0.98 |

Table 5.2. Relationship between mean thickness of light and dark increments on East African large herbivore species. Thicknesses are given in microns.

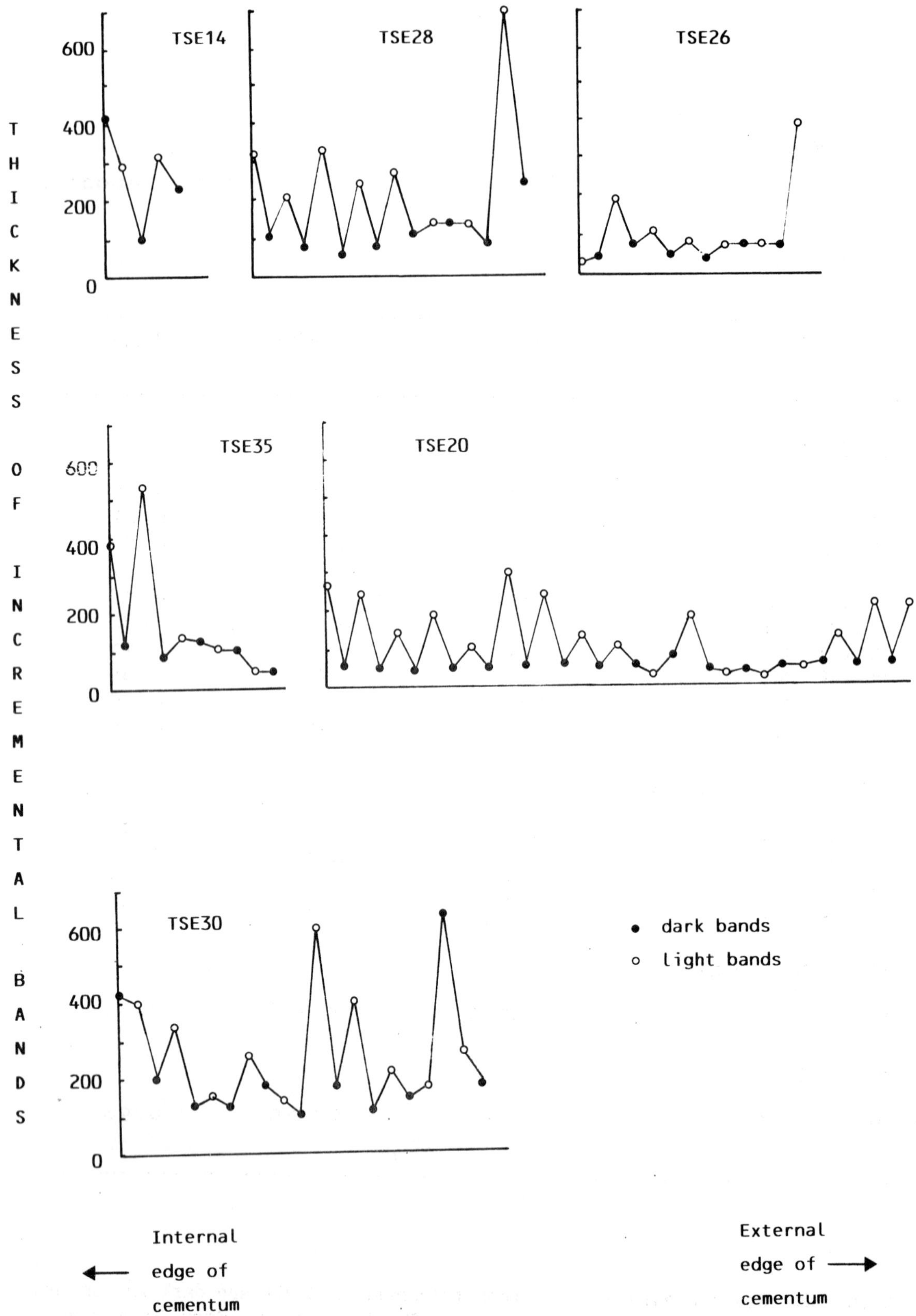


Figure 5.7. Pattern of band thickness for various African buffalo from Tsavo National Park (East).

successive light and dark band from the interior (youngest) to the exterior (oldest) part of the tooth. In some cases these oscillate in a saw-toothed way; at other times there is relatively little variation; and occasionally there is very marked variation. According to the model described above regular oscillation should reflect the coming and going of the rainy seasons. Very thick light bands might be expected to indicate prolonged "good" conditions, while limited increments would indicate prolonged dry conditions and only ephemeral growth (Sinclair 1977). All these Tsavo East specimens died during or just after the prolonged droughts of the early seventies (Figure 5.8) (Phillipson 1975), and TSE 35, TSE 26, and TSE might reflect this. TSE 20, a very old individual, is interestsing in that the earlier bands reflect a regular pattern of seasonal change, switching to a less predictable environment in later life. Regrettably the exact date of death of these animals is not known, and so the rate of cementum growth and its relationship to environmental conditions cannot be pinpointed more accurately.

However, while this simple environmental interpretation of cementum band thickness, similar to that of tree-ring growth, is attractive, several compounding factors are liable to interfere and lead to difficulties of interpretation. For example, a consideration of Figure 5.9 shows that for the same individual, TSE 35, left and right P4s cannot be said to show the same pattern. The same holds true for the M1 and P4 of TSE14. In view of the differences noted above for left and right teeth it might well be that resources are allocated differentially for left and right teeth. Furthermore, even without a single ecosystem, as Phillipson (1975) has shown for Tsavo, conditions can vary considerably locally, so that not all individuals experience the same environment. The pattern of cementum band width variation also holds true for other species (Figure 5.10).

## CONCLUSIONS

At this stage conclusions must remain tentative. This paper has suggested that while the variability in cementum band among tropical African ungulates is such that ageing is problematic, this very variability may act as an indicator of environmental conditions and life history. Broad seasonal trends can be seen in the cementum deposition, but these are likely to be overlain by other factors. Further research is necessary with animals of known age and exact date of death to determine how much palaeoecological information is contained in the cementum of fossil animals.

## ACKNOWLEDGEMENTS.

Collection of field data was supported by grants from the British Academy and the University of Durham. I should like to thank the Ministry of Wildlife and Tourism in Kenya for permission to work in the National Parks, and to the Wardens and rangers of these parks for their assistance and co-operation. Facilities were also provided by the National Museums of Kenya. I am also grateful to Dr. E. Long and the SERC for the loan of a vehicle while in Kenya. Assistance in the field was provided by Dr. Louis Jacobs and Jill Goudie.

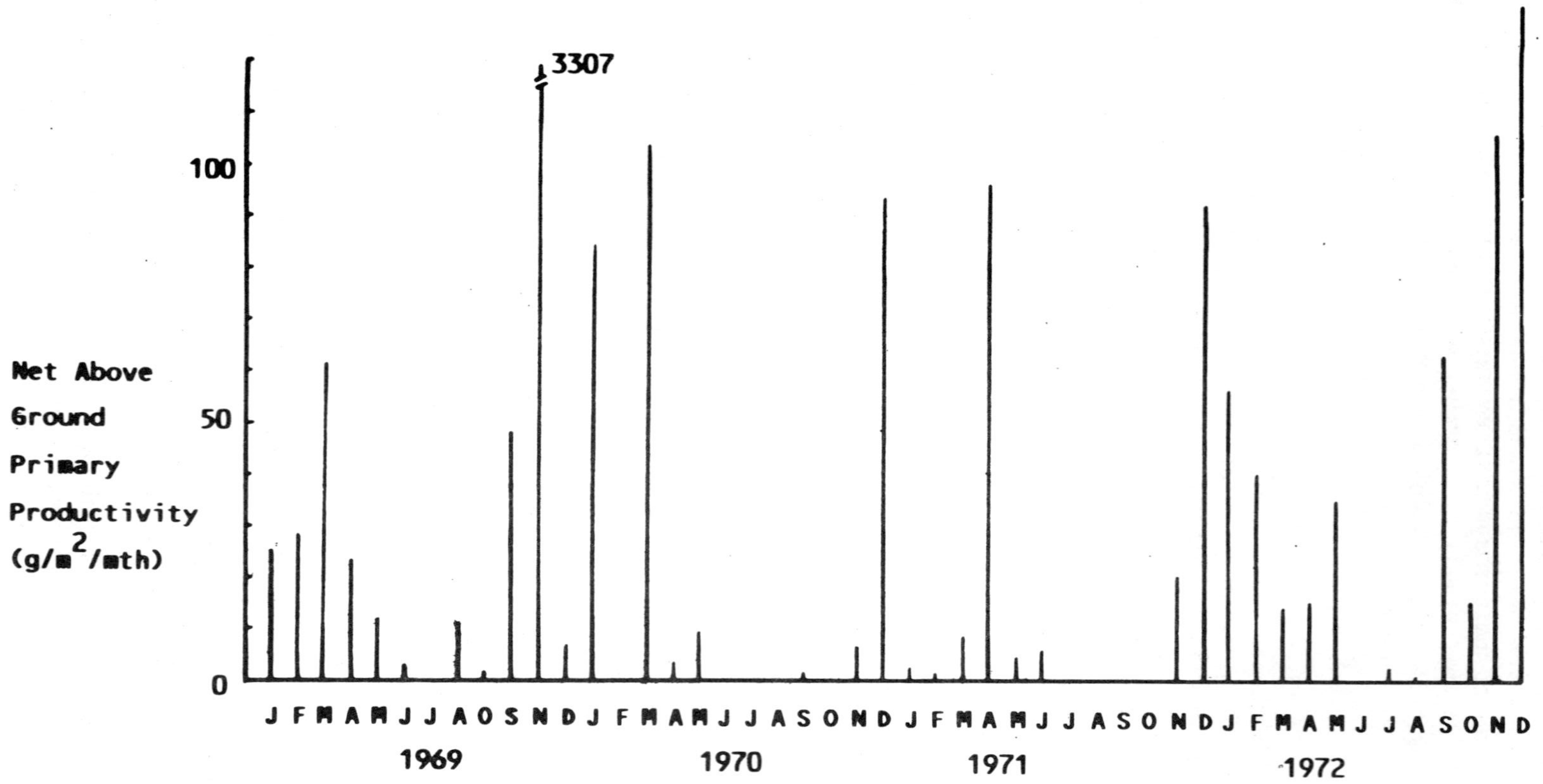


Figure 5.8. Variation in net above ground primary productivity for a four year period in Tsava National Park East. Data from Phillipson 1975.

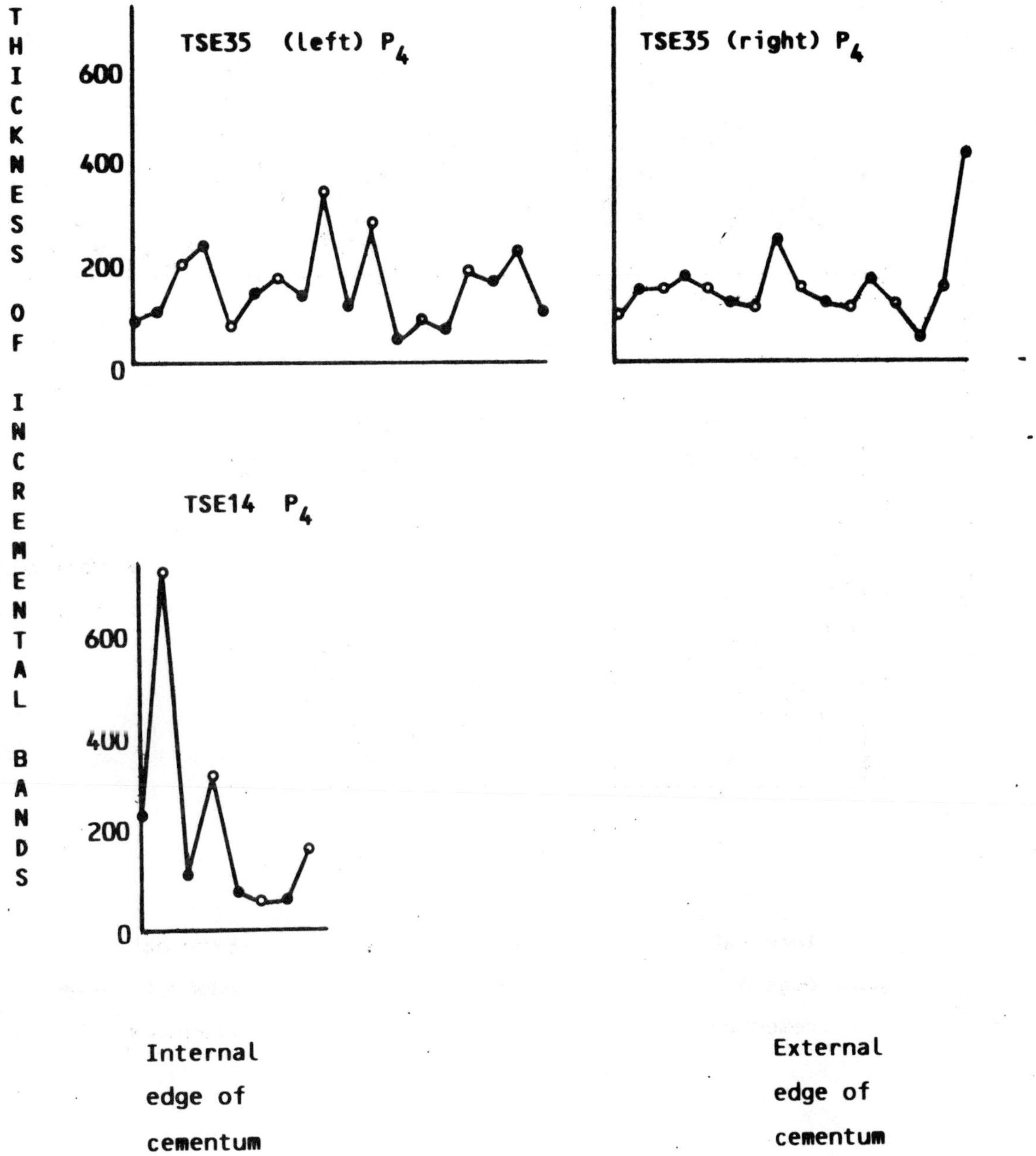


Figure 5.9. Pattern of increment thickness for P4 from two specimens of Cape buffalo from Tsavo National Park (East).

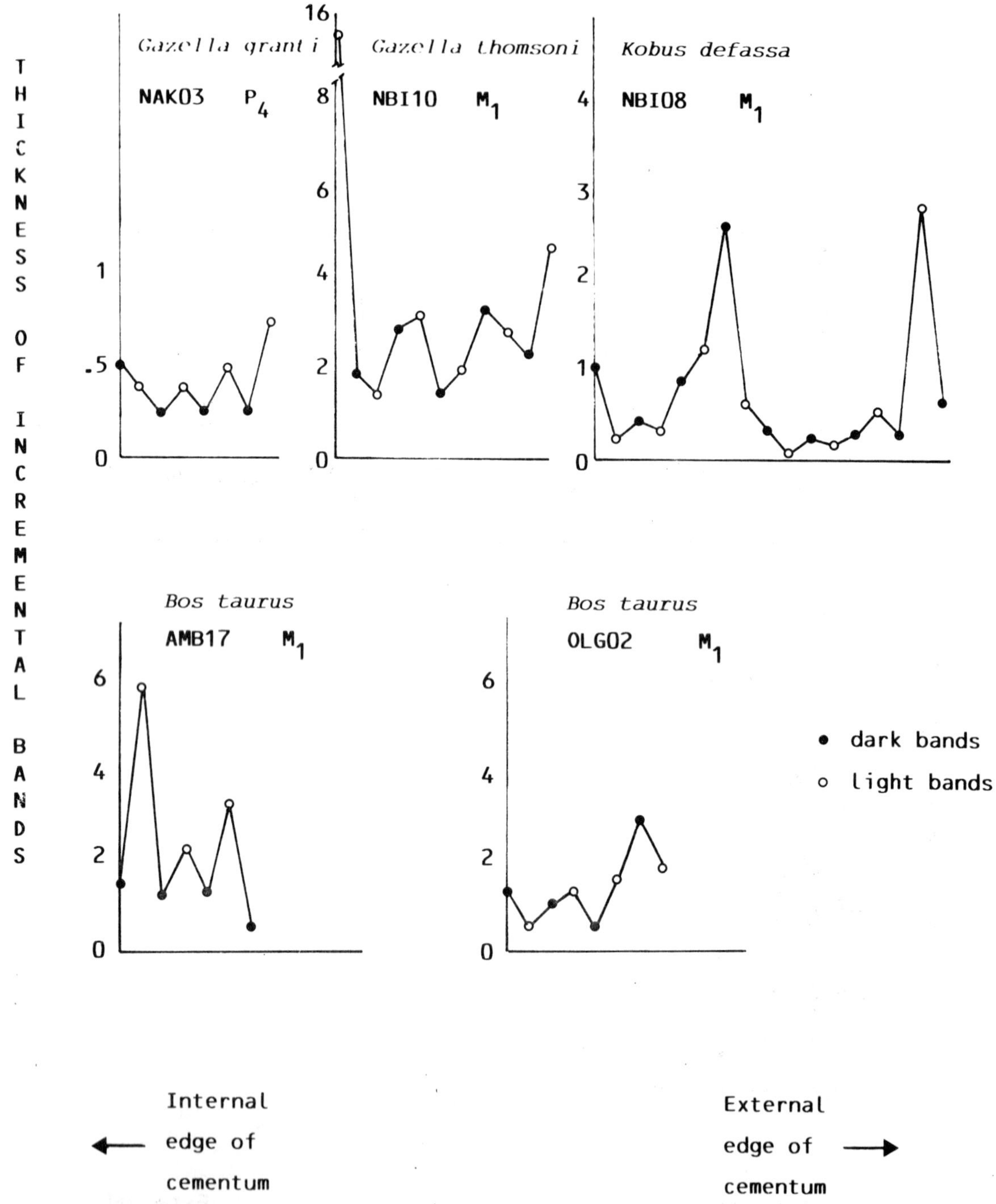


Figure 5.10 Pattern of cementum increment thickness for various species from East African National Parks.

REFERENCES.

Borque, B.J., Morris, K. and Speiss, A. (1978). Determining the season of death of mammal teeth from archaeological sites: a new sectioning technique. Science 199: 530-1.

Casteel, R.W. (1976). Incremental growth zones in mammals and their archaeological value. Papers of the Kroeber Society 47: 1-27.

Klein and Cruz Uribe, K. (1984). The Analysis of Faunal Remains from Archaeological Sites. Chicago University Press, Chicago.

Klevezal, G.A. and Kleinenberg, S.E. (1967). Age determination of mammals from annual layers in teeth and bones. Academy of Sciences, U.S.S.R.

Laws, R.M. (1952). A new method of age determination for mammals. Nature 169: 972-973.

Morris, P.A. (1972). A review of mammalian age determination methods. Mammal Review 2(3): 69-104.

Phillipson, J. (1975). Rainfall, primary productivity and "carrying capacity" of Tsavo National Park (East). Kenya. East African Wildlife Journal 13: 171-201.

Sinclair, A.R.E. (1977). The African Buffalo. Chicago University Press, Chicago.

Spinage, C.A. (1973). A review of the age determination of mammals by means of teeth with especial reference to Africa. East African Wildlife Journal. 11: 165-187.

Stallibras, S. (1982). The use of cement layers for absolute ageing of mammalian teeth: a selective review of the literature, with suggestions for further studies and alternative applications. In: Ageing and Sexing Animal Bones from Archaeological Sites edited by R. Wilson, C. Grigson amd S. Payne. B.A.R. (British Series) 109. pp. 109-126.

<u>Chapter 6</u>

# AN EVALUATION OF SCOTT'S METHOD FOR SCORING DENTAL WEAR

J.F. Cross, N.W. Kerr* and M.F. Bruce

Department of Anatomy
Marischal College
University of Aberdeen

*Department of Dental Surgery
Aberdeen Royal Infirmary

Studies of dental wear, or attrition, in human populations have concentrated on two main areas. Firstly, attempts have been made to correlate attrition patterns with the way in which teeth have been used during life (Leigh, 1925; Molnar, 1971, 1972; Smith, 1972; Taylor, 1963). Significant inter- and intra-population differences in wear have been found. The rate and pattern of attrition has been shown to be affected by a combination of factors such as diets containing a high proportion of fibrous or unprocessed food; the presence of abrasive substances such as sand or grit which may have been introduced to the food during its collection or preparation; and cultural practices such as hide chewing by Eskimos to soften animal skins.

The second area of research has been concerned with the relationship between the degree of attrition and the biological age-at-death of an individual. Miles (1962) devised a system of ageing skeletal material which was based on the analysis of the rate of attrition of the molars. Using a series of Anglo-Saxon crania, he developed a wear chart showing the amount of attrition characteristic of a particular age group. Other workers (Brothwell, 1981; Miles, 1962, 1963; Nowell, 1978) have also assessed age-atdeath using the degree of dental wear.

Most studies on attrition are not directly comparable because different scoring techniques have been used. Unfortunately, many of these methods fail either to discriminate satisfactorily between stages of wear or to describe objectively the amount of dentine exposure. Often, a single score is given to the entire occlusal surface (Brothwell, 1981; Leigh, 1925; Miles, 1962; Molnar, 1971; Murphy, 1959; Taylor, 1963). This method results in considerable loss of information on the differential wear patterns of the teeth. Furthermore, most scoring techniques consist of a small number of broadly defined grades, thereby forcing the classification of attrition into categories which may fail to reflect accurately the amount of enamel present on the occlusal surface.

Scott (1979) devised a scoring technique which appeared to offer both a more objective and a more detailed description of dental wear. The method was originally designed for molar teeth but it could be modified for use on premolar teeth. The system is based on a 4 - 40 point ordinal scale which registers the amount of enamel present on the occlusal surface of a tooth.

The molar teeth are visually divided into four sections and each quadrant is given a score on a 1 - 10 scale. If the tooth is not in

| | | N.W.K. | J.F.C. | | |
|---|---|---|---|---|---|
| | n | mean + sem | mean + sem | r | |
| M1 | 84 | 26.9 + 0.88 | 27.3 + 0.84 | 0.95 | ns |
| M2 | 80 | 17.6 + 0.77 | 18.0 + 0.88 | 0.96 | ns |
| M1 & M2 | 164 | 22.3 + 0.69 | 22.8 + 0.71 | 0.96 | $p>0.05$ |

Table 6.1. Mean, standard error of the mean and correlation coefficient (r) for the scores assigned to the first molar, the second molar and the combined first and second molars by the two observers (N.W.K. and J.F.C.).

occlusion, is damaged or has been lost, either ante- or post-mortem, it is given a score of 0. The score of the tooth is equal to the sum of the four quadrant scores and so ranges from 4 - 40.

Scores 1 to 4 assess the condition of the major occlusal features and are associated with the presence of non-carious pits, with the development of wear facets and with the flattening of the cusps.

Scores 5 to 10 record the amount of dentine exposed in relation to the amount of enamel present in the quadrant area. Score 5 describes a quadrant that has been worn flat and on which dentine is visible on one fourth or less of the quadrant area.

Score 8 indicates the presence of a thick to medium band of enamel on only one side of the quadrant, usually on the outer rim, with dentine exposed on the remainder of the quadrant.

A score of 10 is given to a quadrant in which no enamel is evident. The complete exposure of dentine may be associated with the extension of attrition to below the amelo-cemental junction into the root.

Scott's technique was found to be straightforward and easy to use. The inclusion of a separate score for each quadrant takes into account the differential wear on various parts of the occlusal surface. The large number of scoring categories appears to reduce the subjectivity of the assessment of the degree of attrition.

In order to test the reliability of this technique, it was decided to compare the scores of two independent observers on a series of molar teeth.

Thirty three adult dentitions were selected from the Aberdeen Carmelite collection, which is housed in the Department of Anatomy, University of Aberdeen. The material has been dated as Late Medieval (c. 1300 - 1600). Only the first and second molars were scored by two of the authors (N.W.K. and J.F.C.). A total of 164 teeth were used: 84 first molars and 80 second molars.

The means and standard errors of the means of the attrition scores were calculated for the first molar, the second molar and the combined scores for the first and second molars. The results are shown in Table 6.1.

They show that the second observer (J.F.C.) tended to give slightly higher scores than the first observer. No significant difference between the scores for the first or the second molars was observed but there was a significant difference between the results of the combined first and second molar scores (Student's paired t-test, $p > 0.05$, Table 6.1).

Nevertheless, the high positive correlation ($r = 0.95 - 0.96$, Table 6.1) between the pairs of data suggest that the scores given by the two observers vary in a similar manner. The significant difference between the two observers' scores may be related to the difficulty of distinguishing between the early stages of wear.

The scores of the first observer (N.W.K.) were plotted against the scores assigned by the second observer. Figures 6.1, 6.2 and 6.3. show the inter-observer plots for the first molar, the second molar and the combined first and second molar scores, respectively.

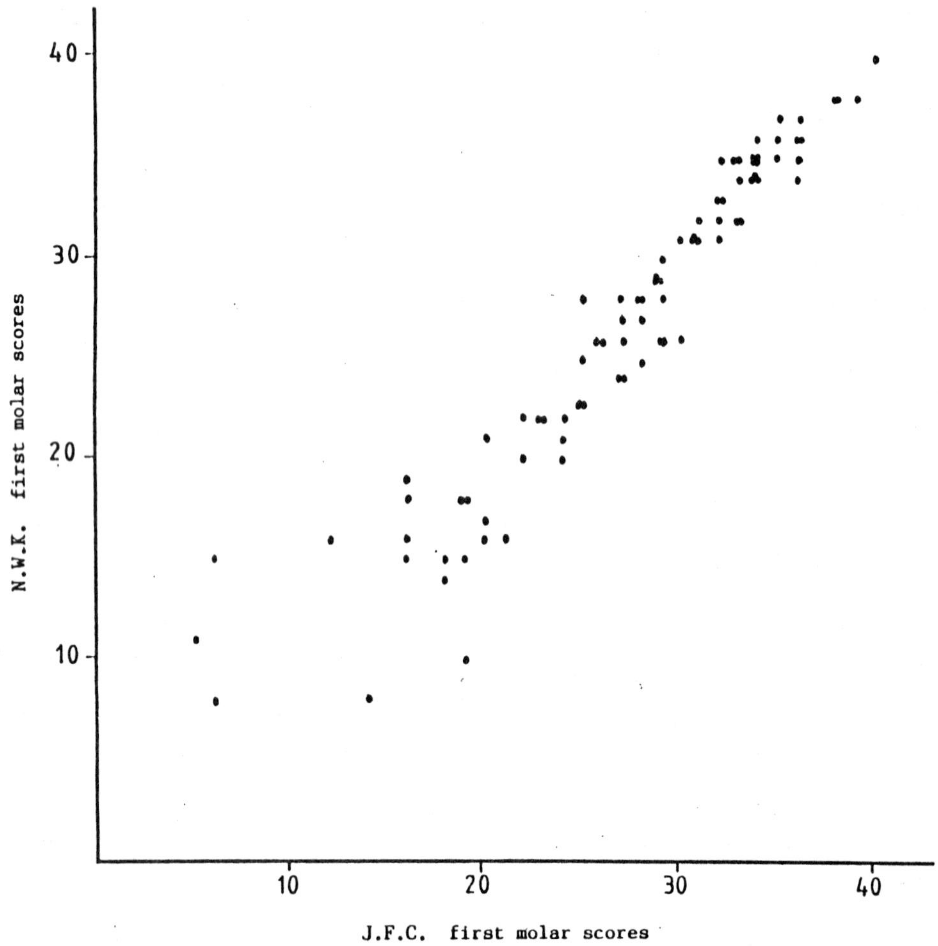


Figure 6.1. Inter-observer comparison of first molar scores.

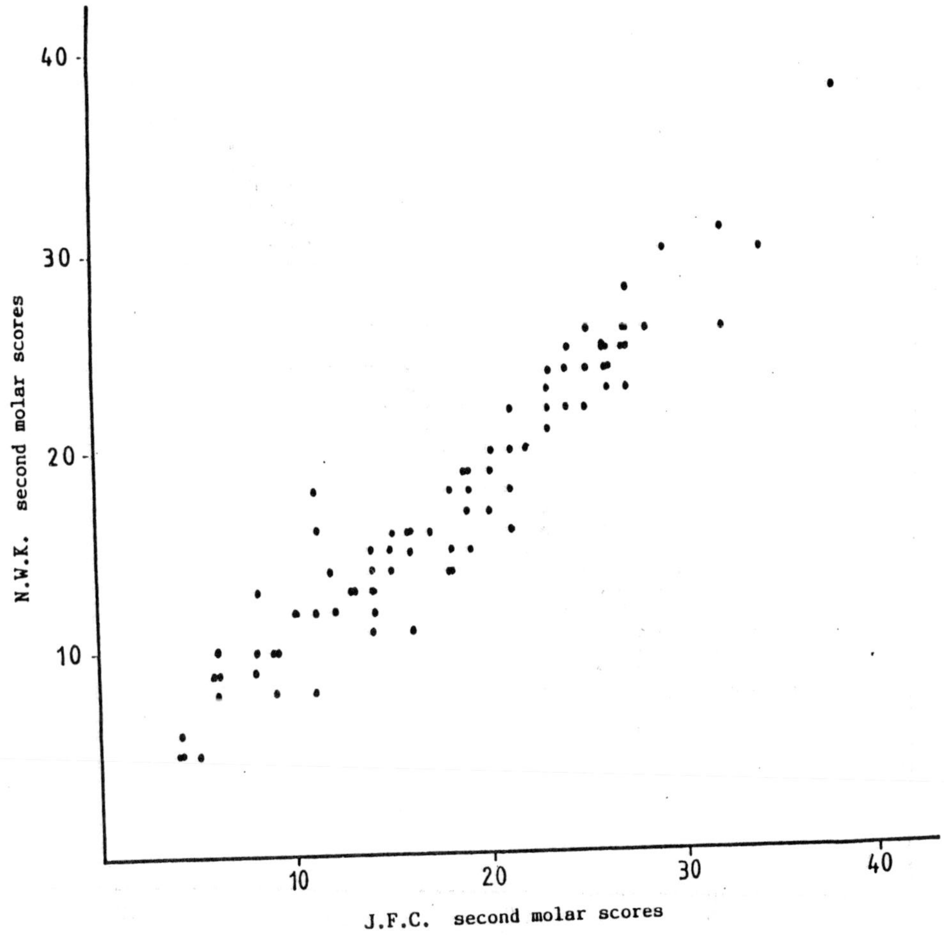


Figure 6.2. Inter-observer comparison of second molar scores.

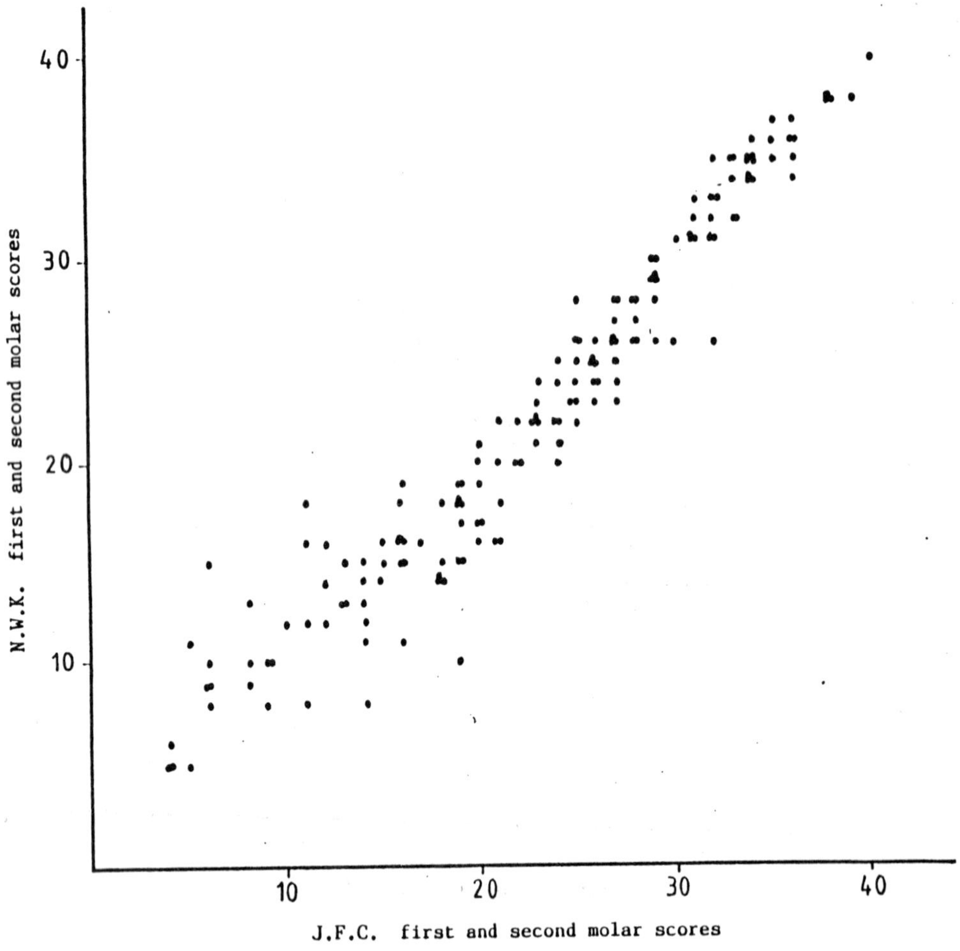


Figure 6.3. Inter-observer comparison of first and second molar scores.

The figures show that there is a fair amount of scatter at the lower end of the scale. This suggests that Scott's quadrant scores of 1 - 4 are not being assigned by the two observers in a consistent manner. These score categories deal with the early wear processes which include the appearance of wear facets, the rounding of cusps and the gradual disappearance of other surface features such as non-carious pits and fissures.

The discrepancy is interesting and may be partly due to the difference in the amount of dental experience between the two observers and partly due to the somewhat subjective description of the 1 - 4 quadrant scores.

From the occlusal scores of 16 upwards, the points on the plot lie very close together (Figs. 6.1, 6.2 and 6.3), indicating that the two observers are giving comparable scores. Quadrants with scores of 5 - 10 are more easily identified as they reflect the amount of enamel present and because Scott's descriptions of the scores are accompanied by a wear diagram.

It therefore seems that the more severe attrition lends itself to accurate and objective assessment by any observer, regardless of previous experience. However, it would also seem advisable for anyone attempting to use the method to have a period of training under the supervision of a dentally experienced person in order to eliminate the problems of distinguishing between the low quadrant scores.

In conclusion, Scott's method of scoring dental wear provides an objective, repeatable and detailed description of the relationship between enamel wear and dentine exposure. It is therefore suggested that in future studies on attrition, whether for the purpose of relating wear to the use of teeth or to the estimated age-at-death, such a system should be used.

## ACKNOWLEDGEMENTS

The authors gratefully acknowledge the financial support from the Scottish Development Department (Ancient Monuments Division) (J.F.C.) and from the Wellcome Trust (N.W.K.).

## REFERENCES

Brothwell, D.R. (1981). Digging up Bones. Third Edition. British Museum (Natural History), Oxford University Press.

Leigh, R.W. (1925). Dental pathology of Indian tribes of varied environmental and food conditions. Am. J. Phys. Anthrop. 8: 179-199.

Miles, A.E.W. (1962). Assessment of the ages of a population of Anglo-Saxons from their dentitions. Proc. Roy. Soc. Med. 44: 881-886.

Miles, A.E.W. (1963). The dentition in the assessment of individual age in skeletal material. In: Dental Anthropology edited by D.R. Brothwell. Pergamon Press: 191-209.

Molnar, S. (1971). Human tooth wear, tooth function and cultural variability. Am. J. Phys. Anthrop. 34: 175-190.

Molnar, S. (1972). Tooth wear and culture: A survey of tooth function among some prehistoric populations. Curr. Anthropol. 13: 511-526.

Murphy, T. (1959). The changing pattern of dentine exposure in human tooth attrition. Am. J. Phys. Anthrop. 17: 167-178.

Nowell, G.W. (1978). An Evaluation of the Miles method of ageing using the Tepe Hissar dental sample. Am. J. Phys. Anthrop. 49: 271-276.

Scott, E.C. (1979). Dental scoring technique. Am. J. Phys. Anthrop. 51: 213-218.

Smith, P. (1972). Diet and attrition in the Natufians. Am. J. Phys. Anthrop. 37: 233-238.

Taylor, R.M.S. (1963). Cause and effect of wear of teeth. Acta Anat. 53: 97-157.

## Chapter 7

## 'ATTRITION' - A CONTEMPORARY DENTAL VIEWPOINT

D.R. Williams and C.M. Woodhead

Department of Prosthetic Dentistry
University of Bristol Dental School

Dentists have traditionally described the loss of tooth substance in their patients after the presumed cause. Thus three conditions are recognised, being the result of erosion, a chemical process involving dissolution, or chelation of enamel constituents at a near-neutral pH; abrasion, the physical removal of tooth substance by agents introduced into the mouth, (e.g. toothbrushes and dentifrices); and attrition, a physical process whereby tooth surface is removed by the movement of the teeth against each other, possibly with an abrasive substance intervening (Eccles 1982).

Latterly, the dental literature has contained papers referring to 'tooth tissue loss' rather than to the more specific erosion, abrasion or attrition. This would seem to make more sense, since it is most likely that all three mechanisms are active simultaneously, the differing wear patterns reflecting only the relative ascendancy of each component. Thus 'attrition', which formerly meant much the same in the dental context to a dentist, an anthropologist or to an archaeologist, is gradually becoming considered by dentists to refer to a mechanism rather than a physical condition.

### THE CURRENT PICTURE

Lavelle et al. (1977, p. 170) have pointed out that "Dental attrition (sic) is a complex polymorphism, being dependent upon masticatory function, physical consistancy of diet, timing and sequence of tooth eruption, tooth form, tooth position within the dental arcade, thickness and hardness of enamel and predisposing factors such as enamel dysplasia, and habits such as bruxism."

In the limited context of the modern British population, tooth eruption, tooth form and position, and enamel thickness/hardness (excluding the dysplasias) may be considered as being reasonably constant. The factors to be considered therefore, are masticatory function, diet, habits and, (in addition to Lavelle's list) tooth restoration and the secondary effects of medical conditions.

### Masticatory function

Bates et al. (1975) published a comprehensive review of papers dealing with masticatory function under the headings of (i) the form of the masticatory cycle; (ii) the speed of mandibular movements, chewing rate and forces developed; and (iii) masticatory performance and efficiency.

Essentially their conclusions were:

(a) The form of the chewing cycle (viewed in the coronal aspect) is 'teardrop' shaped with minor variations consistent for the individual, but with wide variation between individuals.

(b) There is a static contact time of about one fifth of the chewing cycle, about 0.2s, but total contact may be double this as a result of gliding contacts.

(c) In the sagittal plane the opening movement is posterior to the closing stroke, but is very variable as chewing proceeds. The "posterior border line element" does not seem to be reached during function.

(d) The speed attained by the mandible varies, with 64 to 135 mm/s being acceptable estimates - the speed is not uniform throughout the cycle.

(e) The rate of chewing with natural teeth varies from about 49 to 120 cycles/min. The rate is affected by the food being chewed.

(f) Forces developed during chewing with natural teeth are reported as being between 0.3 and 7.2 kg., but are subject to a wide variability depending on both the individual and the food. Maximum forces tend to be characteristic of the individual and are generally independent of the food.

They conclude that subjects possess a natural neurophysiology which controls the masticatory pattern and gives each subject a consistent shape, speed and force to the chewing cycle which is as characteristic of the individual as walking or talking. Alterations in the type of food will alter the cycle within limits set by the neurophysiological pattern. There is, therefore, wide variation between individuals, depending on such factors as past habits, age, sex and occlusion. Alterations to the occlusion by extraction will affect the proprioceptive feedback which will alter this pattern.

It would seem reasonable to assume that this individual variation was also a feature of past populations. If this is so, then the general similarity of wear seen in the various examples of attrited dentitions from similar cultural groups implies that the masticatory pattern is not, of itself, a major influence on the wear of teeth. It only becomes a factor when modifed by other considerations e.g. tough or abrasive dietary elements, or tooth loss.

## Habits

The effect on teeth of habits is variable; not all pipe smokers exhibit an area of tooth tissue loss in relation to their pipestem while even infrequent dressmakers may notch their teeth with pins. By and large, the interest of such localised idiosyncracies lies only in their relation to some apparently innocuous behaviours.

The relation of bruxism to tooth tissue loss is not clear. The aetiology of this condition has been described as involving three factors: nervous tension; pain or discomfort; and occlusal interferences, all of which are presumed to act by increasing muscle tonus (Graf 1969). Arnold (1981) cited three similar factors although termed somewhat differently.

Graf (1969) considered that the most important factor was the presence of occlusal interferences, particularly between the positions of centric occlusion (where there is maximum intercuspation of the teeth) and centric relation (the jaw position where the heads of the condyles are in their most retruded position in the glenoid fossae). However, Nadler (1968) had already suggested that the occurrence of bruxism is practically universal, and latterly this view has been supported by Clarke et al. (1984). Arnold (1981) considered it to be almost universal and linked to psychological stress as a necessary component. Clarke and Townsend (1984) in a study of bruxing during sleep considered the aetiology as being of central origin and stated "a direct causal link between occlusal discrepancies and bruxism has not been demonstrated in controlled experiments."

Wear beyond that designated as stage 3 by Molnar (1971) and which can be ascribed to the mechanism of attrition is uncommon among patients with intact dentitions; therefore bruxism alone, except in extreme forms, is not likely to be a significant contributor to attrition.

Diet

There are two aspects of diet which are of significance in terms of tooth tissue loss - (a) the physical consistency and (b) the chemical constitution of the food. In contrast to the diet of earlier populations, the abrasive content of the modern diet has been reduced to negligible proportions. The only dietary factor of significance in the general population today is the pH of the ingested food or drink. For most people this does not constitute a problem. However, there is a small group who adopt a diet which is particularly high in citrus fruits or their derivative juices. The acid content of such diets may be a major cause of loss of tooth tissue.

Examples of such attack usually occur over most of the anatomical crown of a tooth. However, this action is further modified by particular juice-extracting activities such as sucking the juice into the mouth through clenched teeth (resulting in marked labial enamel loss) or pushing fruit segments against the lingual aspects of the upper incisors with the tongue to express the juice (resulting in marked lingual enamel loss).

Consumption of fruits or their juices (fresh, frozen or reconstituted), particularly citrus species, which is relatively innocuous in small quantities may cause severe erosion when consumption reaches levels as high as sixteen oranges per day (Levine 1974). Similar effects may be seen with high consumption levels of low pH soft drinks. A case where there was daily ingestion of 64 fluid ounces (4 pts. US, 3.2 pts UK) of a diet soft drink, to which was added lemon concentrate, has been described by Mueninghoff and Johnson (1982). Such lesions are easily differentiated from attrition as traditionally described by archaeologists and anthropologists.

Tooth Restorations

Dental treatment may lead to iatrogenic attrition. While traditional restorative materials may cause mild attrition modern composite resin restorations may be particularly abrasive (Chapman and Nathanson 1983).

Such modern restorative materials are based on non-abrasive acrylic polymers containing abrasive filler particles of various sizes. The effect of one such material on opposing teeth can be seen in Fig. 7.1. This wear occurred during a four week period.

The increasing use of such tooth-coloured restorations in posterior teeth, may produce patterns of attrition yet to be described.

## Medical conditions

Medical conditions may lead to loss of tooth substance either directly (i.e. by regurgitation, for example in cases of hiatus hernia, alcoholism, and in anorexia nervosa), or indirectly as a result of the necessity of ingesting low pH medicaments (for example dilute hydrochloric acid in achlorhydria), (Hurst et al. 1977).

As might be anticipated, the principal site of such tooth tissue loss is the lingual aspect of the teeth, and as in the case of dietary erosion should be easily distinguishable from attrition.

## CURRENT EXAMPLES OF ATTRITION:

These illustrate the general types of cases curently being referred to Dental Schools by General Dental Practitioners with a request for advice and/or treatment.

Fig 7.2. Shows photographs taken of a 57 year old man. In fig 7.2a there can be seen a generalised attrition with a 'step' in the occlusal level on the patient's left for which there is no obvious explanation. It is particularly interesting to note the difference in vertical wear between upper and lower anterior teeth. We would suggest that this may be due to the effect of a small ring of lower enamel milling against a large surface area of relatively soft upper dentine. Fig 2b shows the state of the upper arch. There is advanced attrition of the anterior teeth exposing secondary dentine but there is no attrition or facetting on the right posterior teeth. It is our presumption that the attrition has resulted from increased functional loading subsequent to loss of the lower right molars and this is illustrated in fig 7.2c. However it may be noted that there is minimal wear on the lower left lateral incisor and canine which again we are unable to explain satisfactorily.

Fig 7.3 shows photographs of a 61 year old woman. In fig 7.3a the generalised attrition can be seen to be accompanied by persistent enamel chipping. There is approximately equal crown loss from both maxillary and mandibular arch teeth, but the pattern of enamel wear is irregular. (c.f. fig 7.2a). The reason for this is uncertain, but it may be related to an initially greater loss of palatal dentine, leaving labial enamel unsupported which in turn is chipped away during protrusive movements of the mandible. Fig 7.3b shows cupped wear of the upper anterior teeth. This is principally palatal on the upper right canine, but it is interesting to note the transition from the vertical/palatal cupped pattern of wear on this tooth to the more horizontal but cupped loss of the upper left canine tooth. Once more there is minimal wear of the unopposed molar teeth which suggests that reduction in the overall occlusal table is a major factor in tooth tissue loss. Fig 7.3c illustrates the cup shaped wear of the lower anterior teeth

CURRENT EXAMPLES OF ATTRITION

Figure 7.1. A 66 year old male patient. See text for details.

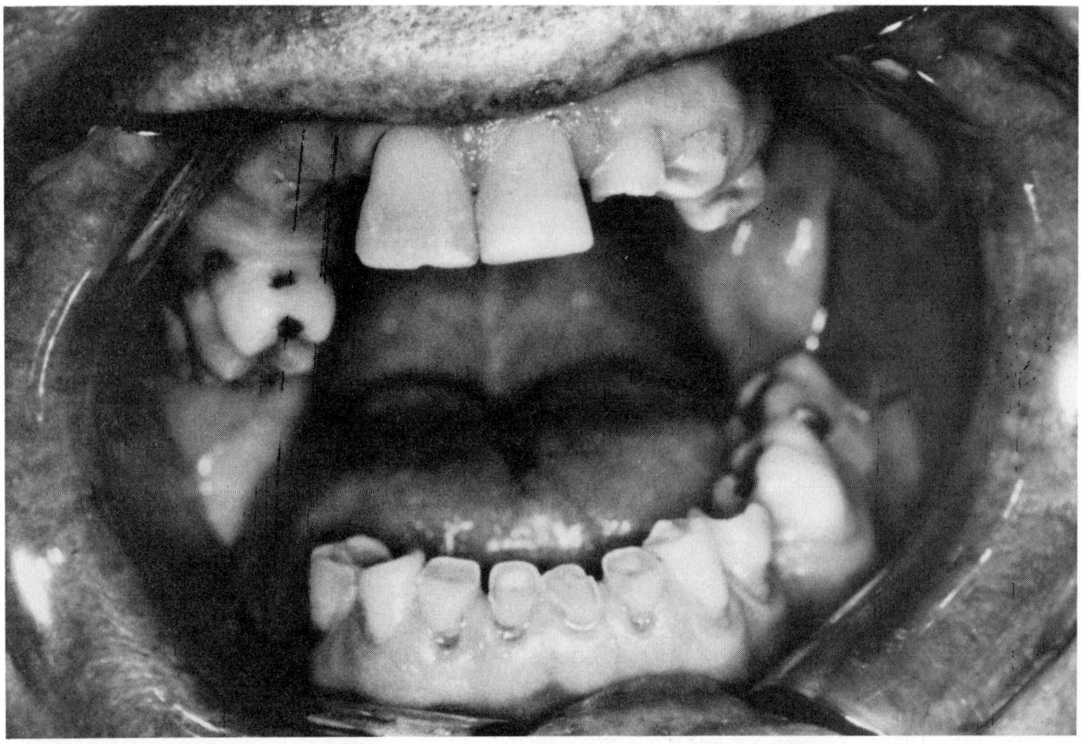

a

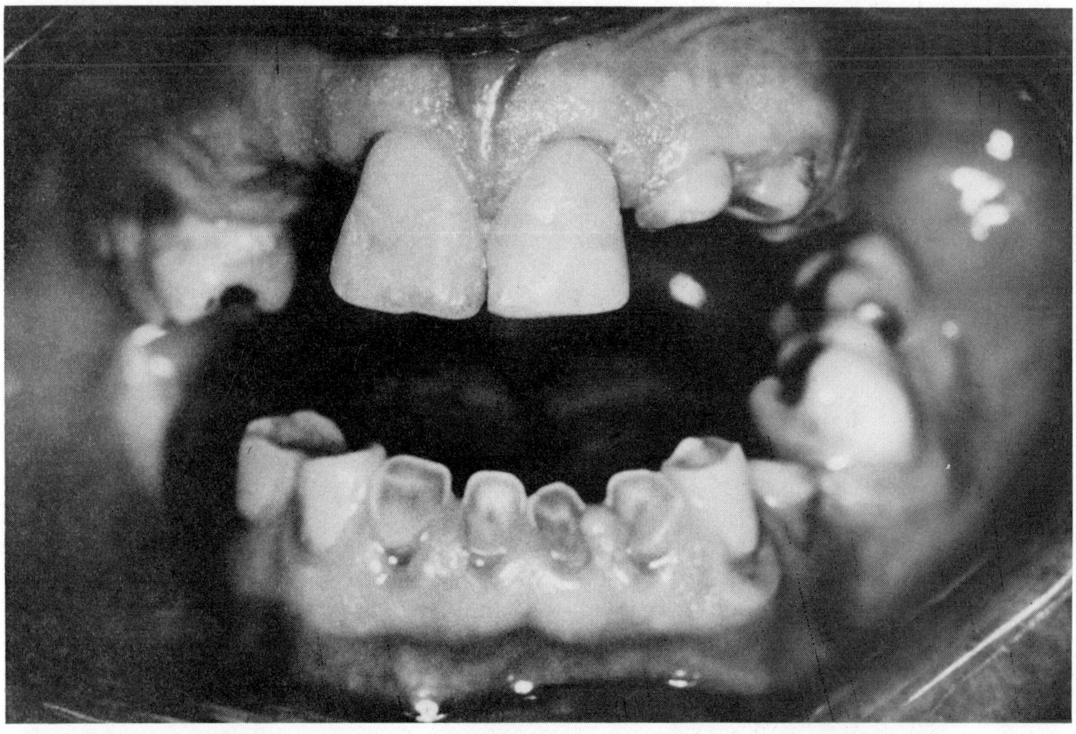

b

Figure 7.2. A 57 year old male patient.

a

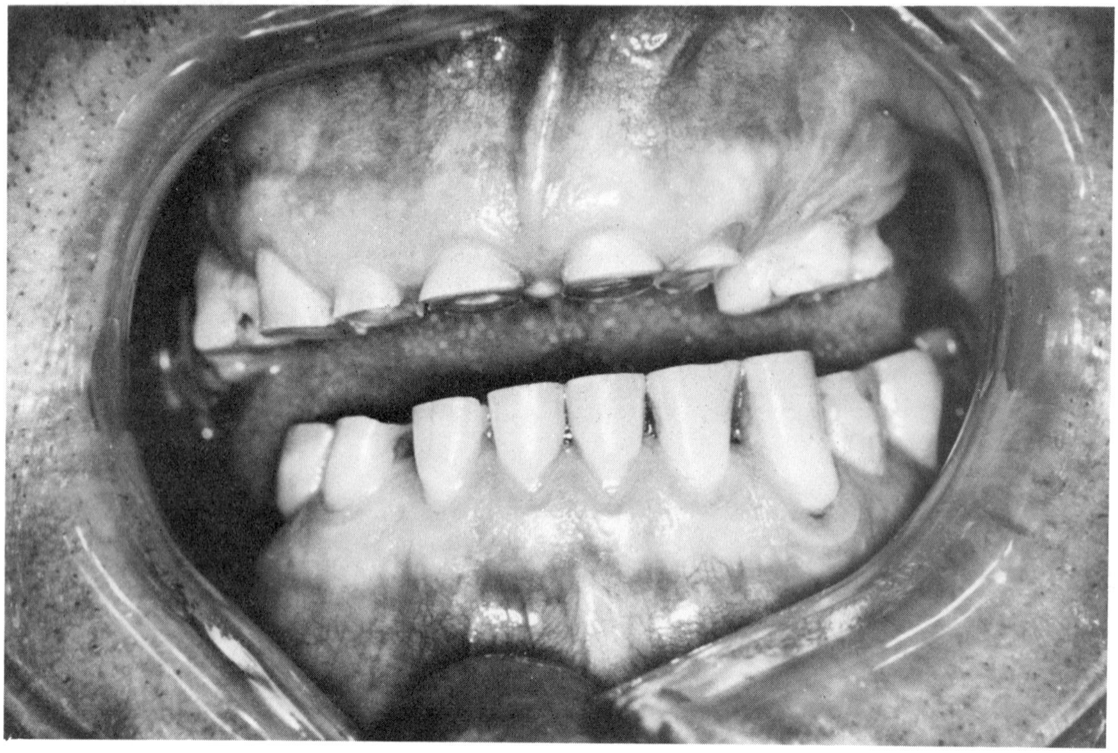

b

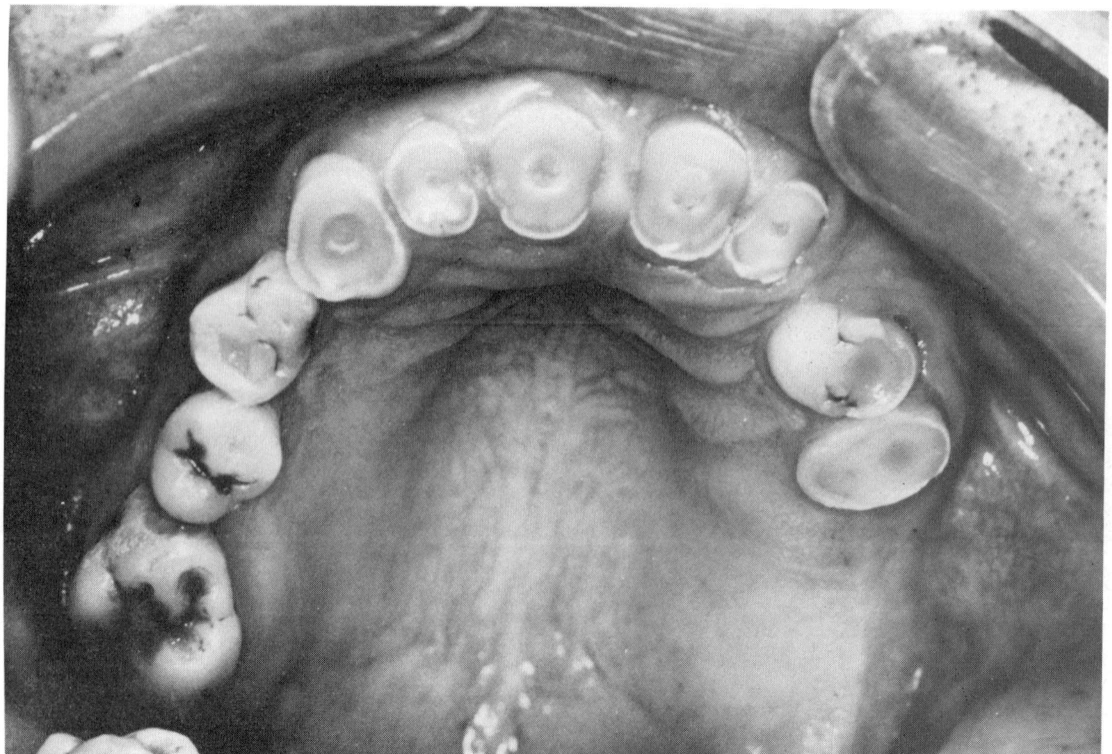

c

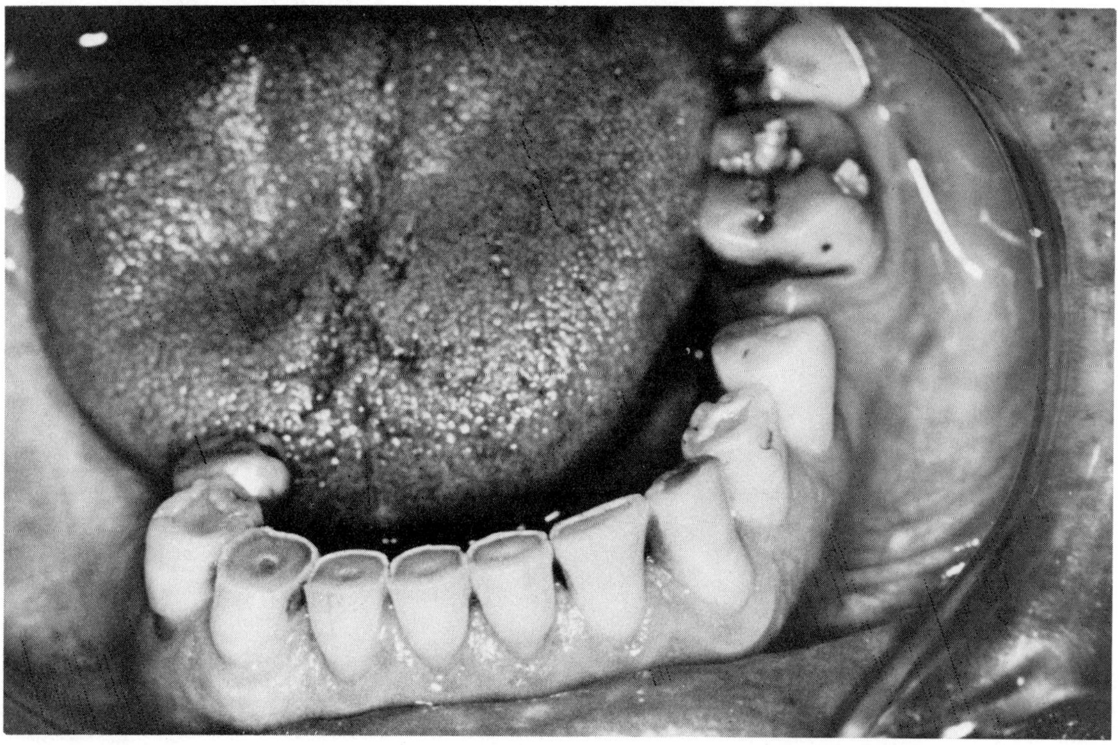

Figure 7.3. A 61 year old female patient.

a

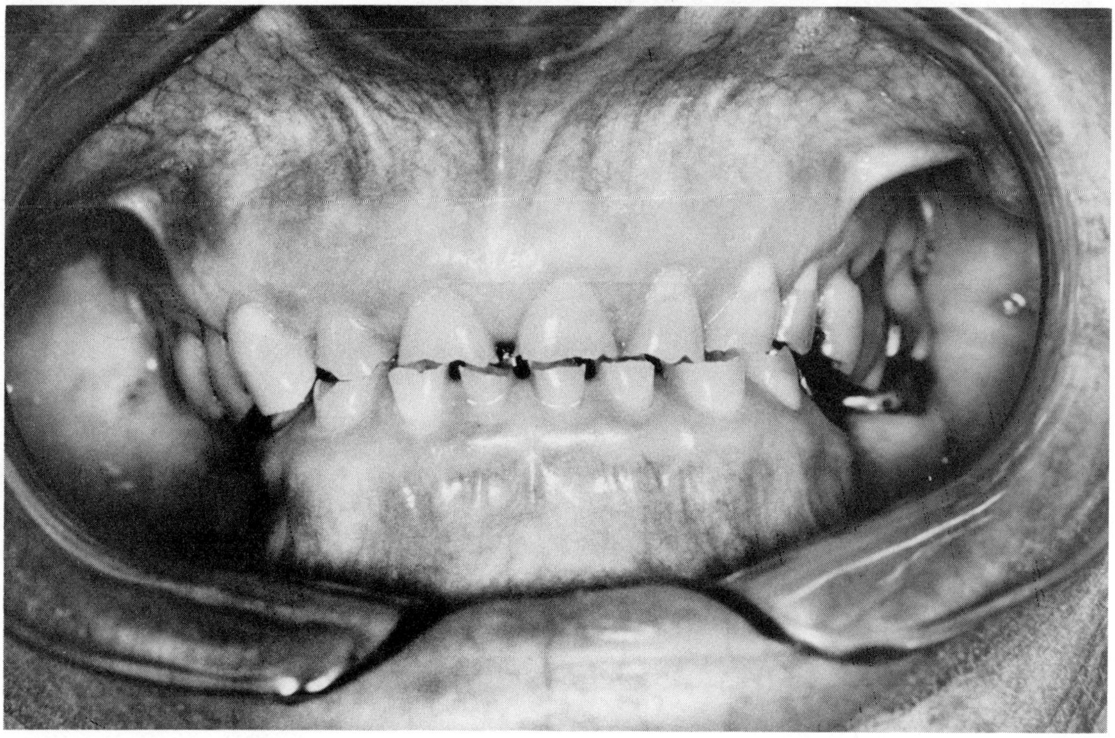

b

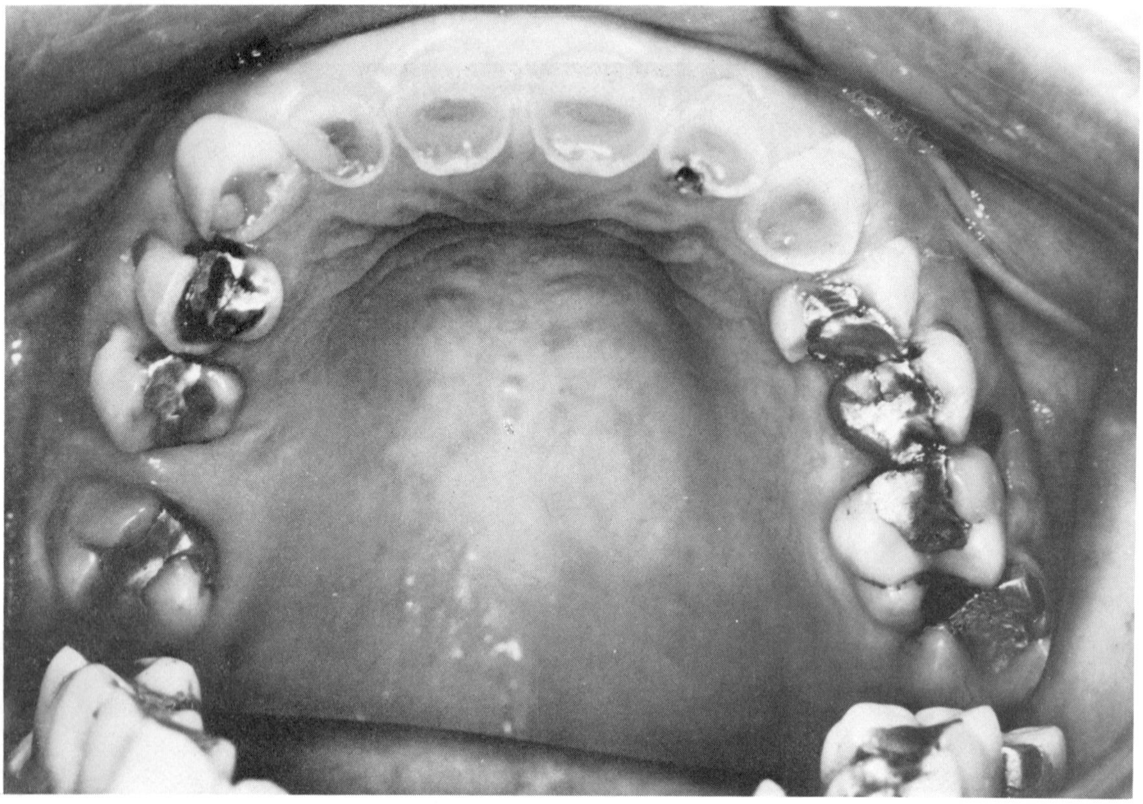

c

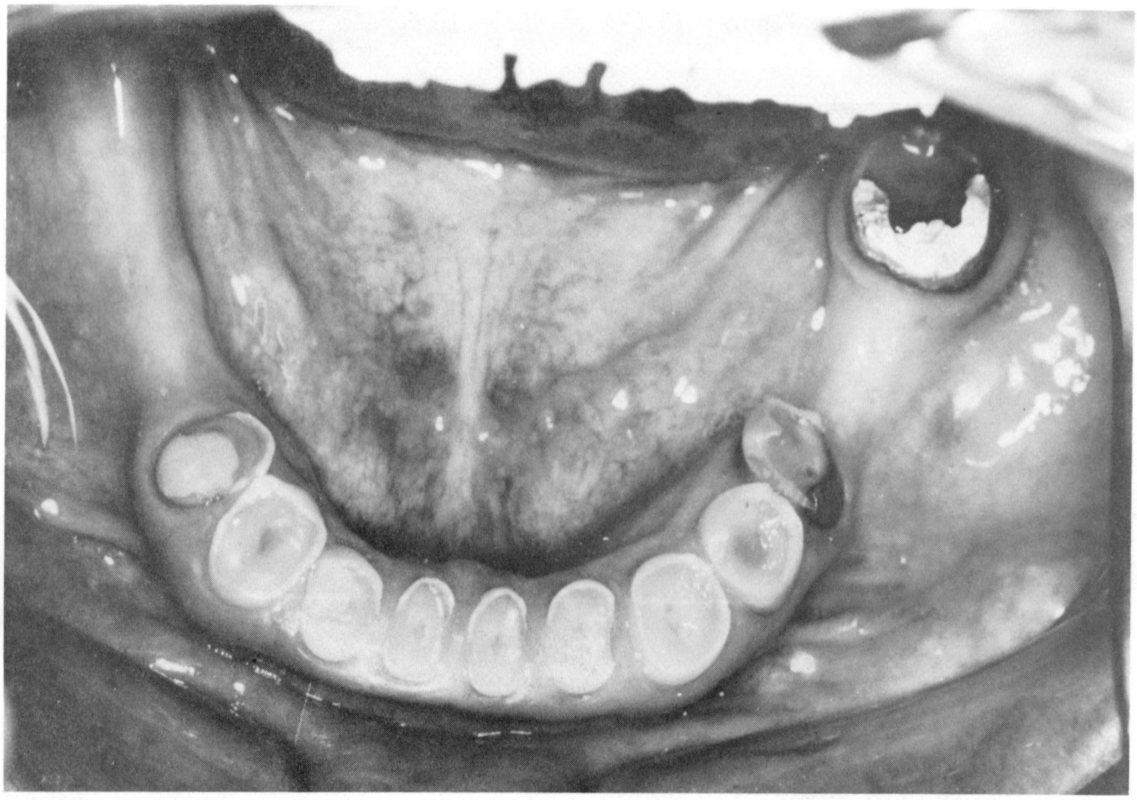

Figure 7.4. A 58 year old male patient.

a

b

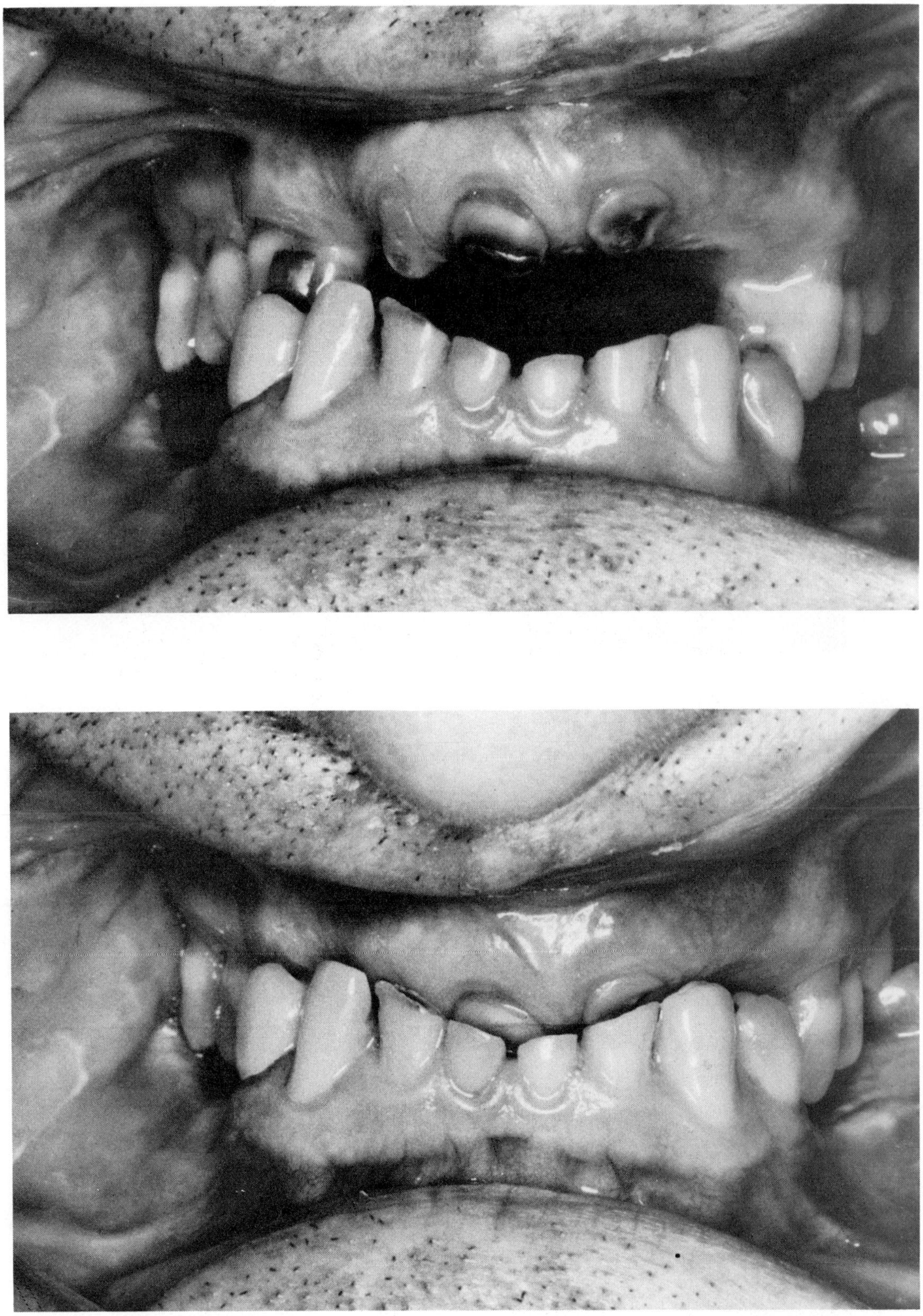

Figure 7.5. A 65 year old male patient.

a

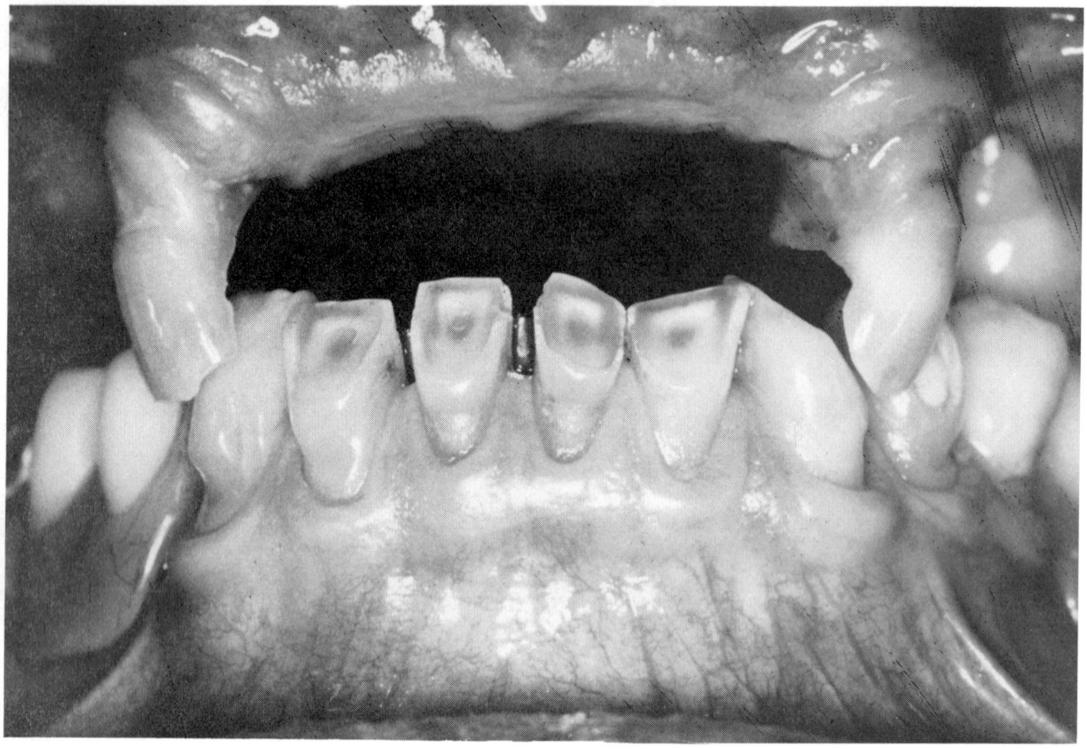

b

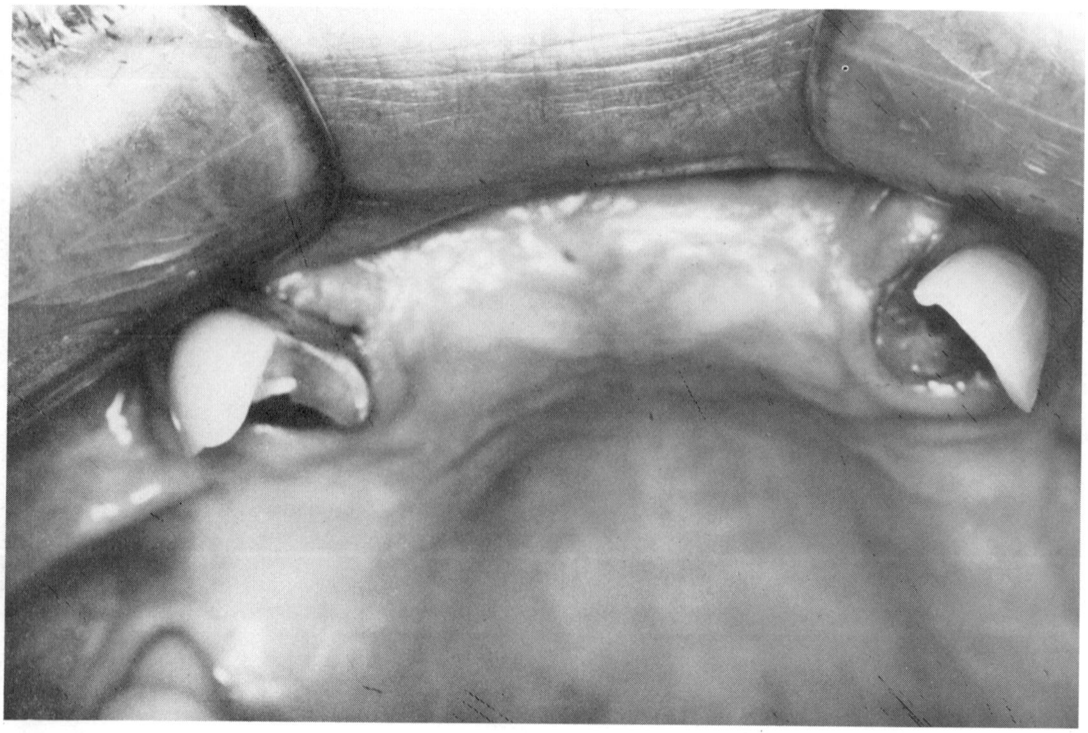

which is sufficient to show the secondary dentine filling the one time pulp chambers. The flattened form of the lower left molar tooth is mirrored by its opposing tooth, the upper left molar.

Fig 7.4 shows photographs of a 58 year old man. In fig 7.4a the patient's teeth are in the initial contact position. It is evident that occlusal support is limited to that provided by the pair of first premolars on each side. In order to function the patient closes into the habitual contact position shown in fig 7.4b where the mandible has been postured forwards and upwards to maximise the tooth contact area. This is only possible due to the loss of molar support. Lateral excursions of the mandible from this position are probably responsible for the V shaped wear pattern seen in the lower anterior teeth, but whether the difference in wear seen here compared with figs 7.2 and 7.3 (essentially horizontal) is due to differences in tooth relation, or differences in temporo-mandibular joint structure is uncertain.

Fig. 7.5 shows photographs of a 65 year old man. In fig. 7.5a the patient is wearing a lower partial denture at the correct vertical dimension of occlusion. There are chisel shaped wear facets on the labial aspects of the lower anterior teeth with corresponding wear on the palatal aspects of the remaining upper anterior teeth (upper left and right canines).

This patient has a 30 year history of heavy bruxing, producing tooth tissue loss which has required increasingly complex restorations. These have failed to withstand the continuing overload, which has led to the loss of the upper incisors and severely compromised the canine teeth. Fig. 7.5b shows the marked palatal horizontal tooth tissue loss with sharply defined vertical limits which has left a thin labial veneer of relatively normal length.

## INTER RELATIONSHIP OF FACTORS AFFECTING TOOTH TISSUE LOSS:

Fig. 7.6 illustrates the complex of factors which may be implicated in tooth tissue loss. The dotted lines represent more tenuous connections between influencing factors. It is evident that while some factors are influential in isolation (e.g. bruxism, oral hygiene) the most gross effects are seen as a result of the interaction of factors in the upper part of the chart (viz. diet, masticatory function and tooth loss). The expression of this is that the upper chart features tend to be the cause of gross tooth tissue loss, whereas the lower features tend to produce relatively localised effects.

## CONCLUSIONS

Tooth wear in the contemporary British population shows a wide variety of forms. These may include patterns similar to those seen in Medieval/Ancient populations but appear to be largely divergent from them.

As far as can be ascertained the principal factor involved is loss of some teeth, added to which may be bruxist, parafunctional and dietary factors. However, the relationship between the loss of specific teeth and the resulting wear pattern is obscure.

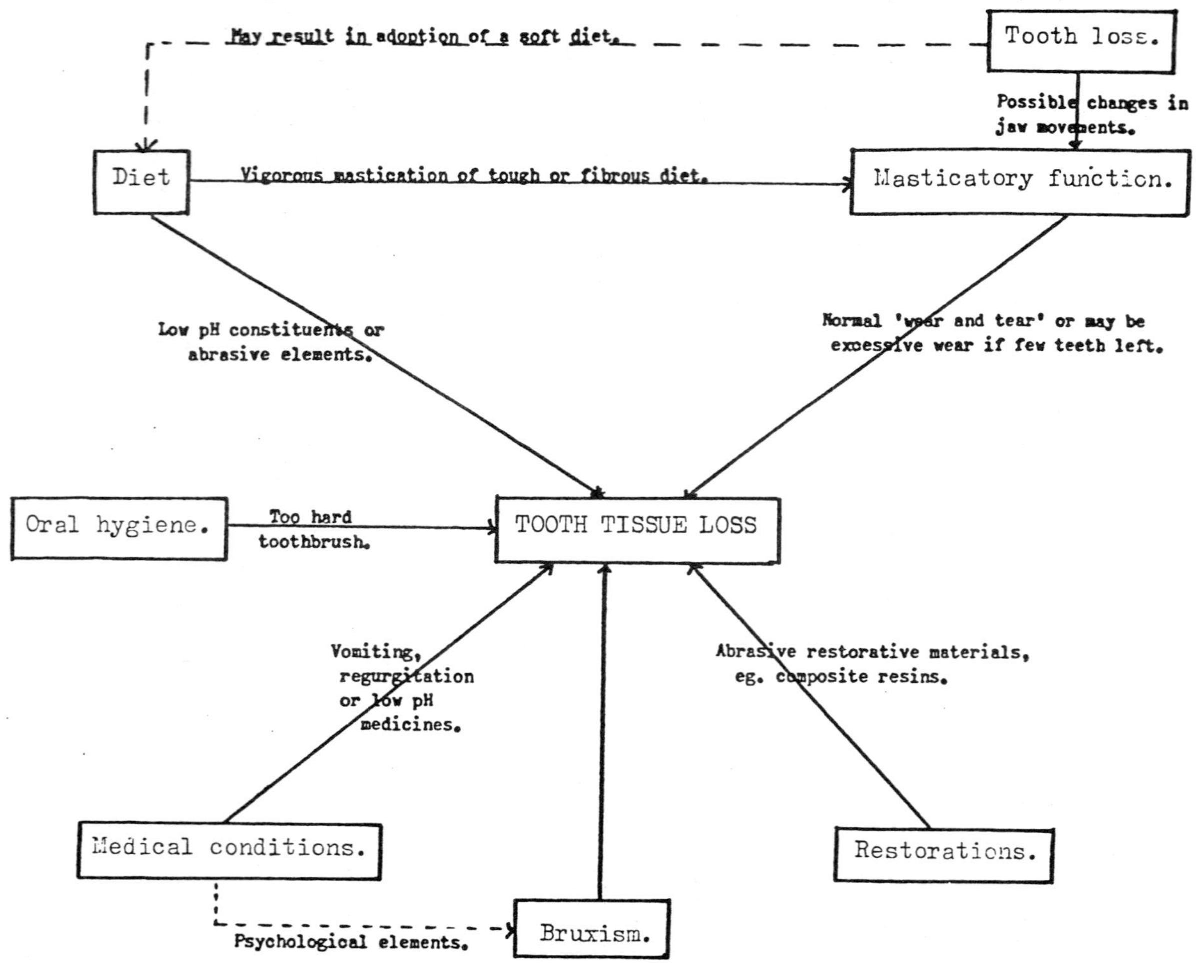


Figure 7.6. Flowchart indicating possible relationships between tooth tissue loss and presumed causative factors.

REFERENCES.


Arnold, M. (1981) Bruxism and the occlusion. Dental Clinics of North America, 25(3): 395 - 407.

Bates, J.F., Stafford, G.D. and Harrison, A. (1975, 1976) Masticatory function - a review of the literature. Part I. The form of the masticatory cycle. Journal of Oral Rehabilitation 2. 281 - 301. Part II. Speed of movement of the mandible, rate of chewing and forces developed in chewing. Journal of Oral Rehabilitation 2. 349 -361. Part III. Masticatory performance and efficiency. Journal of Oral Rehabilitation 3. 57 -67.

Chapman, R.J. and Nathanson, D. (1983) Excessive wear of natural teeth by opposing composite restorations. Journal of the American Dental Association 106: 51 -53.

Clarke, N.G. and Townsend, G.C. (1984) Distribution of bruxing patterns in man. Journal of Oral Rehabilitation 11: 529 -534.

Clarke, N.G., Townsend, G.C. and Carey, S.E. (1984) Bruxing patterns in man during sleep. Journal of Oral Rehabilitation 11: 123 - 127.

Eccles, J.D. (1982) Tooth surface loss from abrasion, attrition and erosion. Dental Update 9: 373 - 381.

Graf, H. (1969) Bruxism. Dental Clinics of North America 13(3): 659 - 665.

Hurst, P.S., Lacey, J.H. and Crisp, A.H. (1977) Teeth, vomiting and diet: a study of the dental characteristics of seventeen anorexia nervosa patients. Postgraduate Medical Journal 53: 298 - 305.

Lavelle, C.L.B., Shellis, R.P. and Poole, D.F.C. (1977) Evolutionary Changes to the Primate Skull and Dentition. Charles C. Thomas, Springfield, Illinois.

Levine, R.S. (1974) Fruit juice erosion - an increasing danger? Journal of Dentistry 2: 85 - 88.

Mueninghoff, L.A. and Johnson, M.H. (1982) Erosion: a case caused by unusual diet. Journal of the American Dental Association 104: 51 - 52.

Molnar, S. (1971) Human tooth wear, tooth function and cultural variability. American Journal of Physical Anthropolgy 34: 178.

Nadler, S.C. (1968) The importance of bruxism. Journal of Oral Medicine 23(4): 142 - 148.

# Chapter 8

## A STUDY OF THE PATTERN OF ALVEOLAR RECESSION

Patricia J.C. Watson
Department of Restorative Dentistry
University of Leeds

Alveolar recession has been used by archaeologists as an indication of the severity of periodontal disease found in populations of former times. The modern clinician looking at archaeological material sees that the pattern of periodontal disease in these populations is very different from that in modern populations, particularly those eating a Western style diet. Bone loss associated with periodontitis simplex, with loss of the interdental crest of alveolar bone is very much less marked with archaeological material, and infrabony pocketing associated with periodontitis complex is rare. There appears to be little association between the amounts of calculus on the teeth and the amount of bone loss, though in modern populations these factors would seem to have a positive correlation (Waerhaug, J., 1952, 1956; Lövdal, A. et al 1956). It may be that such alveolar recession as is found in archaeological material is more indicative of both age change and response to diet, than of disease process, and is possibly directly related to the degree of attrition of the teeth. The occlusal surfaces of the teeth become worn, then passive eruption occurs with the tooth moving further into the occlusal cavity, whilst the level of alveolar bone remains constant. The correlation between attrition and alveolar recession is being investigated and the present study is a first step in this investigation, the purpose being to investigate the pattern of alveolar recession as found in a variety of archaeological specimens.

### Methods and Materials

A total of 83 specimens were examined from a number of sites: Caister, Eccles, Hartlepool, The Hirsel, Jewbury and St. Helens on the Wall York. The dates of these specimens ranged from Anglo Saxon to Tudor. There was no attempt made to match specimens from the different sites, as the numbers available and suitable for study varied.

Modern clinicians generally measure bone loss mesial and distal to each tooth, but in the present study, where bone loss may be more apparent than actual, it was thought relevant in determining the pattern of recession to make measurements at six points on each tooth, mesial, midpoint and distal, on both labial and oral surfaces. (Fig 8.1)

An Omnidepth pocket measuring probe (Whaledent Inc., Brooklyn, New York) was used to measure the distance from the amelocemental junction to the alveolar crest at each of these six points. This probe, whilst a little sharp and with traumatic potential for clinical use, is ideal for archaeological use as the measurement is easily read from a sliding scale on the instrument handle.

The measurements in millimeters were then plotted onto a chart which was devised to be suitable for simple computer analysis. (Fig 8.2) The

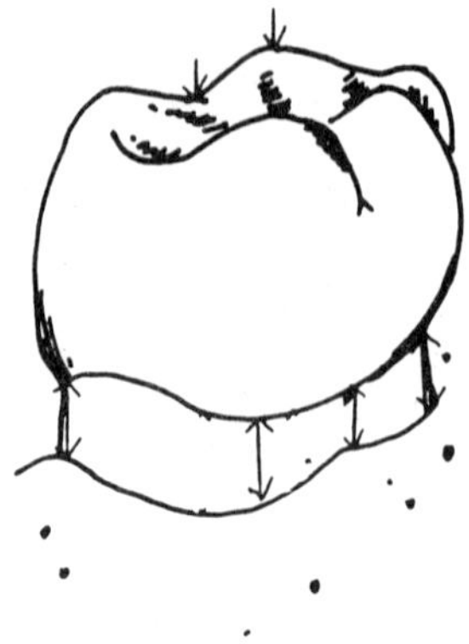

Figure 8.1. Points or measurement on the tooth surface.

STUDY GROUP ______________ REF. NO. __________ SEX ________ AGE ________

MEASUREMENT ALVEOLUS TO ACJ IN MM.

| | | 8 | 7 | 6 | 5 | 4 | 3 | 2 | 1 |
|---|---|---|---|---|---|---|---|---|---|
| LOWER L | L / C | | | | | | | | |
| LOWER R | L / C | | | | | | | | |
| UPPER R | L / C | | | | | | | | |
| UPPER L | L / C | | | | | | | | |

Figure 8.2. Chart used to tabulate the measurements of recession.

specimens were divided into age groups, below 25 (21), 25-35 (24), 35-45 (13), over 45 (19) and indeterminate (6), ageing being from a combination of dental age (Brothwell, 1965, 1982), sutural, epiphyseal union, and pubic symphysis ages.

The mandibles were in general in a better state of preservation than the maxillae resulting in a greater number of mandibular teeth being measured than maxillary, though a reasonable overall distribution of the 1159 teeth measured was achieved. (Fig 8.3) Only teeth which were firm in their sockets were measured to avoid any errors which may have occurred in replacing loose teeth into specimens.

The measurements obtained were analysed using a Gemini Datagem programme on a BBC2 computer. Each quadrant of the mouth was entered and analysed separately, each of the six points on each tooth being analysed as a separate field.

The mean values for each field within each age group were found, also the overall maximum and mean values, and these values were plotted diagramatically using an adaptation of a clinical pocket measurement chart.

## Results and Discussion

The results in tables 8.1 - 8.7 show that in the material examined there was an increase in alveolar recession with age. This increase was not even in its distribution. The first teeth to show signs of significant recession being the premolars and the first molars, this tendency becoming more pronounced with increasing age, and in older age groups the second molars also show significant recession. The incisors in all age groups show less recession than the molars and premolars and the canines show a more gradual increase than the molars and premolars.

The pattern of the recession also changes. In the younger subjects bone is evenly distributed around the tooth whereas with increasing age the recession becomes greater at the midpoints, labially and orally, of the tooth. Recession is somewhat greater on the labial rather than the oral face so that although there is a "mirror image" appearance to the bone loss the greatest degree of recession on any tooth is usually at the midpoint of the labial surface.

These results would seem to indicate that the recession found in archaeological specimens probably stems as much from response to occlusal forces and attrition as it does from any form of periodontal disease as we know it in modern times. The nearest equivalent to the harder diet of former times is probably found today in isolated primitive tribes and Schamschula, et al (1972) investigating populations in Luga, New Guinea found that alveolar and gingival recession were prevalent in older individuals in these tribes.

The molars and premolars carry the greatest occlusal load as they are the teeth used to grind food. One would expect the first molars to be involved early in any apparent recession which was the result of occlusal trauma, attrition and passive eruption, as they are the first permanent teeth to erupt into the oral cavity at about six years. The premolars probably show a greater degree of recession as they have a large and unfavourable crown to root ratio and are particularly vulnerable to trauma

| | 8 | 7 | 6 | 5 | 4 | 3 | 2 | 1 |
|---|---|---|---|---|---|---|---|---|
| Lower Left | 30 | 53 | 51 | 51 | 52 | 45 | 42 | 30 |
| Lower Right | 30 | 51 | 48 | 52 | 52 | 53 | 39 | 32 |
| Upper Right | 20 | 35 | 37 | 37 | 35 | 30 | 16 | 21 |
| Upper Left | 14 | 36 | 35 | 38 | 33 | 32 | 20 | 19 |

Figure 8.3. Numerical distribution of teeth in the sample.

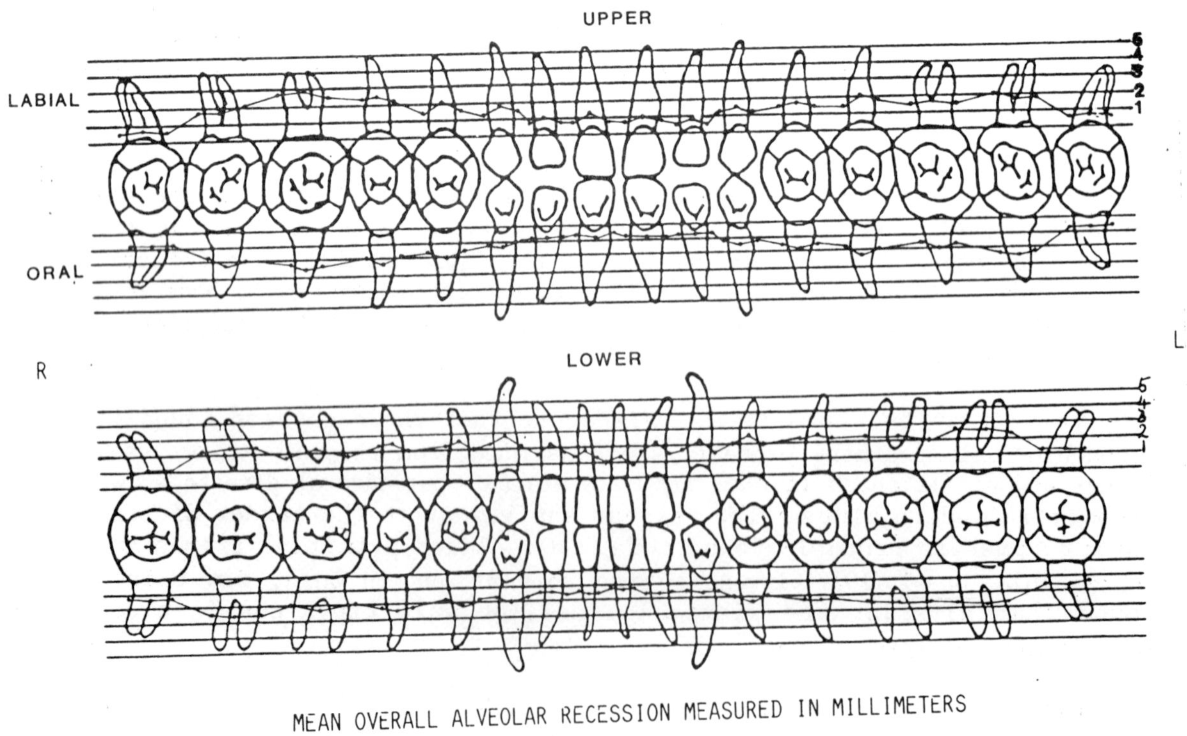


Table 8.1.

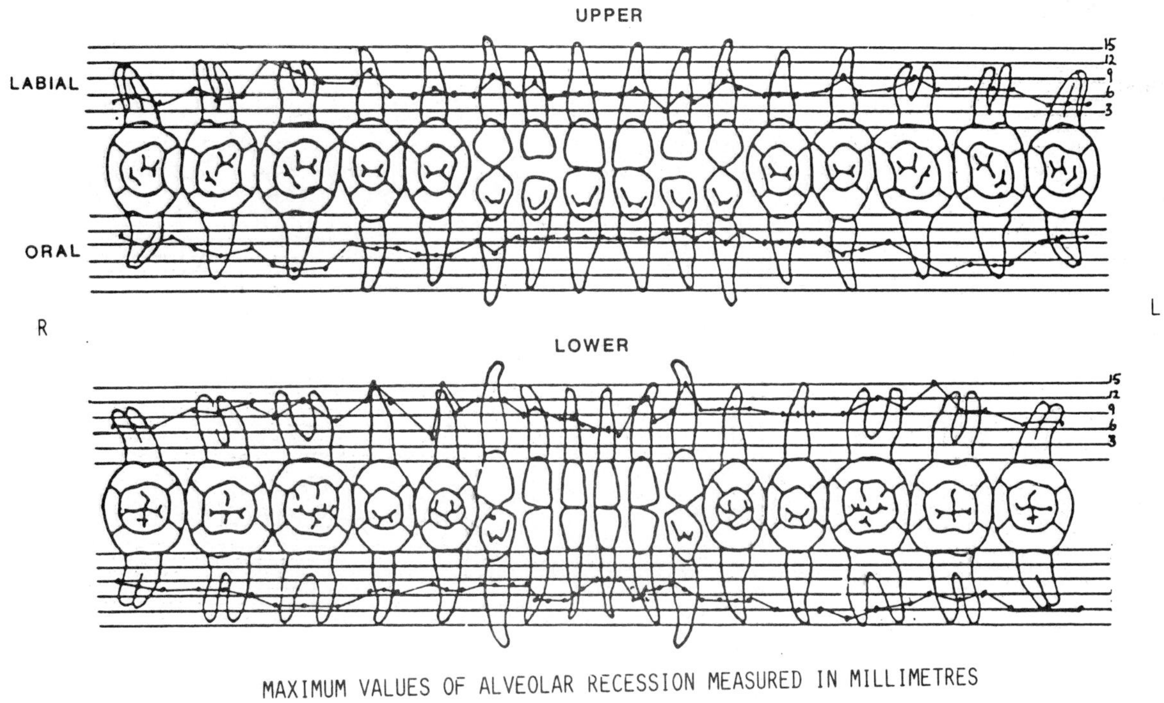


Table 8.2.

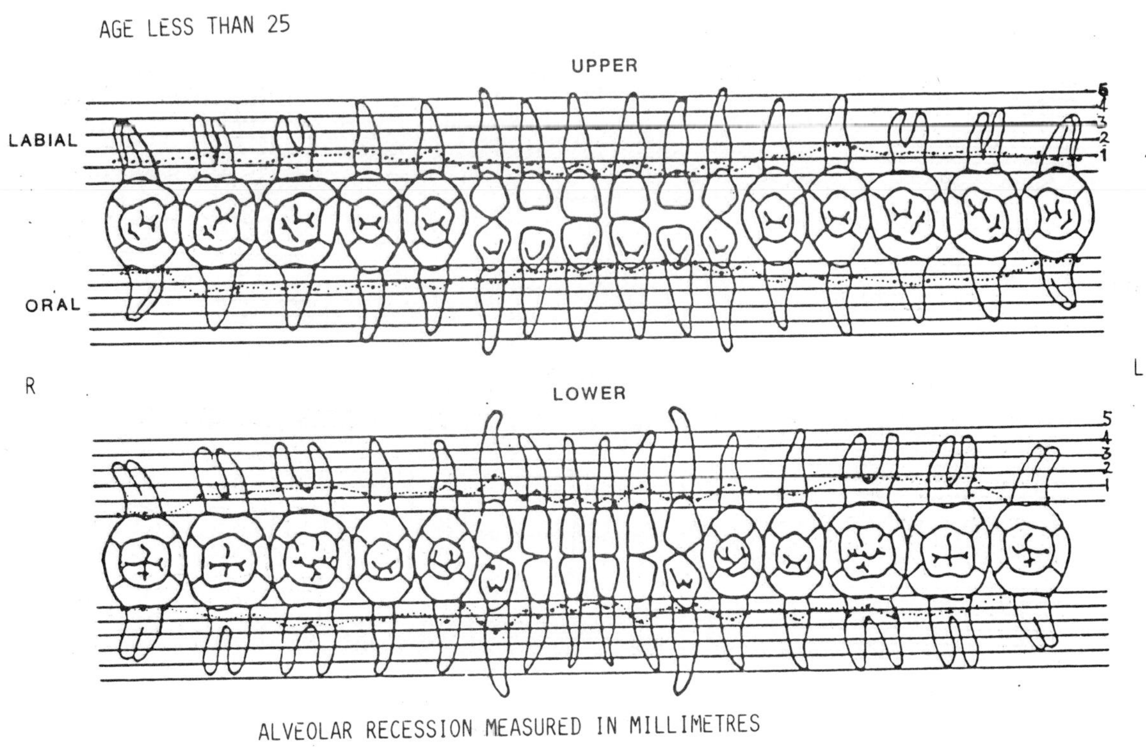


Table 8.3.

AGE 25 - 35

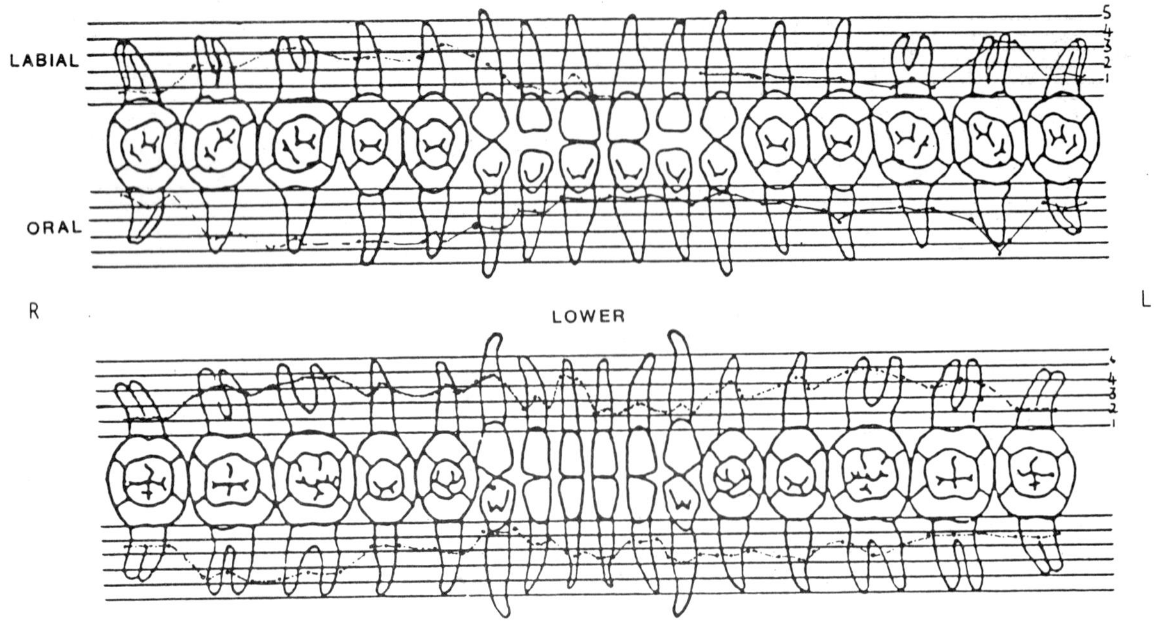


ALVEOLAR RECESSION MEASURED IN MILLIMETRES

Table 8.4.

AGE 35 - 45

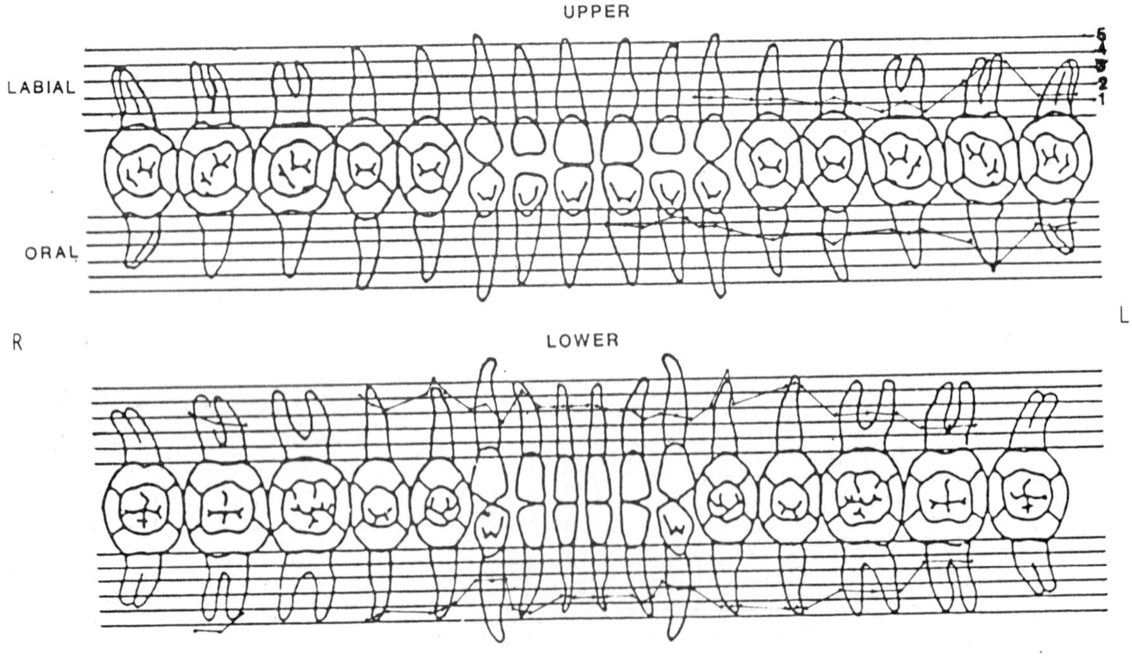


ALVEOLAR RECESSION MEASURED IN MILLIMETRES

Table 8.5.

AGE GREATER THAN 45

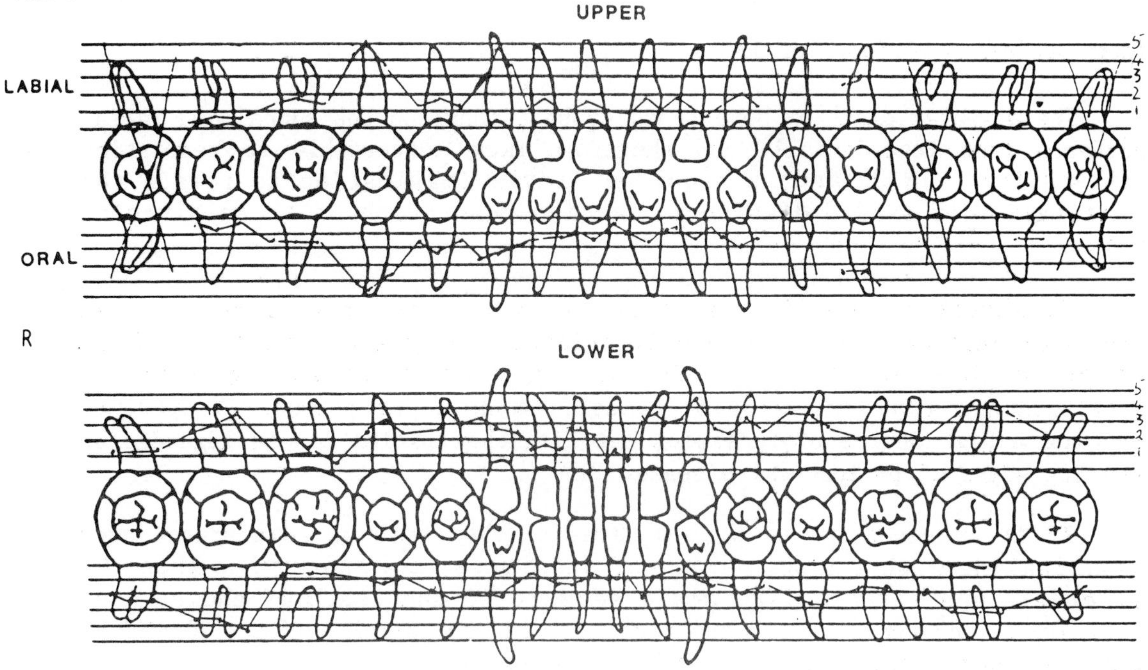


ALVEOLAR RECESSION MEASURED IN MILLIMETRES

Table 8.6.

AGE INDETERMINATE

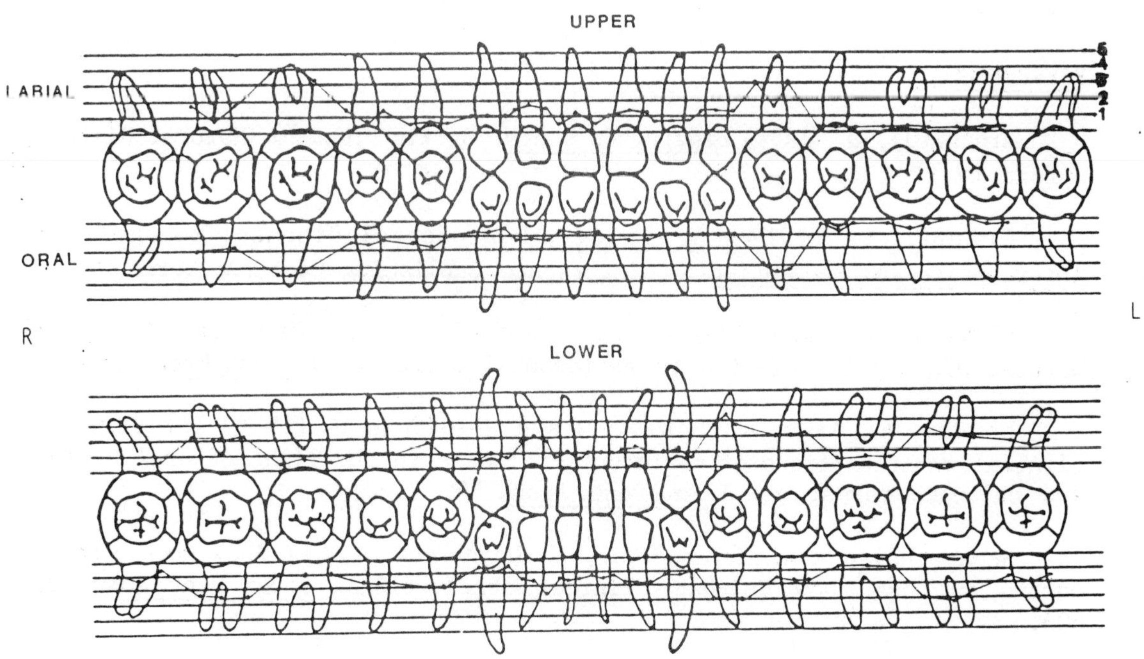


ALVEOLAR RECESSION MEASURED IN MILLIMETRES

Table 8.7.

from occlusion (Cripps, S. 1984).

The alveolar plate of bone tends to be thinner on the buccal and labial surfaces than interdentally and therefore more susceptible to resorption (Hirschfield, 1923) and it requires little imagination to relate the mastication of a hard diet to a reactive resorption of these alveolar plates.

If alveolar recession is to be taken as a measure of anything in archaeological material, it should be related to degree of attrition and age as well as disease. It is probable that a specimen showing a high degree of attrition and alveolar recession comes from an older person. A specimen showing a high degree of recession but little attrition can be regarded as showing signs of periodontal disease.

If it is necessary to pick an area of the mouth as a reference area when dealing with a large number of specimens in a short time then the premolars and first molars would seem to be the teeth of choice, and contrary to common practice, the midpoints of the labial surfaces should be measured when looking for the greatest recession.

## ACKNOWLEDGEMENTS

Thanks are due to Mr. I. Smith, Miss J. Collier and Miss B. Wardman, Department of Restorative Dentistry, University of Leeds, for technical and clerical assistance. Many thanks also to all those who allowed access to specimens, particularly the York Archaeological Trust and Dr. K. Manchester, University of Bradford.

## REFERENCES

Brothwell, D. (1981) Digging Up Bones, British Museum (Natural History) Oxford UP.

Cripps, S. (1984) Aetiology, Periodontal Disease, Recognition, Interception and Prevention. Quintessence Publishing Co., New York.

Hirschfield, I. (1923) A Study of skulls in the American Museum of Natural History in relation to periodontal disease. J. Dent. Res. 5:241.

Lövdal, A., Arno, A., Schei, O. and Waerhaug, J. (1956) Incidence of clinical manifestations of periodontal disease in the light of oral hygiene and calculus formation. J. Am. Dent. Assn. 56: 21-23.

Schamschula, R.C., Keyes, P.H. and Hornbrook, R.W. (1972) Root surface caries in Luga, New Guinea: clinical observations. J. Am. Dent. Assn. 85: 603.

Waerhaug, J. (1952) The Gingival Pocket. Odontologisk Tidsckrift 60, Supplement.

Waerhaug, J. (1956) Effect of rough surfaces upon gingival tissues. J. of Periodontology, 26: 26-29.

Computer Analysis - Gemini Data Gem
24K ROM Based Random Access Database Management System for BBC Micro (Mod. 2)

Chapter 9

# INFORMATION FROM TEETH ON THE GROWTH AND DEVELOPMENTAL HISTORY OF INDIVIDUALS

Simone K. Bullion
Department of Classics and Archaeology
University of Lancaster

The aim of this project is to develop a number of methods whereby the history of growth and development of individuals from past populations can be established from studies of their dental enamel. Research has been carried out initially on modern dental material and then is to be applied to archaeological specimens, mainly from the mediaeval cemetery of St. Helen on the Walls, York.

A detailed study is being carried out, in particular, on disturbances in growth of the dental enamel and the positions in which they manifest themselves. These disturbances are a type known as systemic enamel hypoplasia and are characterised by a reduction in thickness of enamel and a pattern of interference corresponding to the teeth forming at the time of the disturbance (Pindborg, 1970). The clinical appearance of enamel hypoplasia may vary from discrete pitting to single or multiple bands of irregular enamel on the tooth surface (Sarnat & Schour, 1941, 1942; Nikiforuk & Frazer, 1981). The causes of enamel hypoplasia remain unclear but have been associated with dietary disorders such as vitamin D deficiency (Mellanby, 1934), gastro-intestinal disorders (Lindemann, 1958), exanthematous diseases (e.g. measles, chicken pox, scarlet fever) (Shafer et al., 1983), prematurity, congential syphilis and fluorosis (Pindborg, 1970).

In order to study the location and morphology of growth disturbances affecting the crown it is necessary to have a knowledge of the normal development of enamel. In this study this was achieved by means of thin sections examined by polarised light microscopy. For each of the eight morphological types in the permanent dentition and from both upper and lower jaws, five to ten unworn teeth were selected from an overall sample of about five hundred modern teeth. Sections of about 100 micrometres thickness in the bucco-lingual plane of each tooth were produced by standard techniques of sectioning, polishing and grinding. Silicone rubber casts were also taken of the buccal surface of each tooth. These were examined using a stereoscopic microscope and a toolmaker's measuring microscope. Archaeological material and also developing enamel was found to be too fragile to be subjected directly to the sectioning process. These specimens were embedded in a polyester resin using standard techniques and then sectioned, ground and polished as before.

There is an overlapping sequence of crown development for the permanent teeth of man from around birth until the completion of crown formation in the second molar at about eight years. If the third molars are included then this sequence can be extended up to sixteen years, although these teeth can vary a great deal in their development between individuals. If the pattern of the enamel incremental growth lines, the striae of Retzius, are matched from teeth with overlapping developmental times then a chronology could be constructed from the point of birth, or close to this event (depending on the existence of a neonatal line in the first permanent molar) up to the completion of crown formation in the jaws. The feasibility of cross-matching straie of Retzius has previously been tried with success by Fujita (1939) and Boyde (1963).

In this current research it was found that the pattern of the striae of Retzius is more or less mirrored within teeth of the same morphological type from an individual. This is particularly easy to see if there is a prominent series of lines which has been termed a 'signature' pattern in this study. Cross-matching between teeth of different morphological type was found to be more difficult to achieve, but was best attempted when a 'signature' pattern could be identified as before. Cross-matching was most successful for canine and incisor teeth. The molars and premolars seem to show prominent incremental lines to a much lesser degree. The actual spacing and width of the striae of Retzius in a 'signature' group is not identical for teeth of different morphological type. Their position within the crown depends on the stage of development of the enamel at the time of their formation, so the group may occupy a different geometric position within each crown. In this case the important factor was found to be the relative spacing and width of each prominent stria in the group.

The relationship between prominent striae of Retzius and surface effect has been studied. Rose (1977) found that the correlation between hypoplasia and 'pathological' bands within the teeth to be small and insignificant. In this current study it was found that in most cases if there is a disturbance on the surface, even in the form of a single enhanced perikymata, than this can be related to a distinctive stria of Retzius within the tooth. However, it was found that many distinctive striae may occur which are unrelated to events on the surface. It is thought that this may be because the physiological causes of a prominent incremental line may sometimes be insufficient to cause a surface effect. Only, perhaps, if a certain threshold level is reached will the surface effect be activated. This study is aimed at providing a non-destructive technique. There may be an additional advantage in using a method based on surface study, as it is felt that this may result in a reduction in a 'noise' efect where it might be difficult to distinguish separate events occurring during development.

Research is currently being undertaken to estimate the number of striae forming 'domed' incremental layers to the number forming 'sleeved' layers which arise on the surface of the teeth to form the perikymata. There appears to be little variation in the number of layers forming domes for teeth of the same morphological type from different individuals. Work is still at a preliminary stage at present, but it is hoped that a constant may be obtained for each tooth type representing the amount of incremental material which formed prior to the 'sleeve' type being laid down. Hence, any surface study can be related to the overall growing period of the tooth as a whole.

A study is also being made of the variation in cross-striation number (presumed to represent a diurnal rhythm) between striae of Retzius within the same individual and also for different individuals. The number of cross-striations between striae did not appear to vary throughout each tooth from an individual. A variation ranging from seven to ten cross-striations was found to occur between individals, seven or eight cross-striations being the most common figure.

It is thought to be possible to divide the surface of the crown into a number of rough zones. Some work has been carried out previously by Hillson (1979) and Goodman et al (1980). It is hoped to expand on this work by estimating roughly how long each zone took to form from studies of the incremental structures in enamel. It should be noted that the striae of Retzius and therefore the perikymata are closest together near the enamel/cement junction than for the rest of the tooth. This indicates that enamel formation is slower towards the completion of crown formation than during the earlier formation of enamel. This should certainly be taken into account when considering the formation time of each zone. This method should allow growth disturbances to be placed within a known developmental period for each tooth.

All these methods are aimed at a quick, effective and reasonably accurate way of recording the history of growth and development of individuals. Greater accuracy could be obtained by selecting the teeth, cross-matching the disturbance and relating them to the point of birth. This will provide a timed series of events that will be accurate to days if counts of cross-striations are included. This is, however, very time consuming and of limited application where large skeletal collections are to be examined.

## CONCLUSION

This work should provide a number of methods to record enamel hypoplasia, enabling information to be gained on the prevalence of growth disturbances that individuals might have experienced in the past and the age at which they occur. Information cannot be provided on the exact cause of the disturbances but can probably be used as an index of health in a population as a whole.

## ACKNOWLEDGEMENTS

I would like primarily to thank my supervisor, Dr. Simon Hillson for all his help and encouragement with this research. I am also extremely grateful to Mr. Dendy of the Royal Lancaster Infirmary for supplies of modern dental material and also the Yorkshire Museum for access to the archaeological specimens for this study. I would also like to thank Dr. Terry O'Connor and the York Archaeological Trust for all their help and advice.

## REFERENCES

Boyde, A. (1963). Estimation of age-at-death of young human skeletal remains from incremental lines in the dental enamel. Third international meeting in forensic immunology, medicine, pathology and toxicology. London.

Fujita, T. (1939). Neue Festellungen über die Retzius'schen Parallelstreifen des Zahnschmelzes, Anat. Anz. 87: 350-355.

Goodman, A.H., Armelagos, G.J. and Rose, J.C. (1980). Enamel hypoplasias as indicators of stress in three prehistoric populations from Illinois., Hum. Biol. 52: 515-528.

Hillson, S.W. (1979). Diet and dental disease. World Archaeology, 11 (2): 147-162.

Lindeman, G. (1958) Forekomstem af emaljehypoplasi hos børn, som har lidt of mavetarmsygdomme. Odont. T. 66: 101-126.

Mellanby, M. (1934). Diet and dental structure in man. Medical Research Council Special Report Series 191. London.

Pindborg, J.J. (1970). Pathology of the dental hard tissues. Munksgaard, Copenhagen.

Nikiforuk, E. and Frazer, D. (1981). The aetiology of enamel hypoplasia - a unifying concept. J. Pediatr. 98: 888-893.

Rose, J.C. (1977). Defective enamel histology of prehistoric teeth from Illinois. Am. J. Phys. Anthropol. 46: 439-446.

Sarnat, B.G. and Schour, I. (1941). Enamel hypoplasia (chronologic enamel aplasia) in relation to systemic disease: A chronologic, morphologic and aetiologic classification. J. Am. Dent. Assoc. 28: 1989-2000.

Sarnat, B.G. and Schour, I. (1942). Enamel hypoplasia (chronologic enamel aplasia) in relation to systemic disease: A chronologic, morphologic and aetiologic classification. J. Am. Dent. Assoc. 29: 67-75.

Shafer, W.E., Hine, M.K. and Levy, B.M. (1983). Textbook of Oral Pathology. (4th Ed.) Saunders. London.

## Chapter 10

# LEPROGENIC ODONTODYSPLASIA

Charlotte Roberts
Calvin Wells Laboratory
School of Archaeological Sciences
Bradford

## INTRODUCTION

Leprogenic odontodysplasia is a term used for the malformation in growth of the human permanent tooth roots. The condition has been noted in teeth from archaeological sites and only in association with the specific infectious disease, leprosy. In addition, the anomaly has a marked tendency to occur in skeletons with the most severe and low resistant form of leprosy, that is lepromatous leprosy. Interestingly, recent observation of leprous individuals today in Ethiopia did not reveal leprogenic odontodysplasia (Keith Manchester, pers. comm.). Study of this condition has stemmed from work initiated by Knud Danielsen in Denmark (1970) on medieval skeletal material. He studied teeth from leprous individuals and isolated 10 skeletons with leprogenic odontodysplasia from a total of 100 (1%). Since then concentrated surveys of teeth for this condition have been lacking.

Interest in this phenomenon forms part of ongoing research into the antiquity of leprosy and tuberculosis at the University of Bradford. A review of the pathological processes involved in lepromatous leprosy will perhaps help to explain why the permanent tooth roots are affected in leprogenic odontodysplasia.

### Leprosy

Leprosy can manifest itself in the human body as one of three types. The type which affects a person depends on his/her resistance to the bacteria Mycobacterium leprae (Jopling, 1978, 18). Figure 10.1 displays this resistance to the bacteria.

Lepromatous leprosy, or low resistant leprosy, is characterised by facies leprosa on the skeleton, a term coined by Moller-Christensen (1953: 123). This condition comprises several features. The person suffers from an erosion of the anterior nasal spine of the maxilla (Figs. 10.2, 10.3 and 10.4). Erosion of the pyriform aperture is accompanied by an absorption, or recession, of the alveolar process of the maxilla (Fig. 10.5). Eventually there is a loss of the incisor teeth (Figs. 106 and 10.7). An osteitis, or infection of the nasal and oral surfaces of the palate develops (Figs. 10.8 and 10.9) with eventual perforation (Fig. 10.10). Facies leprosa is usually accompanied by non-specific inflammatory and neuropathic lesions on the lower legs and extremeties.

Affection of the face in low resistant leprosy is due to an early infiltration by bacteria into the anterior part of the nasal cavity. The mucous membrane is infected and once this infection reaches the bone, the

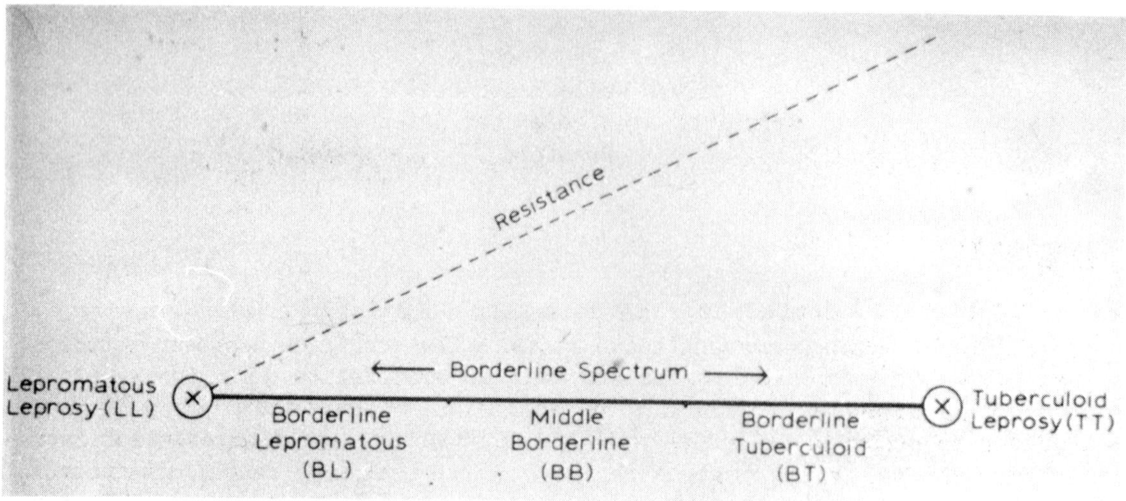


Figure 10.1. Types of leprosy with degree of resistance.

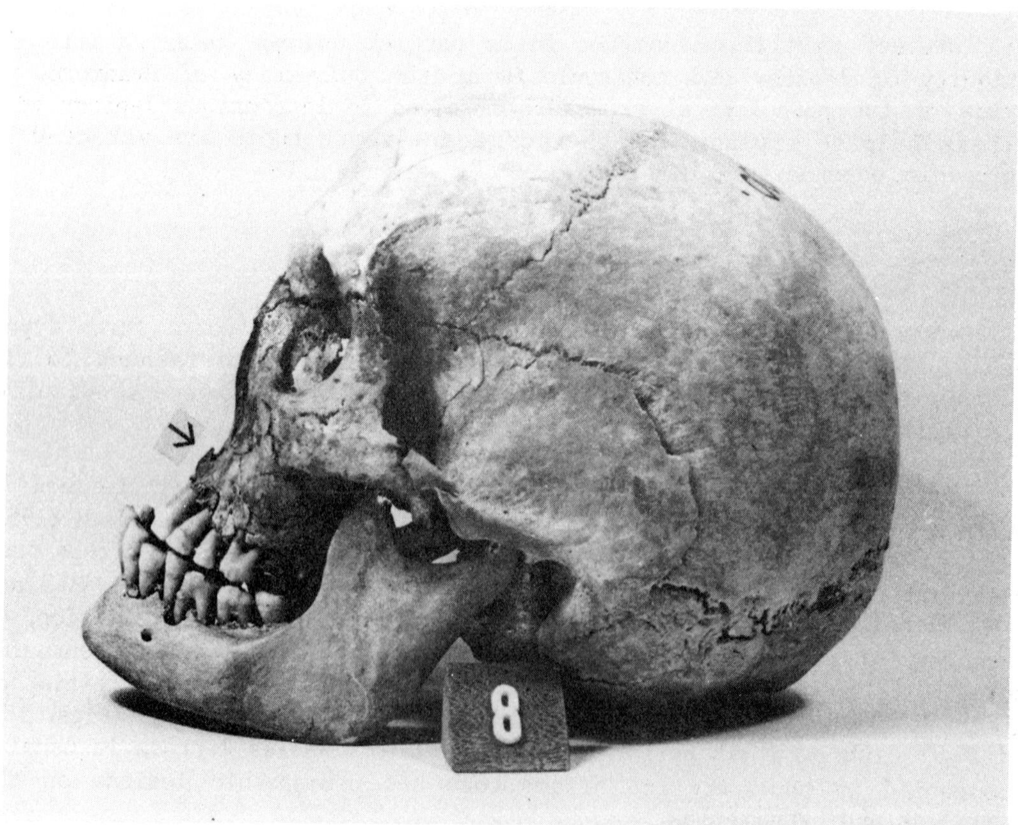

Figure 10.2. Loss of the anterior nasal spine: Danish medieval skeleton.

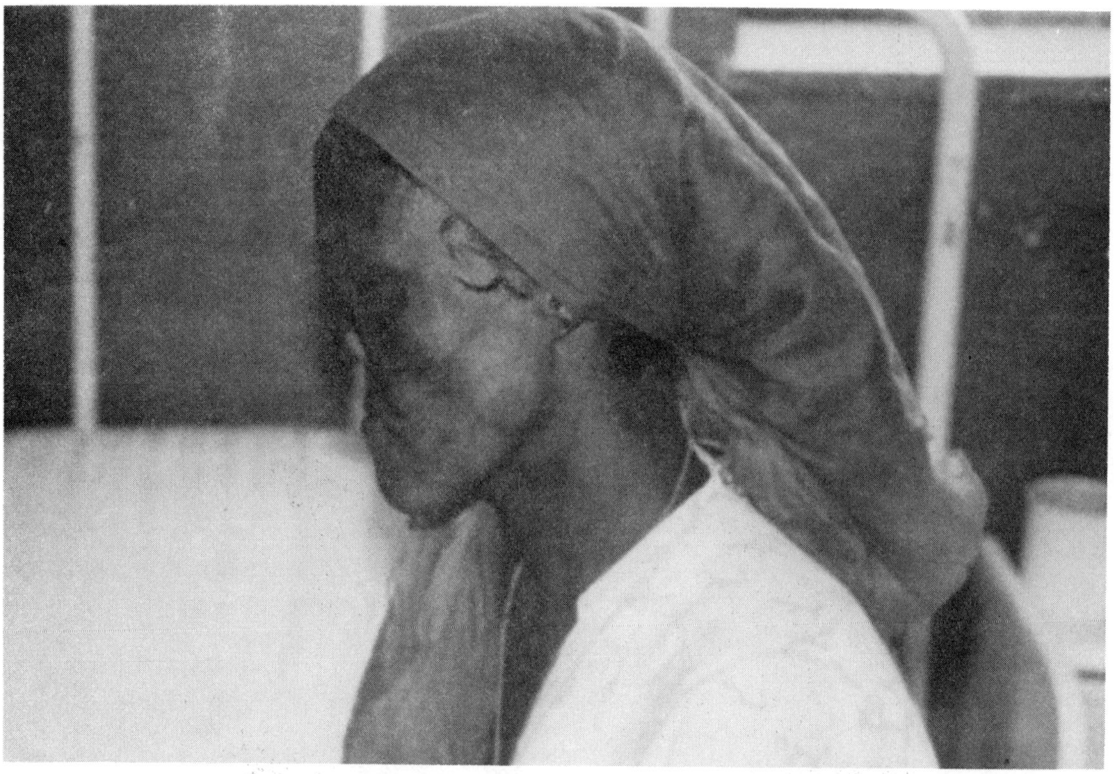

Figure 10.3. Loss of the anterior nasal spine: clinical Ethiopia.

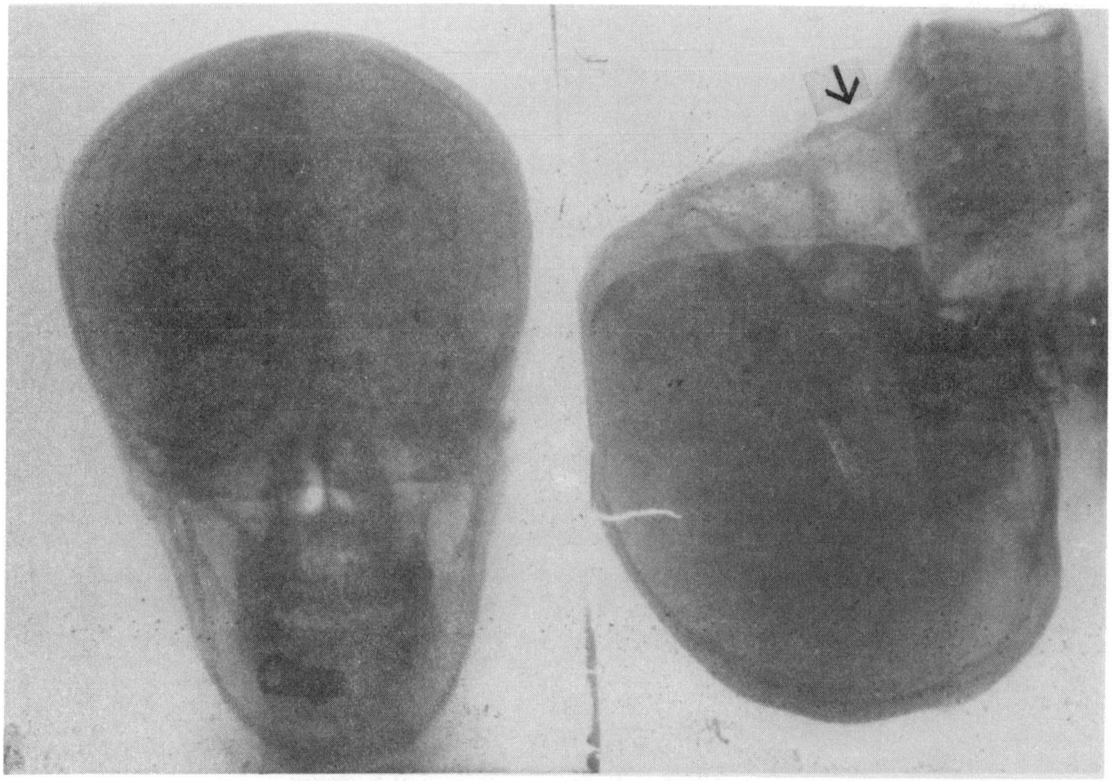

Figure 10.4. Loss of the anterior nasal spine: X-ray Ethiopia.

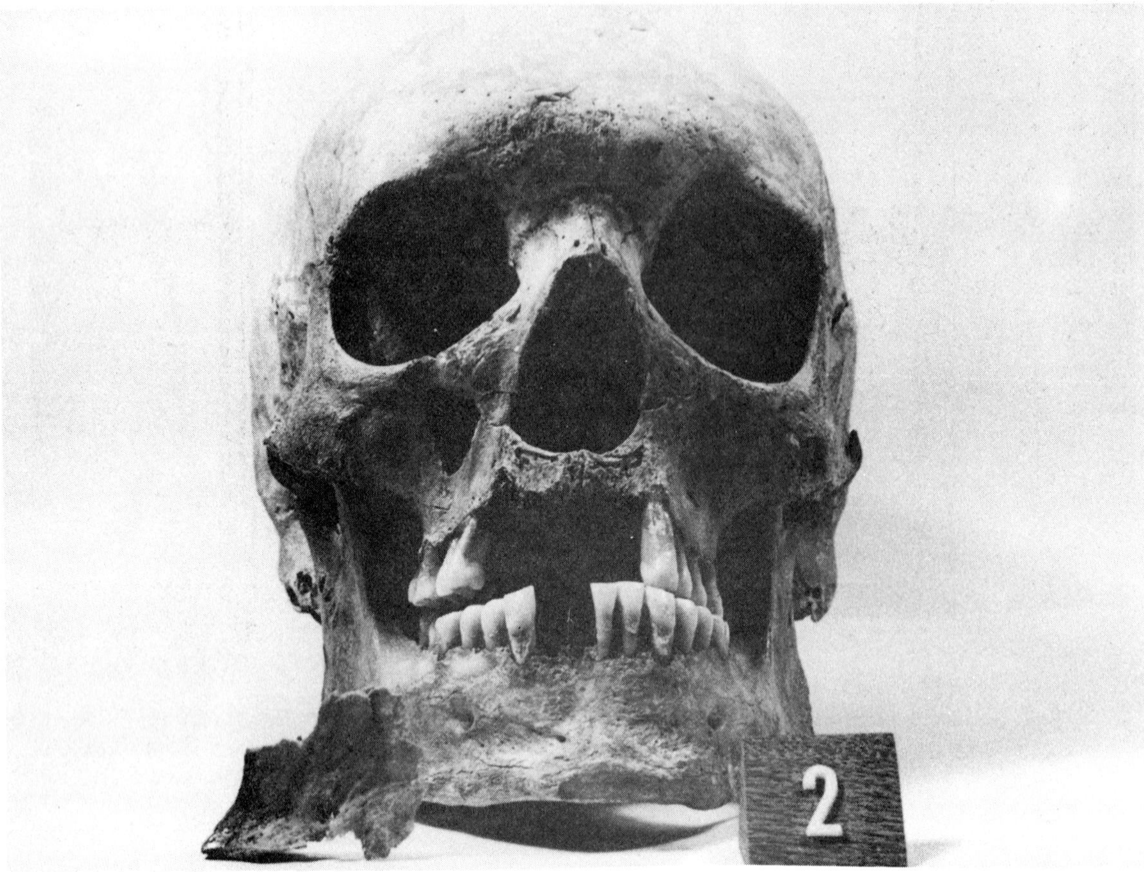


Figure 10.5. Erosion of pyriform aperture and recession of alveolar process of maxilla.

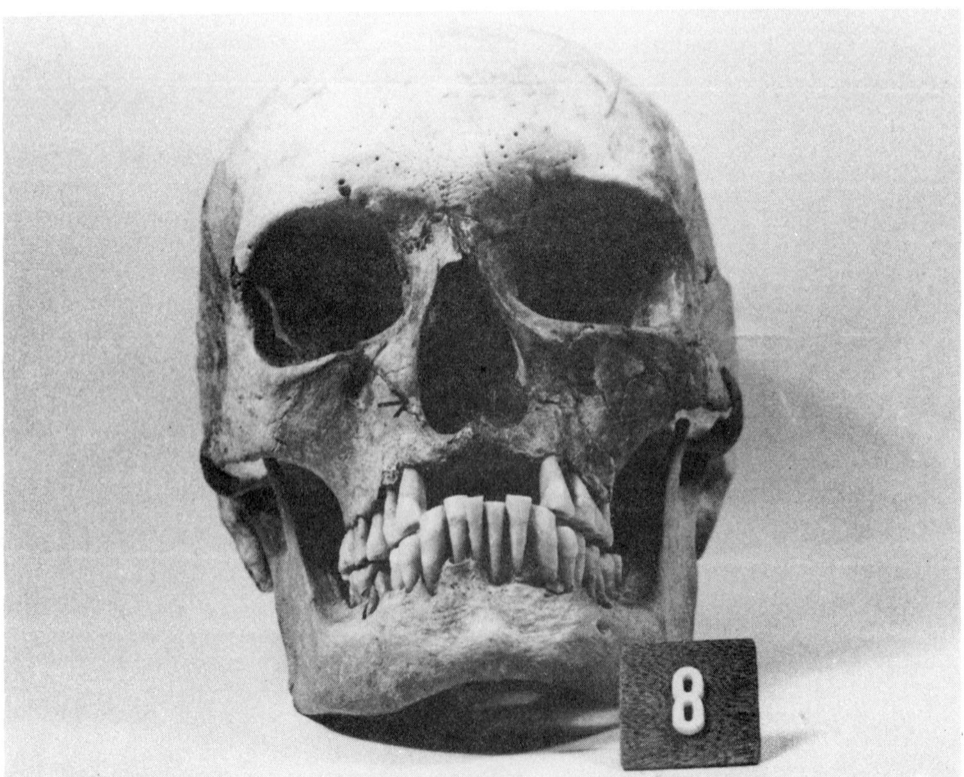


Figure 10.6. Loss of the incisors: Danish medieval skeleton.

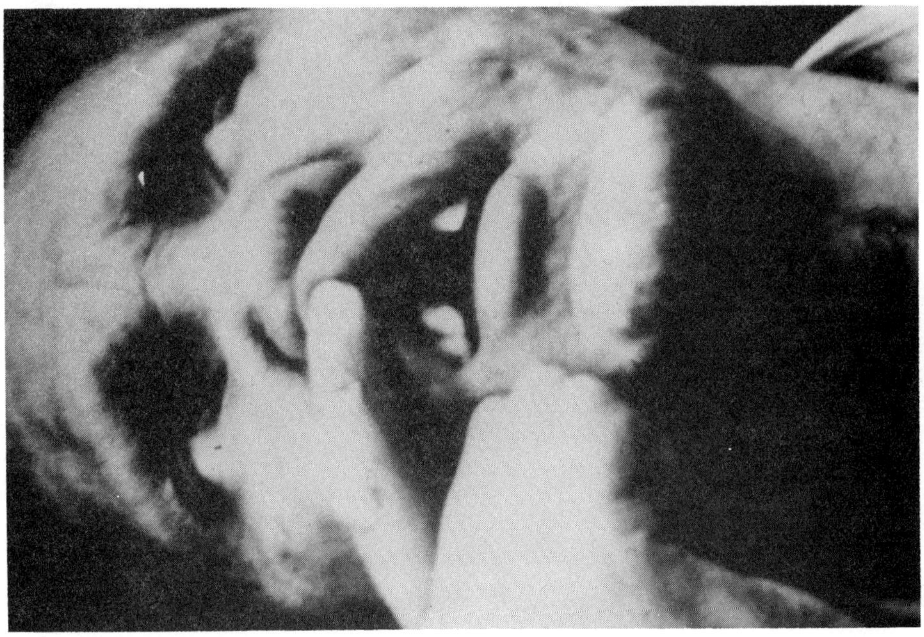

Figure 10.7. Loss of the incisors: clinical.

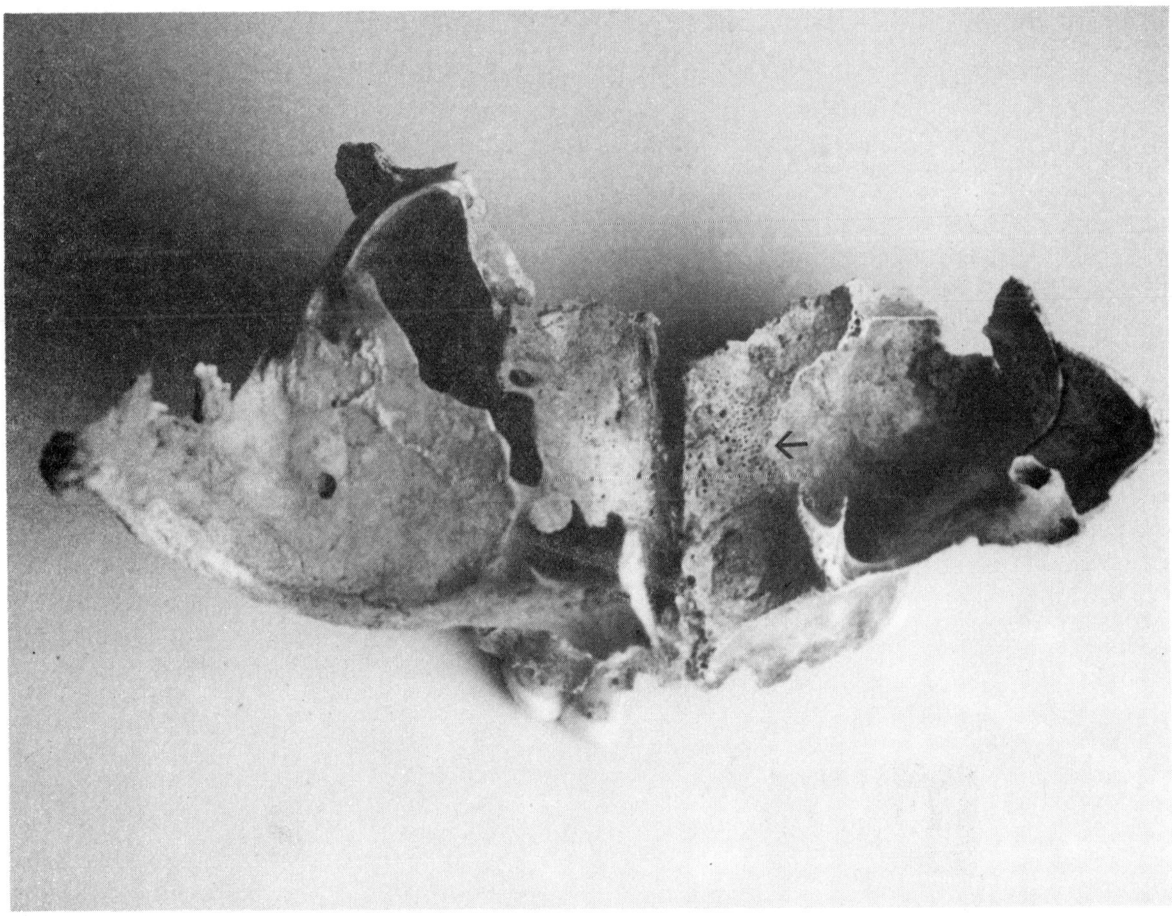

Figure 10.8. Osteitis of palate: Norton Priory, medieval.

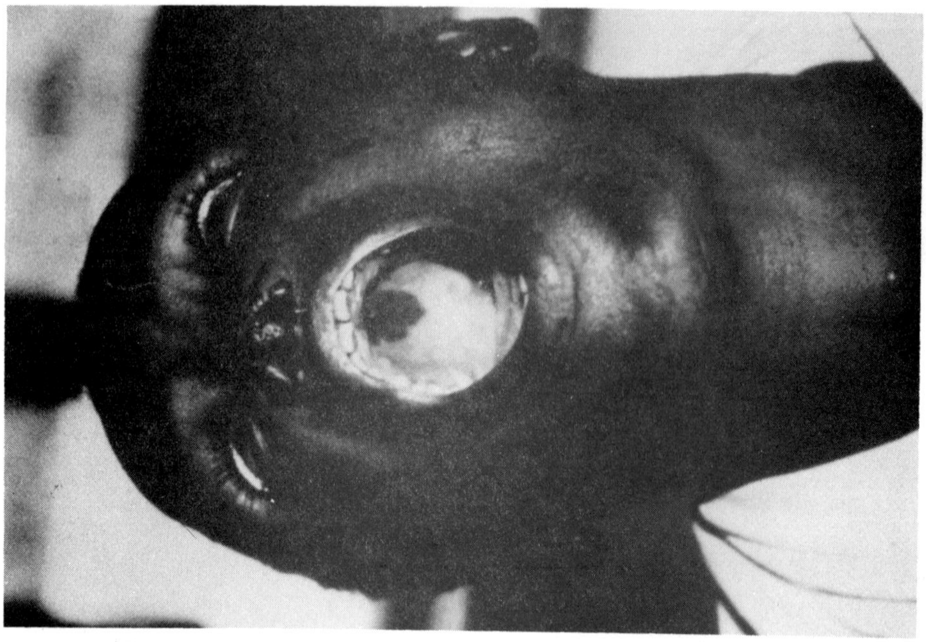

Figure 10.9. Osteitis of palate: clinical Ethiopia.

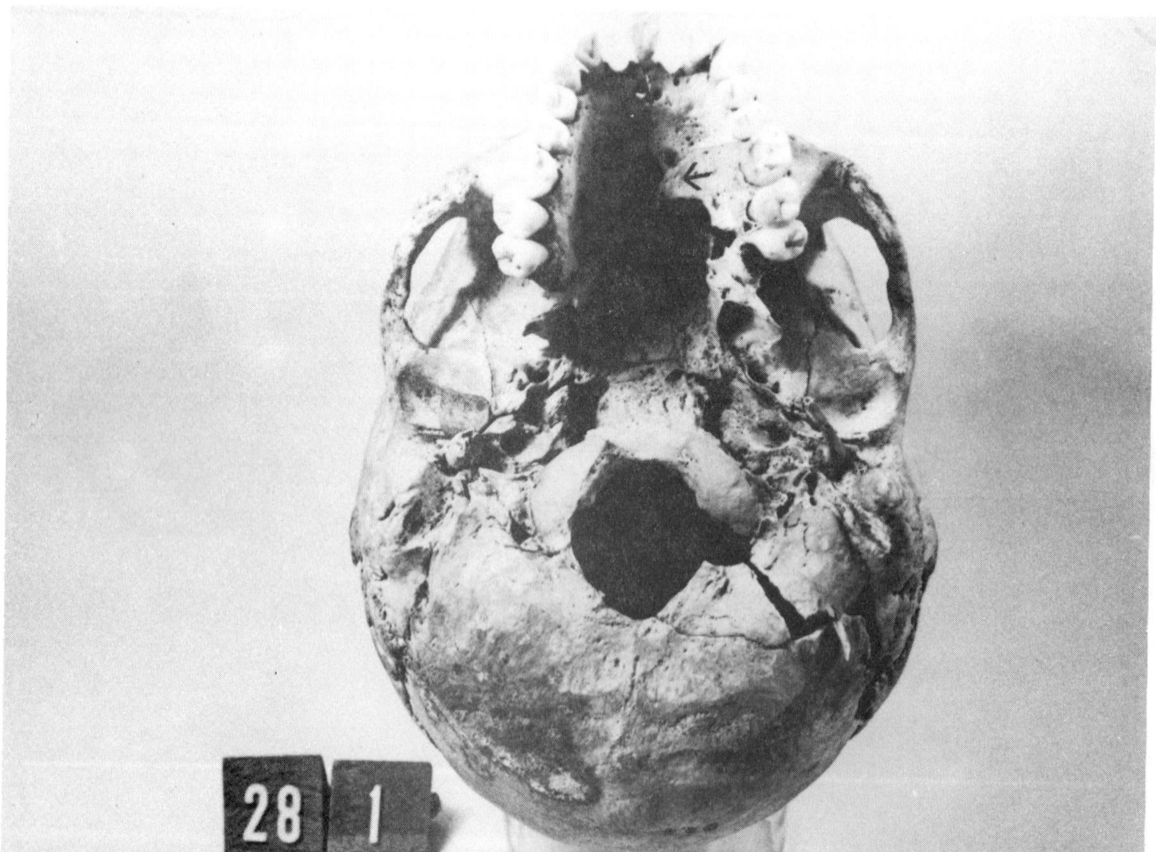


Figure 10.10. Perforation of the palate: Danish medieval skeleton.

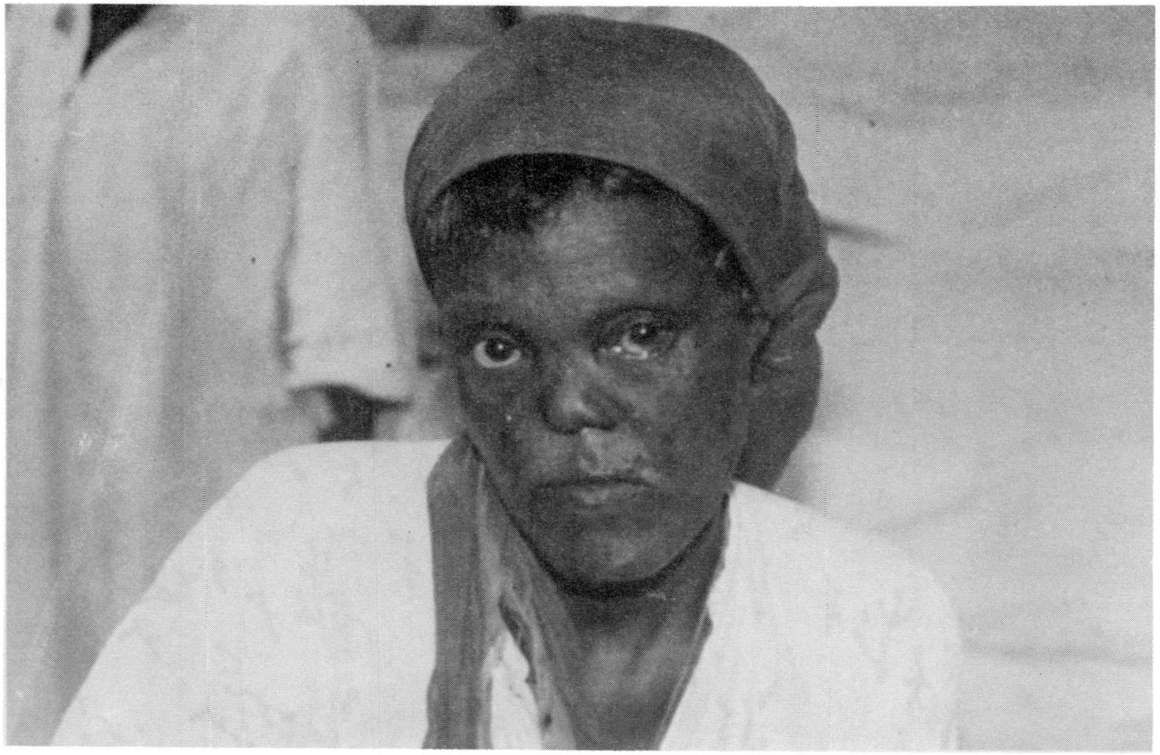

Figure 10.11. Collapse of the nose: clinical Ethiopia.

nose eventually collapses (Fig. 10.11). Difficulty in breathing through the nose leads to mouth breathing and gingivitis.

Leprous change in the nasal and oral cavities tends to occur in the anterior areas, especially in the maxilla. This could be caused by one of the following (Danielsen, 1970, 14f):

1. Lepromatous alteration of blood vessels and nerves passing through the nasal tissues.

2. A low tissue temperature due to mouth breathing which promotes the growth of Mycobacterium leprae.

3. Repeated subclinical trauma.

## Leprogenic odontodysplasia.

Leprosy bacteria are also found in the pulp cavities especially the incisors (Danielsen, 1970:16). They are seen in the premolars and canines less frequently. The molars are unaffected and develop normally.

The features of leprogenic odontodysplasia are found mainly in the incisor teeth especially the maxillary incisors. The condition is usually symmetrical and non-reversible. The teeth show a concentric constriction around the base of the tooth followed by arrested tooth growth (Fig. 10.12). X-ray of these teeth displays the constriction and irregular pulp cavity (Figs. 10.13 and 10.14). The condition has been found to be associated with dental enamel hypoplasia (Danielsen, 1970:13) and crowding of the anterior maxillary teeth with displacement of the lateral incisors (Fig. 10 15). Leprogenic odontodysplastic teeth eventually will be lost due to a combination of loosening of the teeth in the sockets and recession of the alveolar process of the maxilla.

Danielsen found that leprogenic odontodysplasia was associated both with lepromatous leprosy and with people dying before twenty years of age.

## Differential diagnosis.

The following dental pathologies should be considered when diagnosing leprogenic odontodysplasia (Danielsen, 1970:13).

1. Diseases inhibiting or stopping growth and development of the roots of the teeth (e.g. hypoparathyroidism). However, these pathologies usually affect all the teeth and there would be no associated signs such as facies leprosa.

2. Resorptive processes - although size, symmetry and concentric nature of the roots do not conform.

3. Trauma and healing on tooth germs. However, affected roots would not show a symmetrical and concentric appearance.

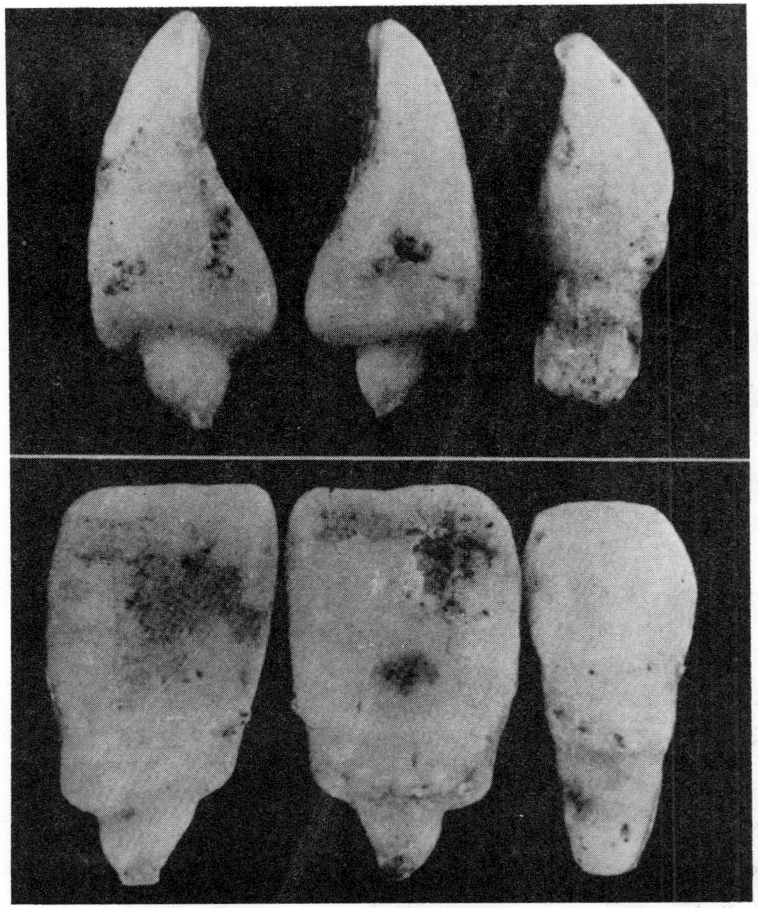

Figure 10.12. Concentric tooth roots in leprogenic odontodysplasia (Danielsen 1970).

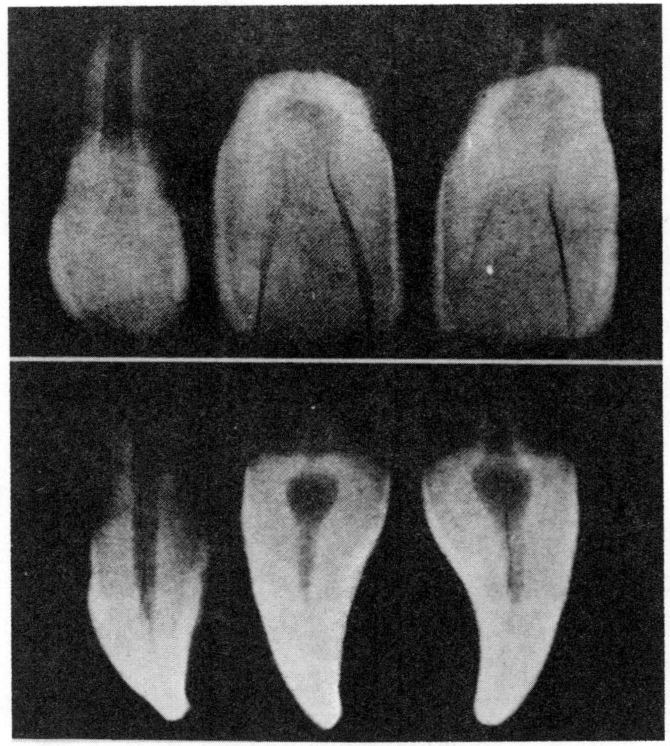


Figure 10.13. X-ray of leprogenic odontodysplastic teeth (Danielsen 1970).

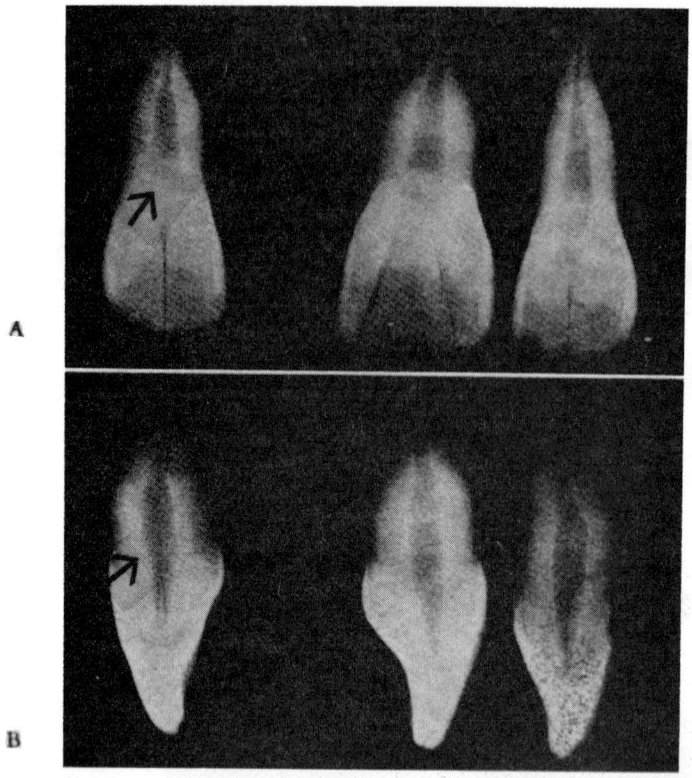


Figure 10.14. X-ray showing irregular pulp cavity in affected teeth (Danielsen 1970).

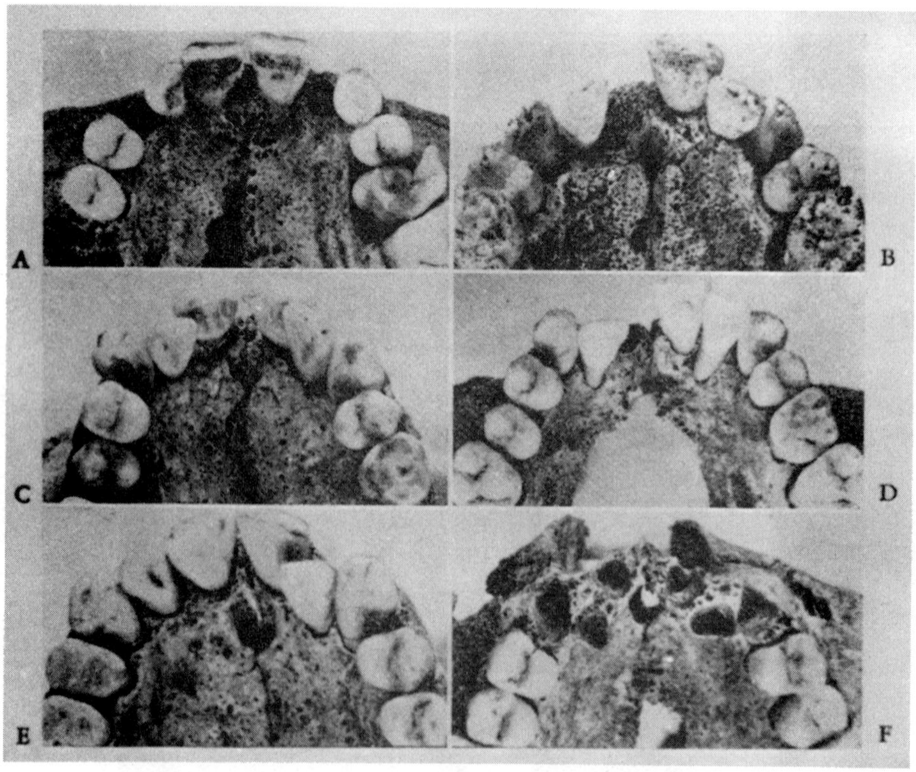


Figure 10.15. Displacement of teeth in maxilla (Danielsen 1970).

## CONCLUSION.

Examination of skeletal material during current research at Bradford has not revealed any leprogenic odontodysplastic teeth. In addition, skeletons with leprous bone change diagnosed in the past have not been seen to be associated with leprogenic odontodysplasia. Several reasons can be forwarded for their apparent absence:

1. All diagnosed leprous indivduals have been adults over 20 years of age. If this is a condition associated with young victims one would not expect to see the feature.

2. Many of the skeletons examined are fragmentary and teeth do not often survive.

3. Lepromatous leprosy sufferers would lose their anterior teeth eventually due to absorption of the alveolar process of the maxilla. Teeth would therefore not survive to be excavated.

4. If leprogenic odontodysplasia is only associated with severe facies leprosa this would restrict observations. Most of the leprous individuals so far diagnosed were not suffering from severe facies leprosa.

This short paper has served two useful purposes. Firstly it indicates to archaeologists the importance of careful excavation of all skeletal fragments however small, including teeth, and secondly by reminding anthropologists and palaeopathologists that leprogenic odontodysplasia may exist in skeletal material excavated and examined in the future.

## ACKNOWLEDGEMENTS.

1. Knud Danielsen for permission to use photographs in Figs. 10.11, 10.12, 10.13 and 10.14.

2. The University of Bradford Department of Photography for reproducing the photographs.

3. Keith Manchester for commenting on this paper.

## REFERENCES.

Danielsen, K. (1970). Odontodysplasia leprosa in Danish mediaeval skeletons. Saertryk af Tandlaegebladet, 74: 603-25.

Jopling, W. (1978). Handbook of Leprosy (2nd edition). William Heineman Medical Books Ltd., London.

Moller-Christensen, V. (1953). Location and excavation of the first Danish leper graveyard from the Middle Ages - St. Jorgen's Farm, Naestved. Bull. Hist. Med., 27 (2): 112-123.

Chapter 11

# A COMPARISON OF METHODS OF AGE DETERMINATION FROM THE MANDIBULAR DENTITION OF AN ARCHAEOLOGICAL SAMPLE OF CATTLE.

D. James Rackham

Department of Archaeology
Durham.

## INTRODUCTION

In the study of human behaviour in both the prehistoric and historic periods the manner of exploitation of both wild and domestic animal resources is of major interest. Often of primary significance in studies of early hominids (Binford, 1984) it often receives less attention in more recent periods, where it is still of major importance to studies of human economies, despite the dramatic increase in the more traditional artefactual material available. Before the wealth of faunal remains from archaeological sites can be realistically utilised in a reconstruction of prehistoric and historic subsistence and market economies, two basic products are required of their analyses. These are the sex structure of the slaughtered population and its age structure. Both are essential to an understanding of the pressures on husbandry and the manner in which domestic species may be exploited both while alive and when dead.

At present few collections allow the realistic determination of the former and the latter are generally assessed within a few broad age categories (Klein and Cruz-Uribe, 1984; Grant, 1984). While this is potentially sufficient for an understanding of the prey selection by paleolithic peoples where work on crown heights have been exploited to group data into 10% of lifespan categories (Klein and Cruz-Uribe, 1984), broad categories can disguise, or even misdirect, when interpreting more recent subsistence economies utilising domestic species. This problem is compounded by inferring the 'real ages' represented by these groups from modern data; an unrealistic model for domestic species. Changes in maturation rate may mean that ages related to developmental stages in modern stock (see Silver, 1969) may not reflect the 'real age' of archaeological material (Rackham, in press) and confound interpretation or make such interpretation ill-founded. The number of wool crops, the years of milking, or the length of time spent fattening or ploughing are significant factors in husbandry and control the basis for selection for slaughter in many communities. Errors in age assessment can lead to grossly different interpretations.

A method by which real or absolute age can be determined is therefore of considerable interest to studies in this area. Similar problems faced modern mammalian ecologists in the 1950's and 60's where age determination was important to the understanding of survivorship and ecology of species. Their studies looked for annual growth patterns that produced recognisable yearly increments (Laws, 1952; Klevezal and Kleinenberg, 1967; Morris, 1972, 1976; Spinage, 1976a) and that with the greatest potential for archaeology are the incremental lines recognised in the cementum of teeth.

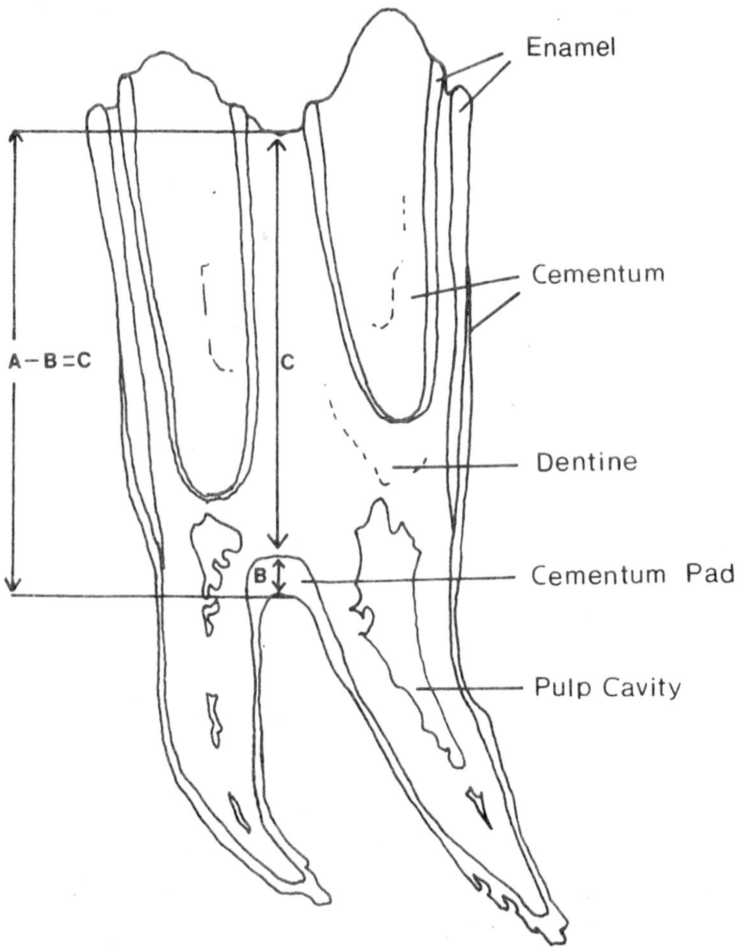


Figure 11.1. Diagram of the longitudinal section of a cattle first mandibular Molar illustrating the measurements used.

This paper discusses a collection of 1st and 2nd century cattle jaws from the Roman settlement at Carlisle. It attempts to assess the potential of studies of cementum annuli and other tooth measures for chronological/absolute age determination of the slaughtered population.

## Method

Four recordable aspects of this sample of jaws, each of which has potential, or has been used, for age assessment are compared and discussed.

Each mandible was recorded for the following information:

1. The tooth wear stage (after Grant, 1975; 1982) was recorded for all surviving teeth. This was computed to a mandibular wear stage (MWS, see Grant, 1982).

2. The crown height of the MI was measured with electronic calipers on the lingual half of the longitudinally sectioned tooth as illustrated in Fig. 11.1.

3. The thickness of the cementum pad between the roots was measured using a binocular microscope and graticule and subsequently converted to millimetres (see Fig. 11.1).

4. True crown height was calculated by subtraction of the cementum thickness from the measured crown height - true crown height (CRHT) is the figure used in all subsequent analyses.

5. Annuli were counted in the cementum on the pad, the roots and on the ventral surfaces of the crown. The latter were often the clearest (Fig. 11.2) and were counted down the tooth to record the maximum number of annuli, but the pads and roots (Fig. 11.3) were in some instances clearer or contained more visible annuli. Four researchers looked at all or part of the series and up to six counts were produced for each tooth. In the analysis below the maximum count recorded for a tooth is the one used.

## Experimental error.

It must first be admitted that the body of data considered below are subject to potentially large experimental error. These fall into the following categories.

1. Crown height and cementum thickness are subject to those errors normally occassioned by measurement, this is potentially the least significant error.

2. Tooth wear stages were recorded by visual comparison using the series illustrated by Grant (1982). This is subject to a certain amount of error (see Levitan, 1982) and in the more advanced wear stages, which coincidentally represent the longest periods chronologically, assignment to a wear stage may be based purely upon individual practice and is likely to be inconsistent between workers (Keiss, 1969) although rarely more than one stage discrepancy. This recording error is potentially significant when endeavouring to assess

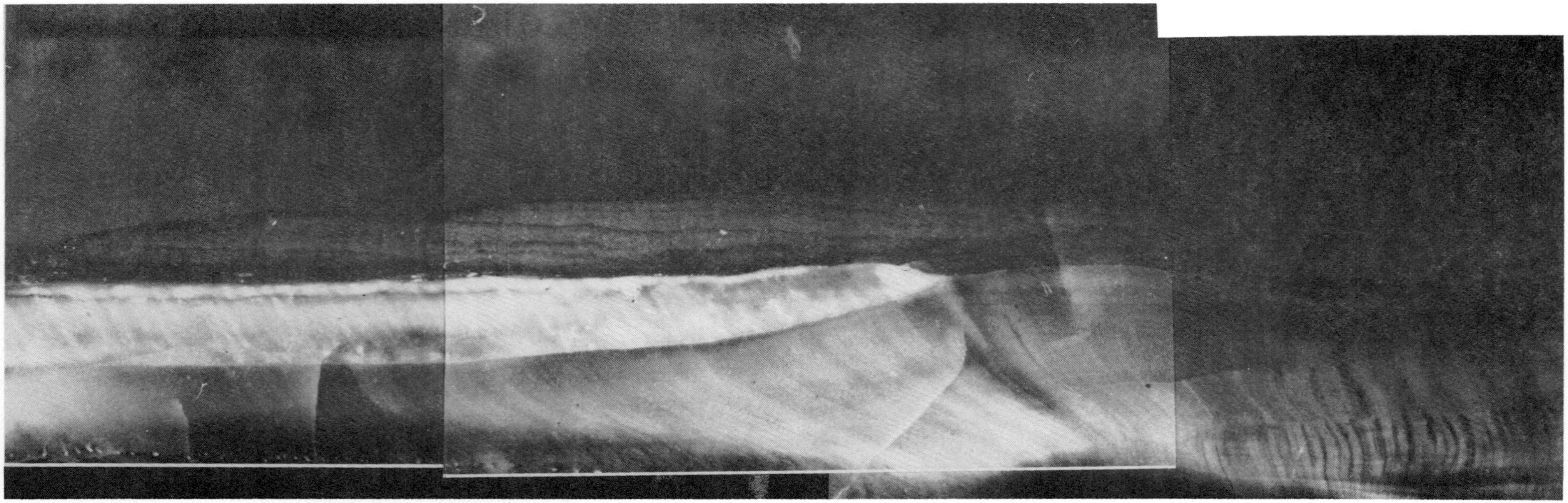

Figure 11.2. Section of cattle molar showing annuli on ventral surface of crown.

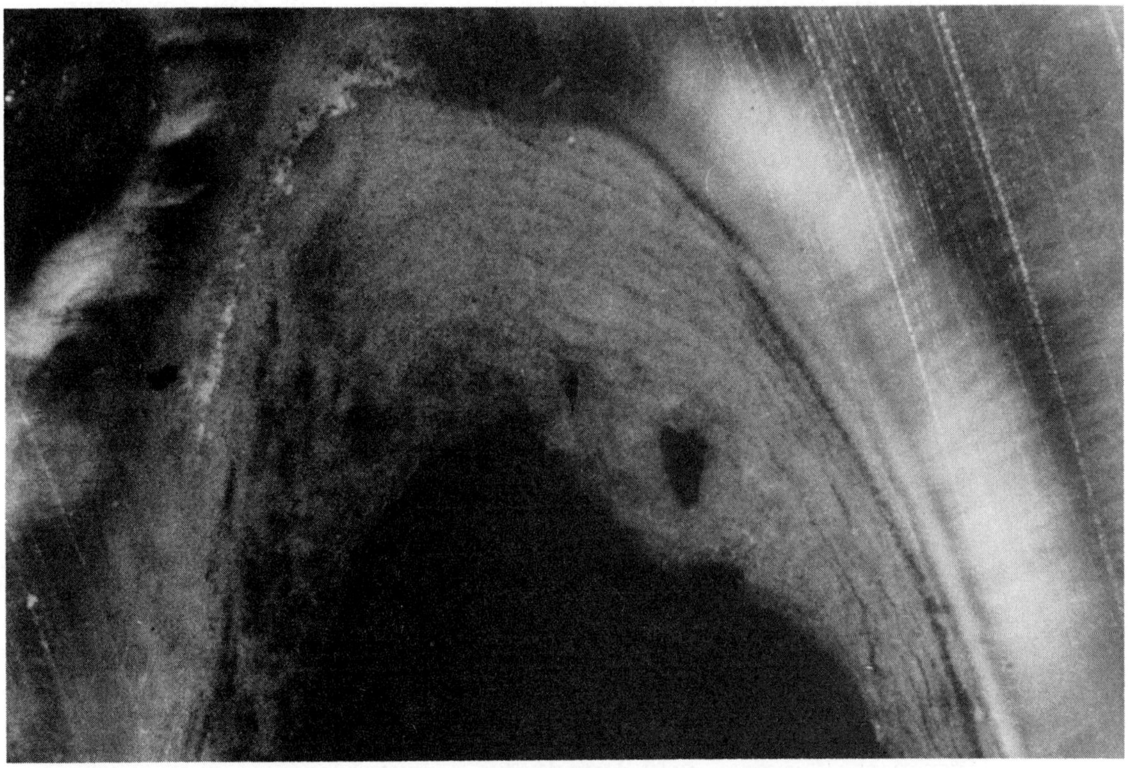

Figure 11.3. Section of cattle molar showing annuli on cementum pad.

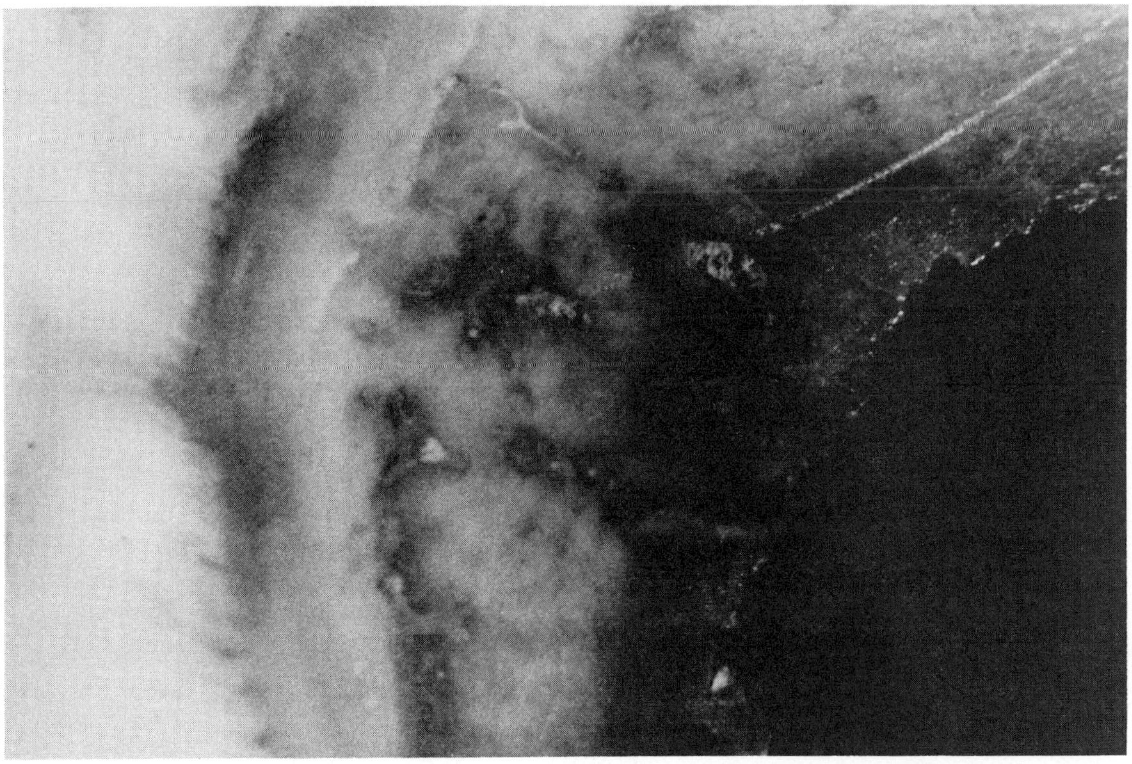

Figure 11.4. Section of cattle molar showing loss of visibility of dental annuli through resorption and redeposition.

the absolute age owing to the relatively long period of time the later wear stages may represent (see Deniz and Payne, 1982).

3. In this article for the sake of comparison assessment of absolute age rests upon the results of the counts of cementum annuli. Therefore the accuracy of the counts is very important. This measure constitutes the most significant experimental error for the following reasons:

a). Although the material discussed here is exceptionally well preserved the clarity of the annuli is extremely variable (Figs. 11.2-4). The counting has relied upon diamond saw cut sections with no artificial staining, the detail visible in the Plates is occasioned by natural staining resultant upon the burial of the teeth in organic rich deposits. The darker stained areas are those strongly calcified and low in cementocytes, and the cellular and lighter areas those traditionally assigned to the summer and fall growth season (Mitchell, 1967; Stallibrass, 1982). This staining is differential between specimens affecting their clarity.

b). It was noticed that in many of the specimens, even those from relatively unworn teeth, sharpeys fibres and resorption and redeposition of cementum had considerably obscured parts of the incremental pattern laid down in the cementum pad and that on the roots (Fig. 11.4). In no specimen was the lower part of the root suitable for counting because of these factors. This contrasts with Stallibrass's (1982) assertion that cementum is very stable and seldom subject to remodelling or resorption.

c). A number of workers (Saxon and Higham, 1968; Mitchel, 1967; Laws, 1952; Low and Cowan, 1963) have mentioned the occurrence of minor or stress lines that they believe are extra to the major banding noted above. These may be associated with pregnancy, breeding, the rut or nutritional factors and increase the number of bands formed each year. The difficulty in following lines in this material meant that many were not visibly continuous and an identification of one line as minor and another as the major increment is somewhat subjective. Where fine lines occurred between strongly stained darker lines these were not counted. A thin sectioning technique would probably improve the definition of these lines.

d). Increasing age generally produced increasing thickness of cementum and in some specimens increasing resorption and redeposition. Therefore annulus counts on some relatively worn teeth were more likely to be less accurate and generally in the direction of underestimation. In Figure 11.5 those counts designated as difficult or likely to be incomplete due to resorption or obscurity are noted by a triangle.

The error deriving from the problems associated with counts of annuli is by far the largest in this data set, and whereas in modern studies the annulus counts have been verified against known age animals, with fossil material this is of course not possible.

Since the sectioning and recording of annuli is a lengthy business and

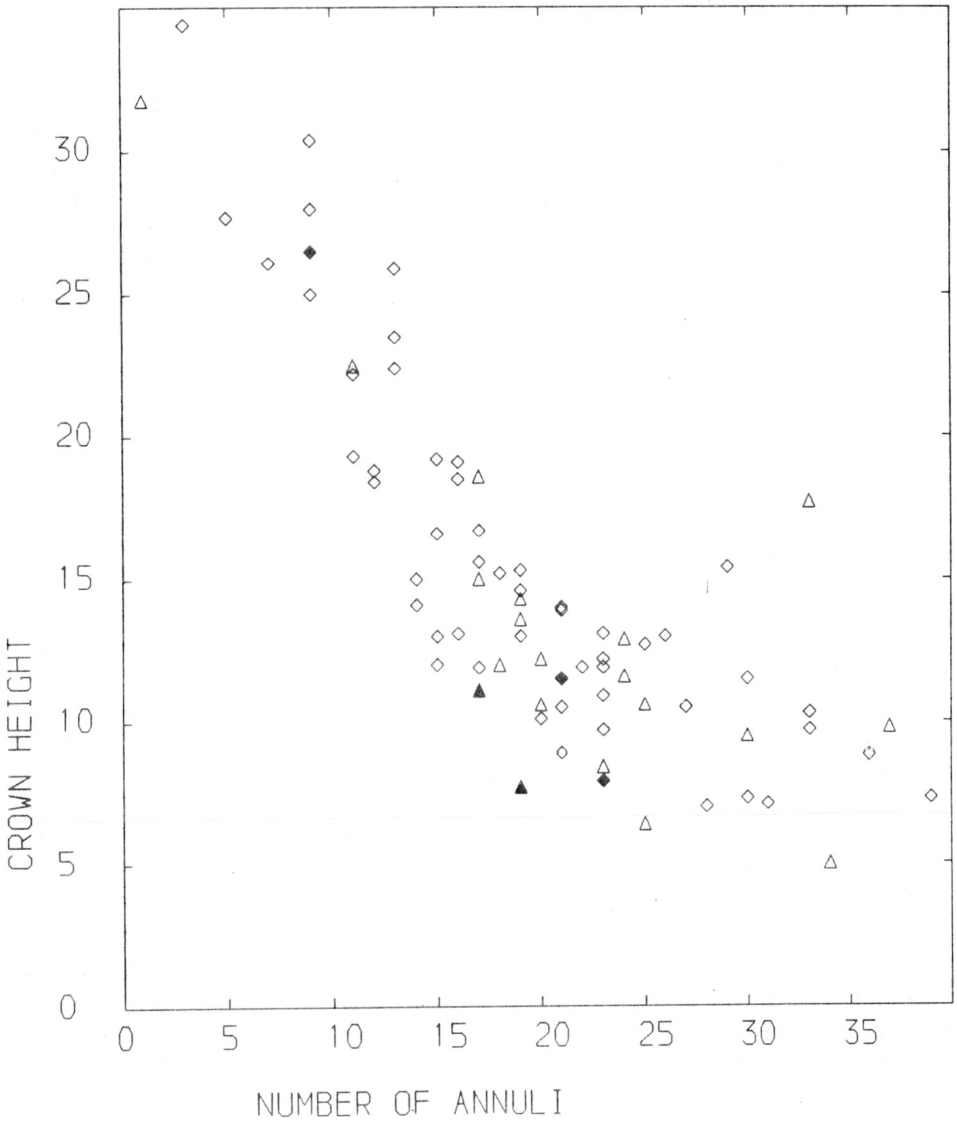


Figure 11.5. Scattergram of crown height against annulus count for 1st and 2nd century cattle mandibular first molar from Carlisle.

anyway only possible in exceptionally well preserved material, it is important to establish from those well preserved collections the limits within which such easily observable or measurable quantities as MWS and crown height (CRHT) can be used for establishing chronological age. Klein and Cruz-Uribe (1984) have indicated that they are not aware of differential wear within populations of a single species except in domestic sheep in New Zealand and Australia (Ludwig, Healy and Cutress, 1966), but Grant (1978) suggests more rapid wear in an Orkney population of sheep owing to bone gnawing and sand ingestion and Weiner and Purser (1957) also report variation in eruption rate associated with different diets and nutrition level and it must be presumed that both these variations will occur between populations feeding on markedly different vegetational communities, those in good pasture by comparison with marginal areas or where high stock density can be artificially maintained. Perhaps in wild animals such differences are less marked. It is therefore likely that the results of this study will not be directly applicable to other geographic areas where a similar study may be necessary to establish the rate of wear in relation to anulus counts. Certainly the work of Coy et al (1982) suggests that age as represented by annulus counts is much younger for a given MWS for Saxon cattle from Southampton than those discussed here.

Estimation of absolute age.

The estimate for absolute age in this sample is based entirely upon the results of the sectioning and annulus counts.

This requires some justification. Stallibrass (1982) recently reviewed the potential of this as a method for absolute ageing of archaeological material. The technique has been applied on archaeological and fossil material with varying success by a number of authors (Saxon & Higham, 1969; Speiss, 1979; Coy et al, 1982; Bourque et al, 1978; Kay, 1974; Rackham, 1982). Coy et al (1982) had some reservations concerning the utilisation of the technique and the failure rate of their archaeological sections was high for a number of reasons. In contrast of the eighty mandibular first molars (M1) sectioned in this study only five specimens were not used in the analysis - one of these because of poor preservation had dematured cementum and in the others poor preservation, resorption or convolution had permitted only a minimum count. Sectioning of material from other sites (Rackham, in press) showed a high failure rate due to poor preservation of the cementum. It would appear that burial in an organic rich environment may be necessary for clarity of microstructure in the cementum. Certainly material otherwise describable as well preserved revealed denatured cementum when teeth were sectioned.

Although most of the work on modern animals has involved wild species some workers (Saxon and Higham, 1968; Klevezal and Kleinenberg, 1967) report incremental lines for domestic species which can be correlated with age. While the biological reasons for the formation of these lines is still unclear (Grue and Jensen, 1979) much work has established from known age animals a correlation between age and annulus number (Mitchell, 1967; Marks and Erickson, 1966; Ransom, 1966;) although some work (Lowe, 1967) has failed to confirm this relationship. The lines have been observed in zoo animals and others where they cannot be attributed to seasonal availability of food and would appear to be a physiological response associated with growth. They occur twice annually in wild ungulates in parts of Africa (Spinage, 1976a) subjected to two dry seasons in the year. The body of evidence would support a conclusion that these annuli are laid down yearly in temperate regions. The clarity of the lines (Figs. 11. 2-4) in most specimens in this study encourages me to use them as a means of determining absolute age.

The annuli in the material under study consistsof broad, light (poorly stained) cellular bands and thinner, dark (stained) acellular lines. The accepted interpretation of these (see Mitchell, 1967) is the light band represents summer and autumn growth and the dark ring the deposition of acellular cementum during the winter and spring.

In this study the tooth chosen for sectioning was the M1. This is the first tooth of the adult dentition to erupt and therefore the annuli will most closely represent the actual age. Modern cattle maxillary molar 1's have fully erupted at approximately one year and one month (Andrews, 1982) although Silver (1969) records this eruption slightly earlier and Grigson (1982) notes the figures used by a number of other authors. Cementum is believed to be laid down during or immediately after eruption and certainly in the least worn teeth in this sample a layer of cementum was already present. Novakowski (1965) however in his study of American Bison suggested that the cementum on the M1 was not laid down in these animals until four and a half years of age, well after the eruption of this tooth. In the present study it is taken that the first pale band is laid down in the summer and fall of the year following birth although we cannot guarantee eruption of the tooth or that this tooth had fully erupted at approximately twelve months in cattle of the Roman period. It may be supposed that if anything this assumption will produce an error biased towards underestimation of real age.

Estimated age in years is therefore taken to be:

$$ANNU/2 + 1$$

where ANNU = total number of light + dark bands.

## Analysis.

The estimate of age based upon the annulus counts is compared with two other commonly used measures for assessing age or relative age, crown height (CRHT) (Spinage, 1972; Klein and Cruz-Uribe, 1984) and mandibular wear stage (MWS) (Grant, 1982).

In 1971, Spinage studying a sample of modern Impala, empirically arrived at an equation that modelled CRHT in relation to an age based upon wear patterns. This gave the equation:

$$Y = Y\emptyset(1 - (T/N)^{k})$$

where Y = the worn CRHT of the M1; YØ = mean unworn CRHT of M1; N = mean age at which Y = 0; T = age in years and k is a constant. Spinage (1972) later studied modern zebra where he applied this curve to data on CRHT and cementum annulus counts giving a most significant fit ($r = 0.959$, $P = <0.05 > 0.02$) with $k = 1/2$. He subsequently applied this model to further ungulate samples (Spinage, 1976a; 1976b). Grimsdell's (1973) study of buffalo arrived at a quadratic function for the relationship between CRHT and cementum annuli for the mandibular M1:

$$Y = 36.283 - 1.191X + 0.009X^2$$

where Y = number of cementum lines; 36.283 = mean unworn CRHT and X = mean CRHT. This regression of his data was for the purpose of predicting the number of annuli from CRHT and is algebraically similar to Spinage's model. Klein et al (1981; 1983; 1984) later adopted Spinage's model for application to archaeological samples. He and others (Klein et al 1981; 1983) analysed a sample of modern known age wapiti in which they used the quadratic regression as the predictive model for age from CRHT on the M1. Klein and Cruz-Uribe (1984) in their recent book advocate an age estimation formula from CRHT based upon an algebraic translation of Spinage's model.

$$T = N - 2(N - Z)(Y/Y\emptyset) + (N - Z)(Y^2/Y\emptyset^2)$$

where Z = the age at which the permanent tooth erupts and the other variables are as above.

In the sample of Roman cattle mean maximum age (N - at which M1 is completely worn down) is not known although records exist for cattle surviving nearly 36 years (Odlum, 1950); most modern cattle in regular use (i.e. for milking and work) survive to an age of approximately 20 years (pers. comm. Peter Reynolds; Grimsdell, 1973). Furthermore no examples existed in the sample with no wear, mean unworn CRHT (YØ) is consequently unknown. Therefore using the model presented by Spinage (1971) the data was analysed iteratively to produce a best fit. The least squares fit (least squares = 718) was produced when k = 0.083, N = 30 and YØ = 169 mm. This figure for YØ is obviously impossible, the maximum measured CRHT was 34.2 mm. Therefore although the maximum age may be appropriate the data for the young age groups is not modelled by this equation. Furthermore substantial changes in the value of k produced fairly small increases in the least squares - i.e. when least squares = 812 k = 0.5, YØ = 32 and N = 18. The relationship of this data to the model was further tested by plotting the residuals (predicted age from model minus estimated age) against the estimated age (Fig. 11.6) when k = 0.5, YØ = 36mm and N = 25 years. The pattern illustrates that this model underestimates estimated age in the young age categories, overestimates in the middle and underestimates again in the old age categories. The data therefore wants to curve more than the model predicts and this is true for all values of k tested.

It is apparent from this analysis that the model is not suitable for the data presented in Fig. 11.5. It is not possible to attribute this discrepancy to any of the errors described above and it is therefore suggested that Spinage's model is inapplicable to this sample of Roman cattle. It is interesting to note that Klein et al (1983) in Fig. 5.2 in which they plot the residuals for true age minus the quadratic prediction of age for the M1 against true age show there is a tendency for the quadratic regression to overestimate in younger animals and underestimate in middle aged animals. This figure suggests that the quadratic model derived from Spinage (1971) does not quite fit the data, and interestingly contrasts with the group understudy by reversing the pattern noted above. Visual observation of Fig. 11.5 suggests that the wear on the M1 may speed up during the early wear period, an aspect not accounted for by the model. This is not unexpected since the rate of wear on the M1 immediately after its eruption is to some extent limited by the rate of wear on the larger deciduous premolar 4 just anterior in the jaw, and until this tooth is lost, diminution of the occlusal surface will be restricted by its rate of wear, although the M1 will continue to erupt after initiation of wear.

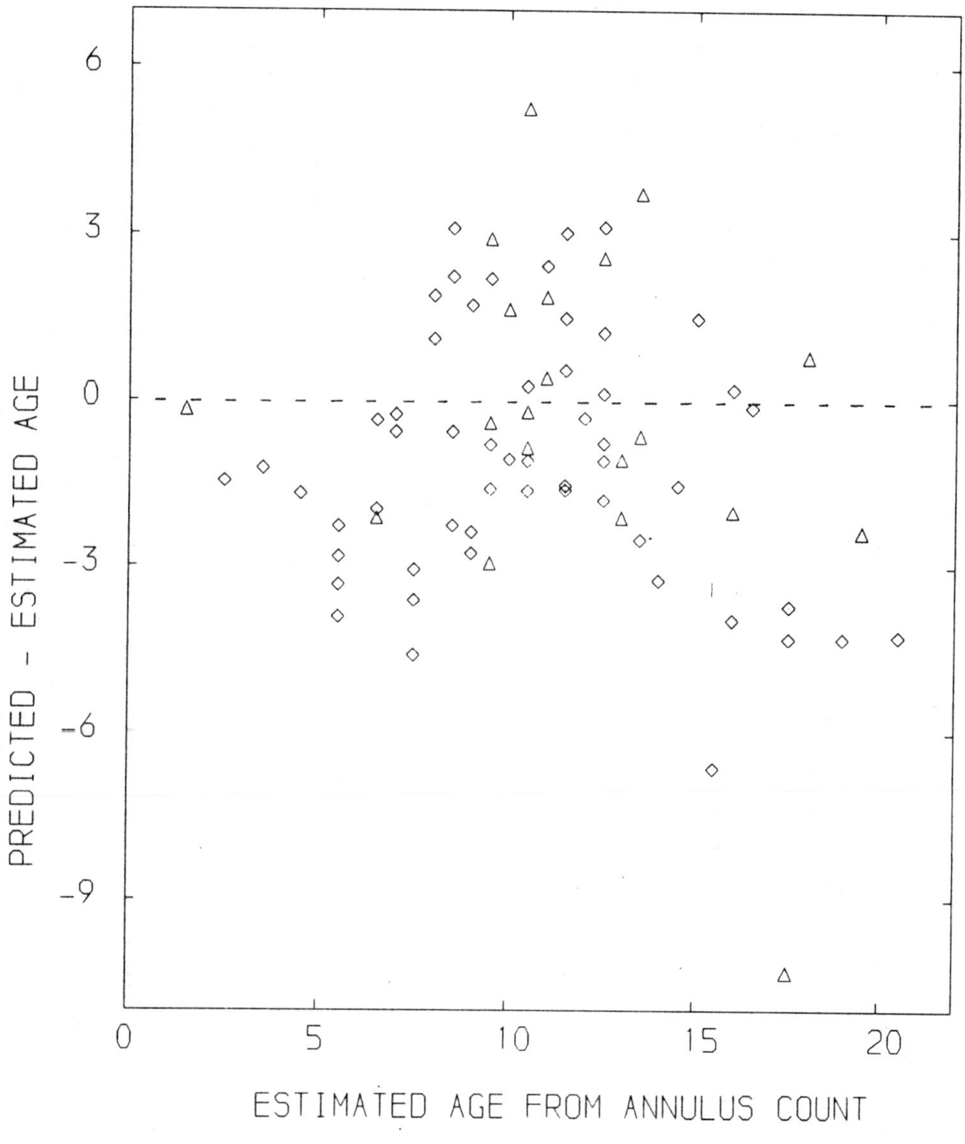


Figure 11.6. Scattergram of residuals of predicted minus estimated age against estimated age for cattle mandibles from Carlisle.

Similarly, by the time the M1 CRHT is reduced to 10-15 mms, all the permanent molars are in full wear and CRHT reduction on the M1 is limited by the overall rate of wear on the whole occlusal surface of the cheek teeth when this is at its maximum surface area. It may therefore be that wear on the M1 is related to age in a sinoidal manner. It is not possible from this set of data to test this, since it has already been noted above that the data allows too much latitude permitting a number of different constants to give 'reasonably good' fits. An accurate estimate for mean unworn CRHT and mean Age at which the M1 wears to zero CRHT in these Roman cattle would simplify the development of a curvilinear model to describe the rate of wear in relation to annulus counts. However in the absence of these data an empirical curvilinear regression is unlikely to accurately describe the biological events. Further discussion is therefore limited to considering the nature of the data rather than producing a predictive model that can be used to age jaws from either CRHT or MWS.

Figure 11.5 illustrates the curvilinear relationship between the number of annuli and CRHT. The filled symbols are specimens in which the posterior cusp of the Molar 3 (M3) is absent or reduced. This reduces the area of occluding surface and may therefore lead to a slight increase in the rate of wear. The sample is small but in the four specimens in which the M3 is fully in wear three certainly have a lower CRHT in relation to annulus count than other examples. The triangles in Fig. 11.5 represent M1's in which there was some evidence to suggest that the annulus count may be an underestimate. If this was true we would expect them to congregate along the bottom edge of the data. Although this has not been tested statistically, it would appear that these counts were not appreciably different from that part of the data set felt to be accurately counted, and any error introduced is presumably fairly small.

In Figure 11.7 number of annuli have been plotted against MWS. These two variables have a positive curvilinear relationship although the scatter is quite wide in the later age categories. This confirms the expected pattern that the larger MWSs represent considerably longer periods than the smaller MWSs. The considerable increase in scatter of data in the older animals indicates that this data is not suitble for regression.

The negative relationship between CRHT and MWS (Fig. 11.8) in contrast to the above figures (11.5 and 7) is essentially linear. The concentration in this figure of a large proportion of the cases into relatively few MWSs and CRHTs contrasts with the pattern observable in Figs. 11.5, 7 and 9. The scale of the variation (in estimated age) of both MWS and CRHT is such that both measures are relatively unreliable as estimates of age after approximately 8 years old. In this sample for example (see Fig. 11.7) an MWS of 45 was recorded for a number of jaws from which the annulus counts gave an estimated age range of 8 years to 20.5 years with a mean age of 12.5 and a standard deviation of 3.62 - i.e. two in every three jaws with an MWS of 45 will lie within an estimated age range of 8.88 and 16.12 years. A similar example may be given for CRHT. A CRHT of 10.11 mm is recorded for a jaw with an estimated age of 11 years, and a CRHT of 10.33 mm for a jaw of 17.5 years. The mean age for M1s with CRHTs between 10.0 and 10.99 mm is 13.07 with a sd. of 2.18 - i.e. two in every three jaws with a CRHT between 10-10.99 mms will lie between 10.89 and 15.25 years. The variability in CRHT in these later wear stages appears to be somewhat less than that for MWS (Figs. 11.5 & 7) and would indicate that CRHT is a more reliable estimate of age in these stages. When considering the pastoral exploitation patterns of prehistoric and early historic populations these

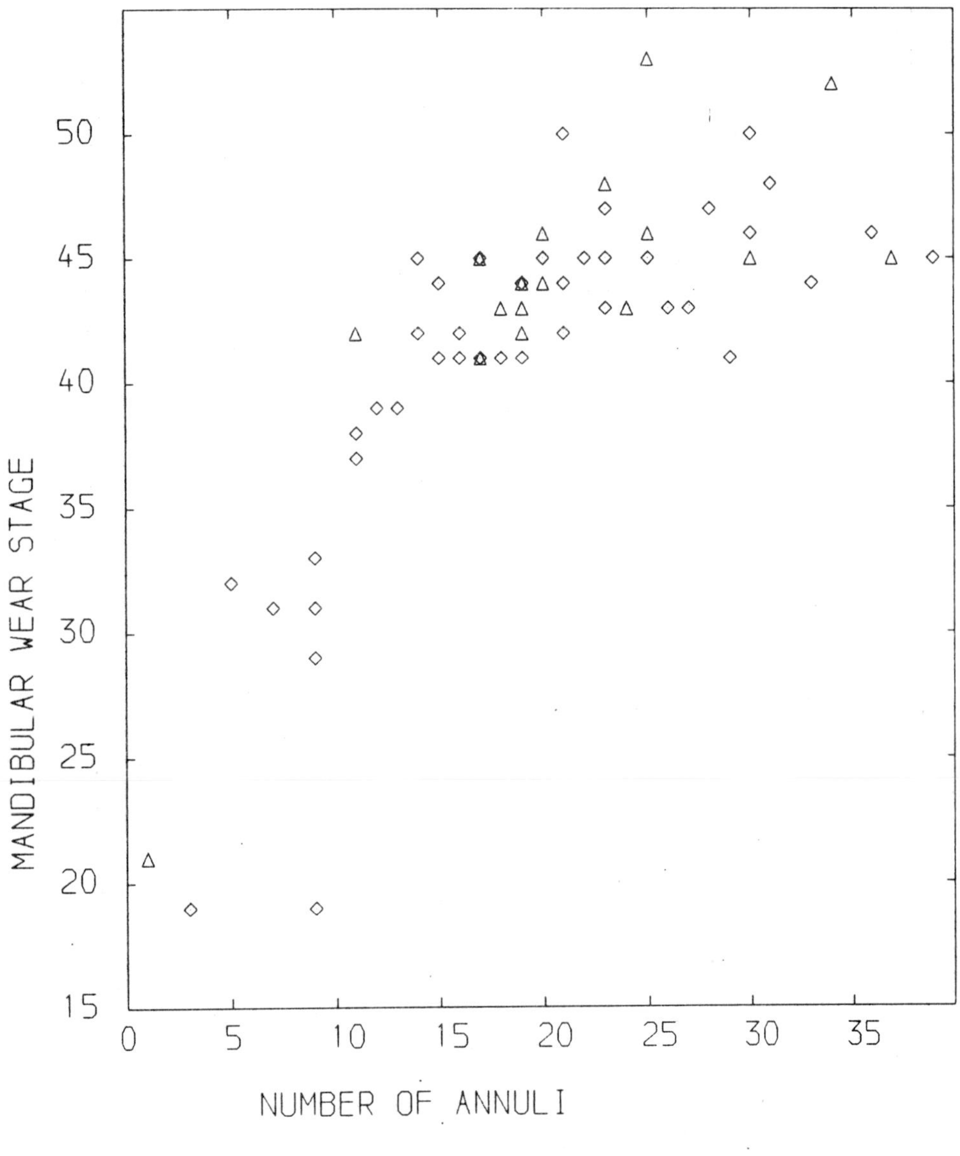


Figure 11.7. Scattergram of mandibular wear stage against first molar annulus count for 1st and 2nd century cattle mandibles from Carlise.

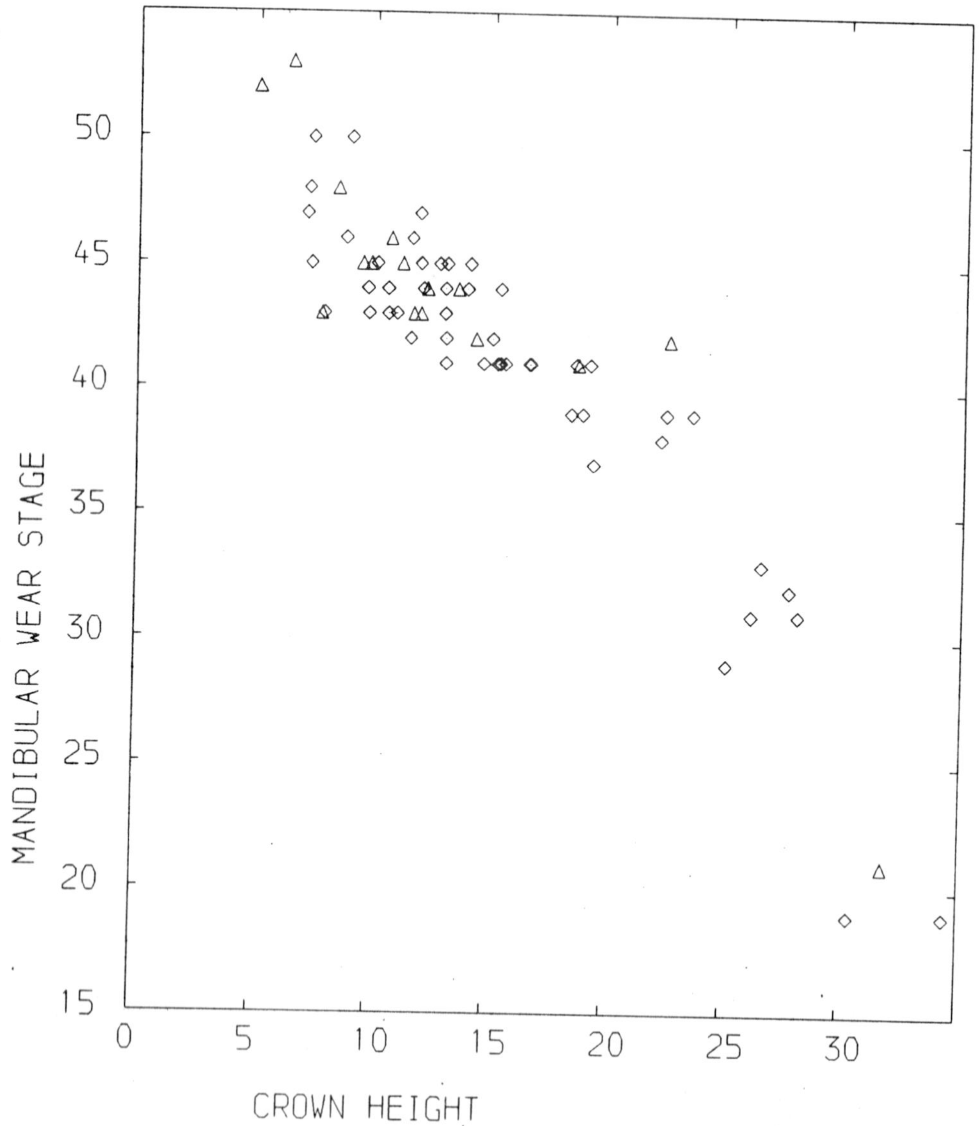


Figure 11.8. Scattergram of mandibular wear stage against first molar crown height for 1st and 2nd century cattle mandibles from Carlisle.

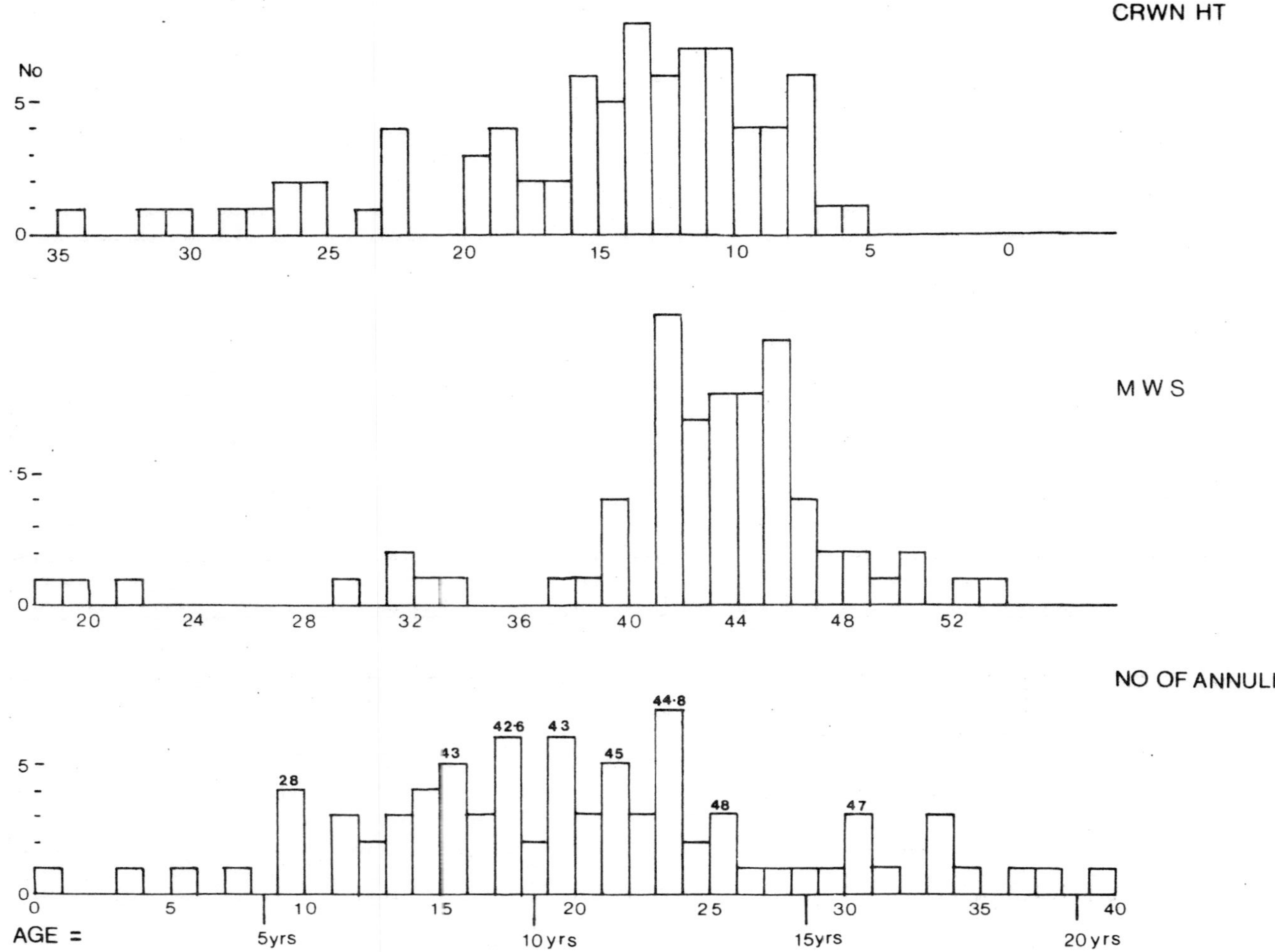


Figure 11.9. Frequency diagram of the occurrence of CRHTs, MWSs and annulus counts for a sample of 1st and 2nd century cattle from Carlisle. The figures on the diagram for annulus count indicate the mean MWS for that count.

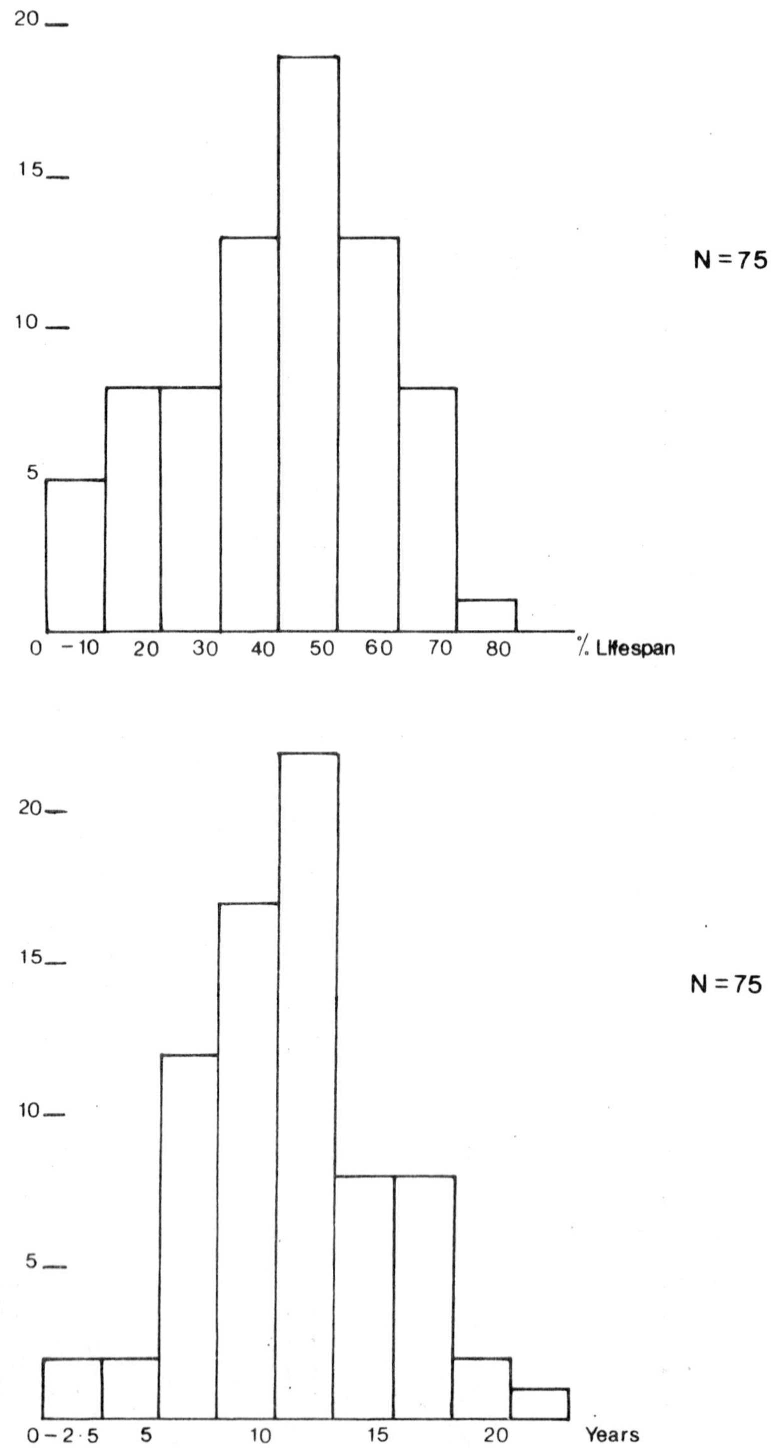


Figure 11.10. Frequency histograms of the age structure of 1st and 2nd century sample of cattle mandibles from Carlisle in 10% units of lifespan (after Klein and Cruz-Uribe, 1984) and 10% units of estimated age from annulus counts using a maximum age of 25 years.

errors are considerable and except where large samples are available, age or even age categories cannot be realistically assigned in the later 50-60% of the potential lifespan of these cattle. This is unfortunate particularly since many samples in Britain (Grant, 1982; Grant, 1984; Maltby, 1981) show that the majority of the cattle are slaughtered within this period of the lifespan or at least when their MWS is in excess of 40.

While the slaughter pattern determined in the manner of Klein and Cruze-Uribe (1984) is not strictly so useful when dealing with pastoral rather than hunting and scavenging economies, it is interesting to compare the results using their formula (in this sample taking k = 0.5, Yσ = 36 & N = 25) and the results from annulus counts in 10% units of lifespan (Fig. 11.10). The effect of the underestimate in the early and later stages of the M1 wear can be seen in Fig. 11.10 where the first two age categories contain a considerably larger proportion of individuals and the later categories contain fewer individuals. The discrepancy is of sufficient magnitude for some misinterpretation.

This study suggests a number of problems in the analysis of the age structure of archaeological samples of domestic species from CRHTs and MWSs. If we can rely on the results of the annulus counts as a realistic measure of true age, then little reliablity can be attached to age predictions based upon CRHT or MWS after about 8 years of age, even when using the model exploited by Klein and Cruz-Uribe (1984). The later wear stages and low CRHTs are subject to such large errors that only large samples may be expected to average out incorrect predictions. Interestingly the range of error found by Klein et al (1983) and Spinage (1972) was also great. Klein et al (1983) admitted that the results could only realistically be used in 10% of lifespan units. Ducos (1968) found fairly wide variability in an index of CRHT and thickness at the base of the crown in a group of modern known age N'Dama cattle. Figure 11.9 illustrates the nature of the variation in these tooth measures and illustrates that information could easily be lost by relying on CRHT and MWS. The results suggest that every opportunity should be taken to study the cementum annuli in samples where preservation is very good if realistic assessment of the age structure is required. Such studies will inevitably assist the interpretation of the MWS and CRHT data for sites where preservation is not good enough for study of the microstructure of the cementum and may result in the development of a more reliable model of first Molar wear. This study has somewhat tacitly accepted that cementum annuli represent annual increments; further supporting work should be carried out on modern domestic material to substantiate this conclusion before results of work such as this are used for indiscriminate interpretation.

ACKNOWLEDGEMENTS

I should like to thank Dr. Judith Finlay, Helen Wilkinson and Sue White for assisting in the counting of the annuli, Sue also assisted with the mathematics and Helen drew Fig. 11.9 and 11.10. Lesley Bailey of the Department of Anthropology, University of Durham sectioned the teeth. Dr. Peter Green, Department of Mathematics, gave me very helpful advice and assistance with the statistics and discourged my initial attempts to simply produce the best fit curvilinear regression through my somewhat inadequate data set. The material utilised for this paper derives from a study sponsored by the Historic Buildings and Monuments Commission.

## REFERENCES

Andrews, A.H. 1982. The use of dentition to age young cattle. In Wilson et al., 141- 153.
4

Binford, L.R. 1984. Faunal remains from Klasies River Mouth, New York: Academic Press.

Bourque, B.J., Morris, K. and Speiss, A.E. 1978. Determining season of death of mammal teeth from archaeological sites: a new sectioning technique. Science 149: 530-31.

Coy, J.P., Jones, R.T. and Turner, K.A. 1982. Absolute ageing of cattle from tooth sections and its relevance to archaeology. In Wilson et al., 127-140.

Deniz, E. and Payne, S. 1982. Eruption and wear in the mandibular dentition as a guide to ageing Turkish Angora goats. In Wilson et al., 155-205.

Ducos, P. 1968. L'origine des animaux domestiques en Palestine. Travaux de l'Universite de Bordeaux, 6.

Grant, A. 1975. Appendix B: the use of tooth wear as a guide to the age of domestic animals. In Excavations at Portchester Castle 1. Roman, B.W. Cunliffe, 437-450. Reports of the Research Committee of the Society of Antiquaries of London, No. 32.

Grant, A. 1978. Variations in dental attrition in mammals and its relevance to age estimation. In Research problems in Zooarchaeology, eds D.R. Brothwell, K.D. Thomas and J. Clutton-Brock, 103-106, Occassional Publication No. 3. London: Institute of Archaeology.

Grant, A. 1982. The use of tooth wear as a guide to the age of domestic ungulates. In Wilson et al., 91-108.

Grant, A. 1984 Animal husbandry. In Danebury an Iron Age Hillfort in Hampshire Vol. 2: The Excavations 1969-1978:1 the finds, Barry Cunliffe, 496-548, CBA Research Report No. 52. London: CBA.

Grigson, C. 1982. Sex and age determination of some bones and teeth of domestic cattle: a review of the literature. In Wilson et al., 7-23.

Grimsdell, J.J.R. 1973. Age determination of the African Buffalo, Syncerus caffer Sparrman. East African Wildlife Journal II: 31-53.

Grue, H. and Jensen, B. 1979. Review of the formation of incremental lines in tooth cementum of terrestrial mammals. Danish Review of Game Biology II (3): 1-48.

Kay, M. 1974. Dental annuli age determination on white-tailed deer from archaeological sites. Plains Anthropologist 19: 224-27.

Keiss, R.E. 1969. Comparison of eruption - wear patterns and cementum annuli as age criteria in elk. J. Wildl. Mgmt. 33, 175-180.

Klein, R.G., Wolf, G., Freeman, L.G. and Allwarden, K. 1981. The use of dental crown heights for constructing age profiles of red deer and similar species in archaeological samples. Journal of Archaeological Science 8: 1-31.

Klein, R.G., Allwarden, K. and Wolf, C. 1983. The calculation and interpretation of ungulate age profiles from dental crown heights. In Hunter-gatherer economy in prehistory: a European perspective, ed. G. Bailey, 47-57, Cambridge: CUP.

Klein, R.G. and Cruz-Uribe, K. 1984. The analysis of animal bones from archaeological sites, Chicago and London: Univ. Chicago Press.

Klevezal, G.A. and Kleinenberg, S.E. 1967. Age determination of mammals from annula layers in teeth and bones Academy of Science, USSR. Translated 1969 from Russian for Dept. of the Interior and the National Science Foundation, US Dept. of Commerce, Clearinghouse for Federal Scientific and Technical Information, Springfield, Virginia.

Laws, R.M. 1952. A new method of age determination for mammals. Nature London 169, 972-973.

Levitan, B. 1982. Errors in recording tooth wear in ovicaprid mandibles at different speeds. In Wilson et al., 207-214.

Low, W.A. and Cowan, I. McT. 1963. Age determination of deer by annular structure of dental cementum. J. Wildl. Mgmt. 27, 466-71.

Lowe, V.P.W. 1967. Teeth as indicators of age with speical reference to red deer (Cervus elaphus) of known age from Rhum. J. Zool., London 152, 137-53.

Ludwig, T.G., Healy, W.B. and Cutress, T.W. 1966. Wear on sheeps teeth. III Seasonal variation in wear and ingested soil. New Zealand Journal of Agricultural Research 9: 157-164.

Maltby, M. 1981. Iron Age Romano-British and Anlgo-Saxon animal husbandry: a review of the faunal evidence. In The environment of Man: the Iron Age to the Anglo-Saxon period, ed. M. Jones and G. Dimbleby, 155-204, BS 87. Oxford: BAR.

Marks, S.A. and Erickson, A.W. 1966. Age determination in the Black Bear. J. Wildl. Mgmt. 30, 389-408.

Mitchell, B. 1967. Growth layers in dental cementum for determining the age of red deer (Cervus elaphus L.). J. Anim. Ecol. 36: 279-93.

Morris, P.A. 1972. A review of mammalian age determination methods. Mammal Review 2 (3), 69-104.

Morris, P.A. 1976. The use of teeth for estimating the age of wild animals. In Development, function and Evolution of teeth, ed. P.M. Butler and K.A. Joysey, 483-94, New York: Academic Press.

Novakowski, N.S. 1965. Cemental deposition as an age criterion in bison and the relation of incisor wear, eye lens weight and dressed bison carcass weight to age. Canad. J. Zool. 43 (1), 173-8.

Odlum, G. 1950. Longevity in dairy cattle. Farmers Weekly, April 14th, 1950.

Rackham, D.J. 1982. Mid-Devensian Mammals in Britain, MSc Thesis, Dept. Geological Sciences, University of Birmingham.

Rackham, D.J. in press. An analysis and interpretation of the sample of animal bones from Thorpe Thewles, Cleveland. In Heslop, D. Excavations at the Iron Age site of Thorpe Thewles. Cleveland. Cleveland County Council.

Ransom, A.R. 1966. Determining age of white-tailed deer from layers in cementum of molars. J. Wildl. Mgmt. 30 (1), 197-99.

Saxon, A. and Higham, C.F.W. 1968. Identification and interpretation of growth rings in the secondary dental cementum of Ovis aries L. Nature. London 219, 634-5.

Silver, I.A. 1969. The ageing of domestic animals. In Science and Archaeology, ed. D. Brothwell and E.S. Higgs, 283-302, London: Thames and Hudson.

Spiess, A.E. 1979. Reindeer and Caribou hunters: an archaeological study. New York: Academic Press.

Spinage, C.A. 1971. Geradontology and horn growth of the impala (Aepycerus melampus). J. Zool., Lond. 164: 209-25.

Spinage, C.A. 1972. Age estimation of zebra. East African Wildlife Journal 10: 273-77.

Spinage, C.A. 1976a. Incremental cementum lines in the teeth of tropical African mammals. J. Zool., Lond. 178, 117-131.

Spinage, C.A. 1976b. Age determination of the female Grant's gazelle. East African Wildlife Journal 14: 121-34.

Stallibrass, S. 1982. The use of cementum layers for absolute ageing of mammalian teeth: a selective review of the literature with suggestions for further studies and alternative applications. In Wilson et al., 109-126.

Wiener, G. and Purser, A.F. 1957. The influence of four levels of feeding on the position and eruption of incisor teeth in sheep. J. Agric. Sci. 49, 51-55.

Wilson, B., Grigson, C. and Payne, S. 1982. Ageing and sexing animal bones from archaeological sites, BS 109, Oxford: BAR.

# PART II

# STUDIES OF PAST POPULATIONS

## Chapter 12

# LEAD, CADMIUM AND ZINC LEVELS IN TEETH FROM ROMANO-BRITISH BURIAL SITES

M.V. Stack[1] & D.K. Whittaker[2]

[1]MRC Dental Unit
University of Bristol Dental School

[2]Dental School
Cardiff.

## INTRODUCTION

Inferences concerning environmental lead exposure of communities living during historic and prehistoric times have been made on the basis of analyses of bones and teeth recovered from archaeological sites. In some circumstances the amount of lead absorbed and subsequently stored may be correlated with living standards (e.g. Aufderheide et al., 1985). The most reliable values are to be expected when burials have taken place in rock shelters (e.g. Rogers and Waldron, 1985) or have been followed by mummification in dry desert sand or in the tombs of Ancient Egypt (e.g. Stack and Fletcher, 1984). Fairly reliable analyses should be possible when site soils show levels of lead similar to those in bones and teeth. Quite unreliable analyses can result when there has been burial in lead coffins or in ground which is traversed by metal-polluted streams. Similar considerations apply to other trace metal analyses.

The use of lead became widespread in Roman times, and mineral deposits in the Mendip Hills, near Bristol in the west of England, provided a source utilised for a considerable distance around during the Romano-British era. Mendip lead was used for the lining of wooden coffins recovered from one of the cemeteries (Poundbury) near the settlement adjacent to modern Dorchester. Mendip mine tailings have been leached for two millenia by streams that traverse these hills by underground courses. One of these streams emerges near the chambered Wookey Hole show cave, and a relatively recent diversion to provide a factory water source resulted in the flooding of a "cemetery" in the fourth chamber, from which Romano-British skeletal material was recovered (Rogers, 1978).

A limited study of levels of lead, cadmium and zinc has been concerned with the contrasted environmental conditions of these two sites. Soil lead levels at Poundbury have been found to be in the same range as have been observed for British soils generally (Waldron et al., 1979). However, the Mendip cave sediments from which skulls were recovered contained lead at high levels (Stenner, 1978), perhaps one hundred times those originally present in the teeth now analysed.

The three metals analysed were lead, cadmium and zinc. Cadmium is more toxic than lead but is present at much lower concentrations, a typical value for modern teeth being 0.1 $\mu$ g/g (parts per million). Zinc is an essential element, but high intakes can interfere with the availability - and toxicity - of other elements.

## MATERIAL AND METHOD

Teeth from immature skulls recovered from the Poundbury site were made available in two small groups. In both there were similar numbers of primary and permanent teeth, but in the second group it was possible to match deciduous teeth with permanent teeth in the same skulls. Thus there was the possibility that a reasonable estimate of a trace metal in a permanent tooth could be made, given that of the corresponding deciduous tooth. Specimens (n = 24) were cleaned mechanically, either lightly, or more thoroughly in the case of the second group - to the extent of sacrificing up to one-tenth of the specimen; lower analytical values resulted from the latter group. Young premolar teeth (n = 10) from the Wookey Hole Cave site (Rogers, 1978) were scrubbed with 2% nitric acid, a milder procedure than the above. Several other ancient teeth from Mendip caves were also analysed by Coles (1979).

Cleaned specimens were dissolved in a high-grade nitric acid or a 1:1 mixture of nitric and perchloric acids by warming gently. They were diluted and partially neutralised for reaction with an organic reagent such that its heavy metal salt could be extracted from the acid phase by shaking with an organic solvent that was only partially miscible with water. The solvent layer containing the extracted trace metals was analysed for lead, cadmium and zinc by atomic absorption spectrophotometry, using background correction of the signals. Standards contained the trace metals in the proportions expected for analyses of modern teeth.

## RESULTS

Levels of lead, zinc and cadmium in the groups of teeth are shown in Table 12.1, and estimates of permanent tooth levels from those found in deciduous teeth of the same skulls, based on linear regression of the actual data pairs, are shown against the observed values (Table 12.2).

The means of Table 1 are based on logarithms of the analytical values, since a symmetrical distribution resulted when this transformation was used with the lead and zinc data. Specifically, nearly all the transformed values were within 70 to 130% of the means, and half of these were within the range 90 to 110%.

## DISCUSSION

The overall means for the levels of trace metals in the Poundbury teeth were in the regions of 15, 0.5 and 150 $\mu$ g/g, respectively, for the analyses of lead, cadmium and zinc. Similar mean values for cadmium and zinc were found for the Wookey Hole cave teeth, but very much higher values were found for all the lead analyses. The mean value for lead in Poundbury teeth matched those found for teeth from another Mendip cave ("The Slitter") occupied during the same era. Concentrations of organic material in teeth from this cave, and from another in the vicinity - also yielding specimens from the same era - were very similar to those typical of modern teeth (Stack, unpublished data, 1955). It may be presumed therefore that the environments in these caves had never become wet for appreciable times. Much lower lead and cadmium levels were, however, found for teeth recovered from another dry Mendip cave ("Aveline's Hole", Burrington Combe, unpublished data, MVS & RPF, 1984) occupied some millenia earlier. The

Table 12.1. Values for lead, zinc & cadmium in Romano-British teeth (log means: $\mu$ g/g).

| Metal | Poundbury Primary Teeth | Poundbury Permanent Teeth | Wookey Hole Cave Teeth |
|---|---|---|---|
| Lead | 20 | 12 | 75 - 80 |
| Cadmium | 0.52 | 0.44 | 0.6 |
| Zinc | 180 | 120 | 160 |

It is possible that two-thirds of this value may be accounted for by contamination during submersion.

Table 12.2. Values for lead in permanent teeth estimated from values found in primary teeth (Poundbury).

| Pb in primary tooth | Pb in permanent tooth | Pb in permament tooth (est) |
|---|---|---|
| 6.3 | 2.8 | 3.0 |
| 8.8 | 5.0 | 4.6 |
| 13 | 8.3 | 7.4 |
| 13.7 | 7.0 | 7.9 |
| 30 | 20 | 20 |

fourth chamber of Wookey Hole Cave has been flooded for at least a century, and the skeletal material exposed to wet sediments.

Explanation of the very high levels in the cave teeth was considered to be afforded by the finding of Stenner (1978) that lead levels in the bone-bearing sediments there were some thirty times as high as those typical of samples from sixteen caves not known to be associated with lead-contaminated streams. There is thus a reasonable presumption that there had been extensive uptake of lead by the bones and teeth since the fourth chamber was flooded. In a discussion of this problem (Stack & Coles, 1983) it was sugegsted that subtraction of an arbitrary 50$\mu$ g/g from these lead analyses would result in a notional mean of 25$\mu$ g/g and a relative standard deviation (RSD) for a group of nearly 30%. This value falls within the range of the RSD values for the Poundbury group and of two other groups representative of archaeological populations. However, the RSD for the original data was below 10%, an unusually low variability.

Even higher lead levels than those of the cave teeth were noted in some teeth from recovered the Poundbury site where burials had been made in lead-lined coffins; the cadmium and zinc levels were not unusual. An extreme example of similar contamination was reported (Maenhaut et al., 1981) following analyses of bones of a skeleton of the Middle Ages recovered from a cathedral crypt. The specimens had the appearance of normal bones (after removal of a reddish-brown patina showing 8-24% lead) but they showed lead levels of 0.6%, a value 100 times higher than would normally be expected. Soil lead levels in the vicinity of the skeleton were 1000 times those of average soils.

It is thus clear that in trace metal analysis of teeth, care has to be taken that the environment has not contributed to the levels present during life, as has been demonstrated for bones in soils of varying lead content by Waldron (1983),

## SUMMARY

Toxic trace metals were analysed in teeth from young individuals buried in contrasted sites. One was a surface cemetery where levels of lead in the teeth were similar to those in the soil, the other a cave "cemetery" where lead levels were high in the teeth, and thought to reflect the very high levels in the cave sediment. Zinc levels were comparable with those of modern teeth but cadmium levels were somewhat higher, as were those of lead, in primary and permanent teeth.

## ACKNOWLEDGEMENTS.

We thank Drs. Theya Molleson (British Museum Natural History) and Juliet Rogers (University of Bristol) for supplying the Romano-British teeth from Poundbury and Wookey Hole Cave sites, respectively. Analyses of cave teeth were reported by Stephen Coles (M.Sc. dissertation, University of Bristol). Thanks are due to Robert Fletcher (MRC Dental Unit) for analyses of the two groups of teeth from the Poundbury site.

## REFERENCES.


Aufderheide, A.C. et al. (1985). Lead in bone III. Prediction of social correlates from skeletal lead content in four Colonial American populations. Amer. J. Phys. Anthropol. 66: 353-361.

Coles, S.G. (1979). The determination of certain trace metals in teeth with special reference to lead as a pollutant that accumulates in calcified tissues. MSc Dissertation, Univ. Bristol.

Maenhaut, W. et al. (1981). Analysis of skeleton remains, ascribed to Mary of Burgundy, and of soil samples recovered from the central tomb of the Church of Our Lady, Bruges. Bull. Soc. Chim. Belg. 90: 1115-1125.

Rogers, J. (1978). The human remains from the Fourth Chamber, Wookey Hole Cave. Proc. Univ. Bristol. Spelaeol. Soc. 15(1): 33-38 (see Stenner, 49-52).

Rogers, J. and Waldron, H.A. (1985). Lead concentrations in bones from a Neolithic long barrow. J. Archaeol. Sci. 12: 93-96.

Stack, M.V. and Coles, S.G. (1983). Concentrations of lead, zinc and cadmium in teeth from a cave used for Romano-British burials: Effect of lead contamination. Proc. Univ. Bristol Spelaeol. Soc. 16(3): 193-200.

Stack, M.V. and Fletcher, R.P. (1984). Trace metals in teeth from Ancient Egypt. J. Dent. Res. 63: 506.

Stenner, R.D. (1978). The concentration of copper, lead and zinc in sediments in Wookey Hole Cave, Somerset. Proc. Univ. Bristol. Spelaeol. Soc. 15: 49-52.

Waldron, H.A. et al. (1979). Lead concentrations in bones and soil. J. Archaeol. Sci. 6: 295-298.

Waldron, H.A. (1983). On the post-mortem accumulation of lead by skeletal tissues. J. Archaeol. Sci. 10: 35-40.

Whittaker, D.K. and Stack, M.V. (1985). The lead, cadmium and zinc content of some Romano-British teeth. Archaeometry 26: 37-42.

## Chapter 13

# OCCLUSAL AND APPROXIMAL WEAR IN ROMANO-BRITISH SKULLS

David Whittaker
Dental School
Cardiff

Occlusal wear of teeth has been extensively studied both in extant (Gjermo et al., 1984) and historic (Griffin, Powers and Kruszynski, 1979) populations. The amount of occlusal wear and its rate of progression have considerable clinical implications not only in relation to possible over closure of the masticatory apparatus and consequent strain on the temporomandibular joints (Mack, 1984) but also in relation to stresses placed upon the periodontal structures (Latcham et al., 1983). From a forensic or anthropological viewpoint occlusal wear has provided the basis for methods of ageing of individuals within a skeletal population (Brothwell, 1963; Miles, 1962). Approximal wear of the teeth has received much less attention and has largely been related to reduction in mediodistal length of the teeth, which coupled with mesio-migration results in shortening of the arch from incisors through to molars (Murphy, 1964). Very little is known about the types of approximal wear occurring in the human dentition and even less about the methods of production of such wear facets.

As well as changes in the dimensions of the teeth as age progresses there has been described frequently a loss of alveolar marginal bone and this has been related to chronic inflammatory periodontal disease occurring throughout the life of the individual (Hull, Hillam and Beale, 1975). Both dentists and anthropologists have a tendency to look at these three parameters of change independently, but they are clearly intimately related and may be dependent upon and influenced by both diet, habits and disease processes.

In seeking to reconstruct the masticatory habits of earlier populations the teeth and surrounding bone must be considered as a dynamic system, complicated by relative movements taking place between the component parts. For example, examination of both clinical and skeletal material from varying populations, ancient and modern, has suggested that as age progresses the alveolar margin moves away from a fixed point on the teeth such as the cervical margin. The very reasonable assumption has been made that bone is being resorbed in response to chronic inflammatory periodontal disease and that horizontal alveolar bone loss is a clinical problem in all populations. However it has long been known, for example in herbivores, that teeth which wear occlusally continue to erupt to exactly compensate for such wear (Poole, 1976) and it was suggested some thirty years ago that a similar event may occur in man (Begg, 1954). If this is the case then measurements from cervical margin to alveolar crest are made against the background of a tooth wearing down occlusally and erupting continuously to compensate for this mechanism as well as perhaps wearing approximally and drifting in a mesial or distal direction. These measurements are therefore extremely difficult to interpret. The only satisfactory method to study changes in alveolar crestal height, for instance, would be to measure not from the teeth but from a fixed point in the jaw.

In the past clinical measurements have been made utilising standard radiographic techniques (Lennon and Davies, 1974) and apparent changes in the height of alveolar crestal bone have been attributed to chronic infection at the gum margins producing osteoclastic resorption. Recent clinical reports have attempted to measure alveolar bone loss by simply measuring from the cervical margin of the teeth to the alveolar crests in young people and comparing these measurements with similar ones in older members of the population (Rohner, Cimasoni and Vuagnat, 1983). However if teeth do indeed continue to erupt throughout life to compensate for occlusal wear, then reports of alveolar bone loss occurring throughout life may have mistaken increasing alveolar crest to cervical margin of teeth measurements as representing loss of bone whereas in fact they may represent movement of the teeth away from the bone.

Fortunately Darling and Levers (1975) demonstrated in modern populations that the inferior alveolar canal running through the mandible is a fixed line throughout life and can therefore be used as a base line for measurements to the alveolar crest and to various points on the teeth. Newman and Levers (1979) tested this suggestion in Anglo-Saxon skulls and concluded that alveolar bone stays static in relation to the fixed line of the canal but that the teeth continue to erupt throughout life to compensate exactly for occlusal wear. A similar study was carried out by Levers and Darling (1983) on a mixed group of skulls and they also showed that with the exception of the mediaeval skulls the alveolar crest seemed to remain more or less static throughout life.

Such studies call into question the assumption that most ancient populations suffered from chronic loss of alveolar bone interpreted as evidence for chronic periodontal disease. It is theoretically possible that alveolar bone is constantly resorbed throughout life due to chronic inflammatory disease but is redeposited at exactly the same rate to compensate for occlusal movement of the teeth. Studies of this complex phenomenon should therefore include histology of the alveolar crestal margins to determine whether bone is being resorbed or deposited.

In so far as approximal wear of teeth is concerned, even less information is available. It has long been known that the mesio-distal dimensions of teeth reduce with age and that the total length of the dental arch tends to decrease as teeth drift mesially to compensate for this wear. The actual pattern of wear was briefly described by Shaw (1931) and Hinton (1982) but little is known about the shape and type of approximal attrition. It has been reported in Australian aboriginal skulls (Campbell, 1925) and also in Anglo-Saxon skulls (Miles, 1969) and in the Bantu races (Shaw, 1931) and Wolpoff (1971) and Hinton (1982) studied both approximal and occlusal wear in defined populations. Shaw described the pattern of wear as being in the form of an open 'S' with the convex aspect of one tooth contacting the concave aspect of an adjacent tooth. No information is available as to the incidence of convex or concave wear facets on molar teeth and for this reason occlusal wear, alveolar crestal bone movements and approximal wear will be considered together in this present communication.

## MATERIALS AND METHODS

Of approximately 1200 inhumations from the Poundbury (Dorset) Romano-British site, 500 relatively intact skulls were studied in the British Museum (Natural History). These skeletons date from about 300 AD and have been described in detail previously (Whittaker et al, 1981). The skulls were placed in ascending sequence of age using the method of Brothwell (1963) based on occlusal wear patterns of molar teeth, the method of Miles (1962) based on differential rates of wear of the molars related to their time of eruption and also using post-cranial evidence of age. It is accepted that none of these methods produce accurate ageing especially in the older age groups but combined evidence of this nature should ensure the skeletons are correctly sequentially aged and this will meet the purposes of the present investigation. The skulls were placed into four groups 1, 2, 3 and 4, the youngest group being 17-24 years and the oldest rather more than 45 years.

Standardised X-rays were taken of right and left sides of the mandibles using a Philips X-ray machine positioned at right-angles to both film and teeth. Exposures were made at 15 milliamps and 40 kv on X-ray film placed lingual to the jaw and parallel to the long axes of the teeth. Using vernier calipers measurements were made from the upper border of the inferior alveolar canal (IAC) to:-

1) the apices of the teeth

2) the alveolar crest

3) the cervical margin of the teeth

4) the occlusal surface of each of the three molar teeth.

This method was based on that of Darling and Levers (1975). Statistical differences between measurements in age groups 1 and 2 and age groups 2 and 4 were calculated using the Student's 't' test. In addition to these radiographs, teeth were extracted along with their surrounding alveolar bone and were sectioned using a diamond inner cutting wheel. The sections were polished to a thickness of approximately 100 $\mu$m and examined at low power in a light microscope. Finally the approximal mesial and distal surfaces of premolars and molars were carefully examined and assessed as having one of four categories of approximal wear pattern. These were: concave facets, convex facets, flat wear or 'S' shaped wear. Both measurements on radiographs and the type of approximal wear were subjected to tests of inter examiner variability, which was usually within 5%. If doubt existed both examiners conferred in making a decision as to measurements or type of wear.

## RESULTS

### 1) Radiographs of mandible

A typical radiograph is shown in Figure 13.2. The opaque soft wire placed in the inferior alveolar canal is to aid localisation of this structure. Measurements from the IAC to the occlusal surface in first, second and third molars showed no change in these measurements as age increased from 17 to more than 45 years (Figure 13.2). However measurements from the IAC to the root apex showed increasing distances as age progressed. These were statistically significant in the case of the first and second molars but not in the case of the third molar (Figure 13.3). Measurements from IAC to alveolar crest (AC) in first, second and third molars showed no statistical changes as age progressed (Figure 13.4). Combined measurements

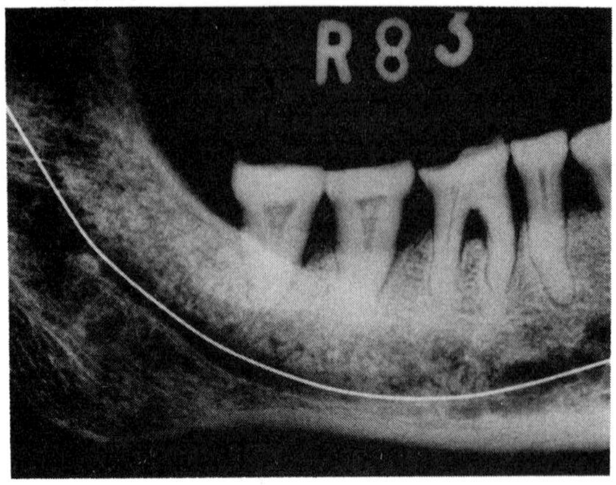


Figure 13.1. Standard radiograph of right side of mandible. The stainless steel wire is to help locate the IAC. Measurements were made from the upper border of IAC to apex, alveolar crest, cervical margin and occlusal surface.

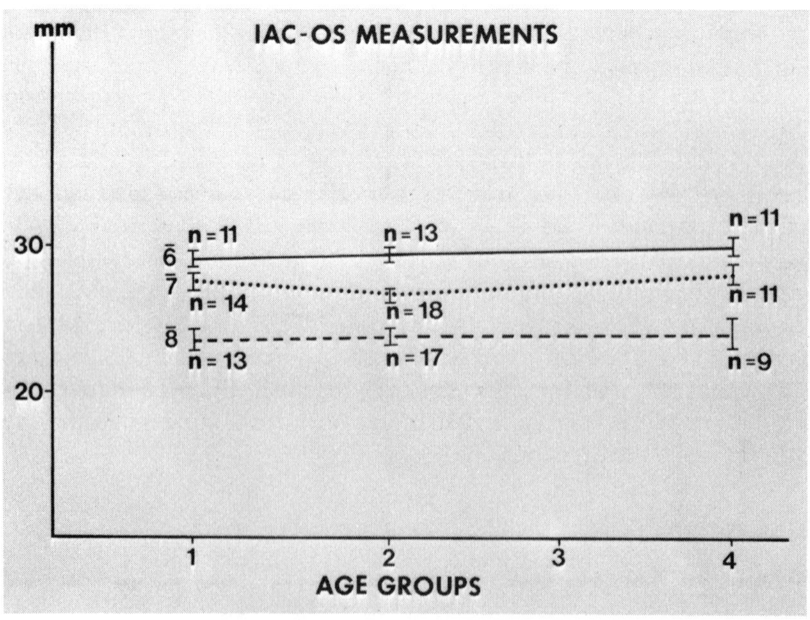


Figure 13.2. Measurements from IAC to occlusal surface in the four age groups. Bar = standard error of the mean.

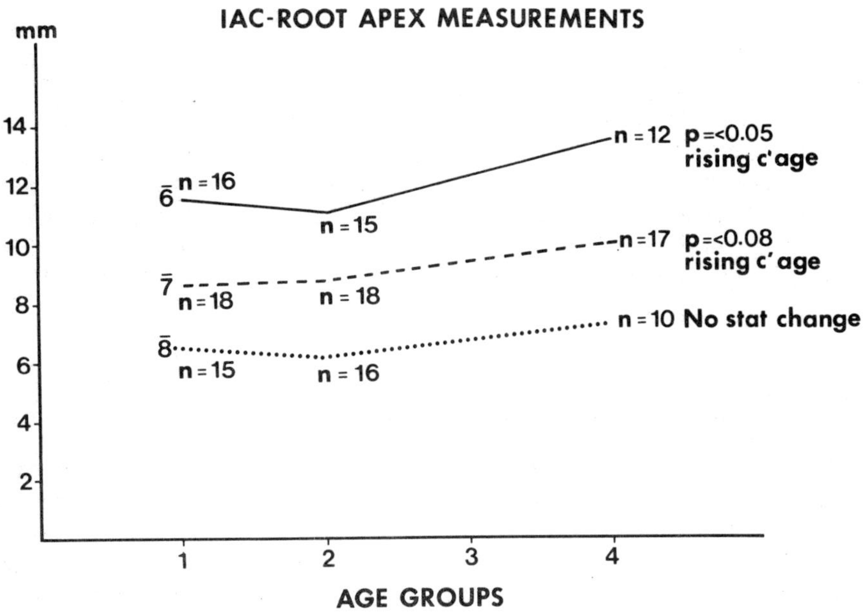


Figure 13.3. Measurements from IAC to the root apices. This distance increased as age progressed.

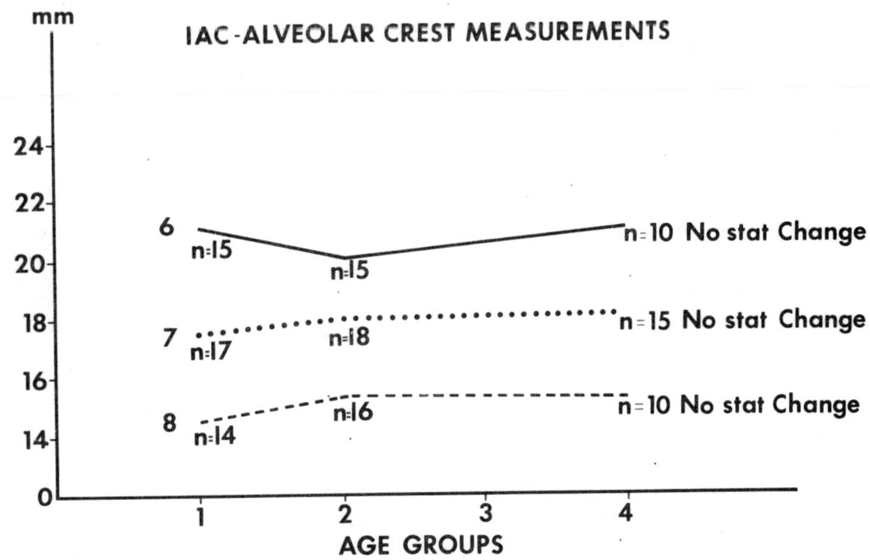


Figure 13.4. As age progressed there was no significant change in the position of the alveolar crest.

from all three molar teeth confirmed these results showing no statistical change in the position of the occlusal surface and the alveolar crest after age group 2 when related to the IAC. There were however statistically significant changes in the position of both the cement enamel junction (CEJ) and the apex of the teeth as age progressed and these two fixed structures on the tooth moved away from the IAC in a parallel fashion with increasing age. Measurements of the relationship of the lower border of the mandible to the IAC showed a slight deposition of bone with increasing age (Figure 13.5).

2) Ground sections through alveolar bone

The most typical appearance on these sections was of addition of bone both on the buccal and lingual aspects of the tooth. On the buccal aspect there was 'lipping' produced by addition of bone at the alveolar crest itself whereas on the lingual side there was often a large exostosis producing bossing and marked ridging of the bone below the alveolar crest. Only in a few cases was there any evidence of bone resorption and even in these specimens there was always evidence of bone deposition occurring concurrently (Figure 13.6).

3) Pattern of approximal wear

A preliminary analysis was carried out to see if there was a pattern of approximal wear when all ages of skulls were grouped together. The results indicated that for both mandible and maxilla and for both right and left sides there was a highly significant difference between the type of wear found on mesial and distal surfaces of the teeth. First molar teeth had a high incidence of concave facets on the mesial surface compared with the distal surface which had a high incidence of convex facets. Similar results were seen in the other molar teeth studied. The percentage of concave, convex and flat faceting in mesial and distal sites in the maxilla and mandible are shown in Table 13.1. Flat facets are evenly distributed both in the maxilla, mandible, right and left and mesial and distal surfaces of the teeth but concave facets were seen much more frequently on the mesial surfaces of premolar and molar teeth whilst convex facets were seen much more frequently on the distal surfaces of the same teeth. This distribution is shown diagramatically in Figure 13.7.

## DISCUSSION

In these studies of occlusal and approximal wear in Romano-British skulls, male and female skulls have been grouped together. In a previous study on this material (Whittaker, Parker and Jenkins, 1982) no significant differences were seen between cervical enamel junction to alveolar crest measurements in males and females and there was also some doubt about the accuracy of sex determination in this material. For these reasons the sexes were combined. There have been many studies of alveolar crest measurements on dried skulls previously (Lavelle and Moore, 1969; Sagnae and Olsson, 1977) but clear relationships between tooth wear and axial movement of teeth have not emerged. Clinical studies using bitewing X-rays and measurements of cement enamel junction to alveolar crest (Latcham et al, 1983; Rohner, Cimasoni and Vuagnat, 1983) have failed to take into account possible axial continuing eruption of the teeth. The present method, based

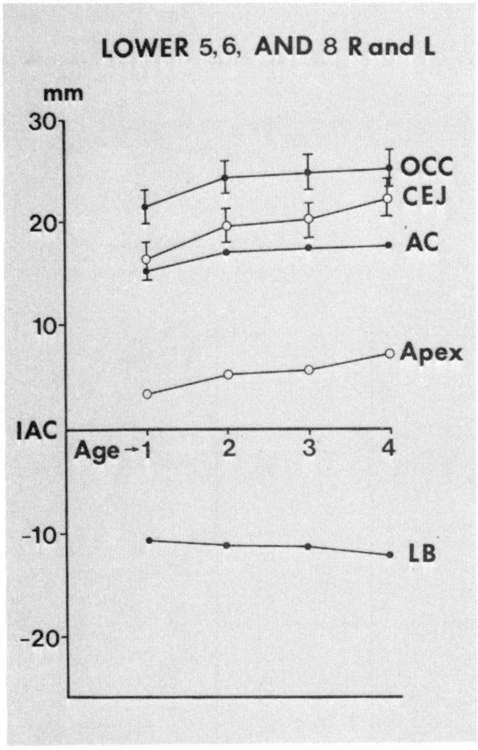


Figure 13.5. Mean measurements for lower second premolars and molars are shown. From age groups 2 to 4 the occlusal surface, alveolar crest remained ar a constant distance from IAC. Apex and cement enamel junction moved away from IAC as age progressed.

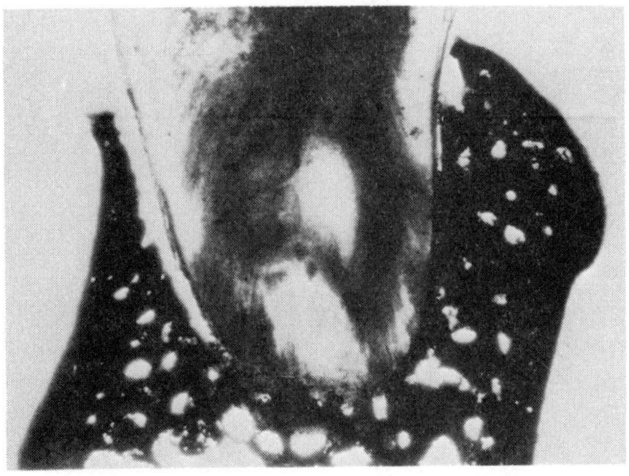

Figure 13.6. Ground section of molar tooth in situ. There is no evidence of bone loss at the alveolar margins.

Table 13.1 Incidence of wear on approximal surfaces of upper and lower teeth.

| | | % CONCAVE | | % CONVEX | | % FLAT | |
|---|---|---|---|---|---|---|---|
| | | Mesial | Distal | Mesial | Distal | Mesial | Distal |
| MAXILLA | Left | 55.9 | 23 | 16.1 | 45.6 | 28 | 31.4 |
| | Right | 52.4 | 23.2 | 18.1 | 44.1 | 29.5 | 32.7 |
| MANDIBLE | Left | 46.9 | 33.3 | 26.5 | 38.3 | 26.6 | 28.4 |
| | Right | 50.6 | 25.1 | 21.5 | 46.9 | 26.9 | 28 |

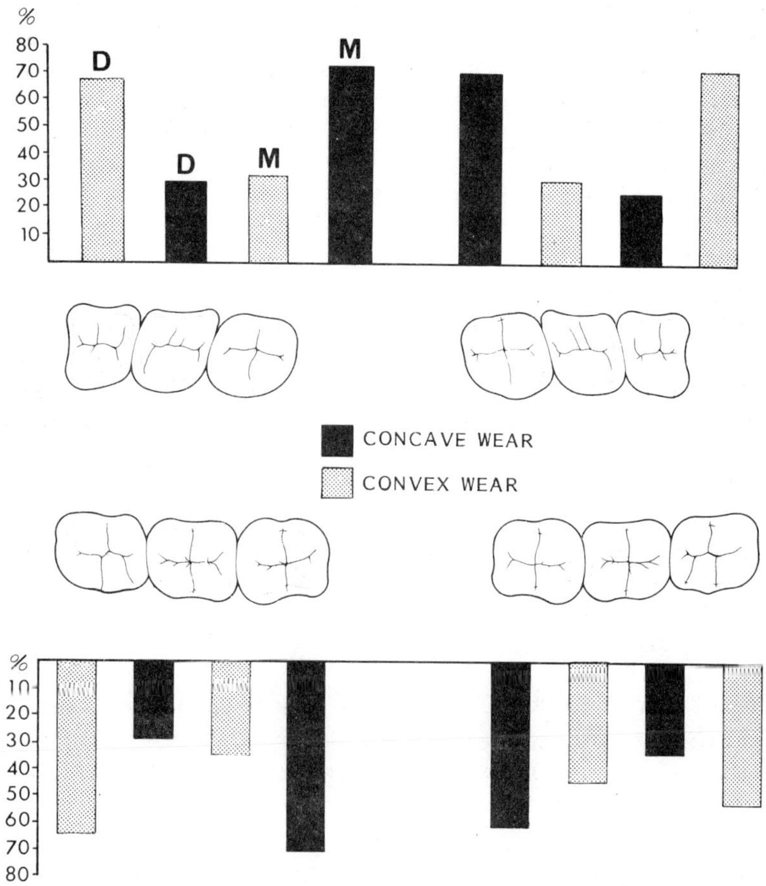


Figure 13.7. Percentage of teeth with concave or convex wear facets on both mesial and distal surfaces. In each quadrant conxex wear is more common ditsally and concave wear mesially (M = mesial, D = distal.)

on the finding of Darling and Levers (1975) that the inferior alveolar canal is a fixed line, overcomes these difficulties and allows direct measurements to be made in the varying age groups.

Newman and Levers (1979) used a similar method in an Anglo-Saxon population of skulls and showed that teeth continued to erupt to compensate for wear. In addition they found no evidence in changes in the relationship of IAC to AC. The present study using measurements from the fixed line of the IAC has confirmed these views and demonstrates the movement of teeth from the IAC appears to be true eruption and not due to increased CEJ-AC measurements occasioned by loss of alveolar crestal bone during chronic inflammatory periodontal disease. It appears that the level of the alveolar crest remains more or less static as age progresses and this finding seriously calls into question the conclusion that many early historical populations suffered from periodontal disease as estimated from apparent loss of alveolar crestal bone.

This present work does not necessarily imply that there was no loss of crestal bone throughout the life of these individuals but it does imply that this bone was replaced by lipping or bossing thereby making conclusions about periodontal bone loss extremely unwise. Anthropologists and dentists should be wary of commenting upon previous periodontal disease processes in skeletal material unless measurements from the fixed line of the IAC have been employed. In so far as approximal wear is concerned, it is accepted that there are difficulties in surveys of this nature on material 1500 years of age. For example the assessment of wear on the mesial surface of the first maxillary premolar is difficult because of the concavity already present in the form of the canine fossa on this tooth. Where there are high levels of occlusal attrition, assessment of approximal wear becomes even more difficult.

In spite of these difficulties there are highly significant differences in the distribution of concave and convex facets in this material and further studies of this distribution may well indicate differences in masticatory activity, for example, between apes and man. There are a number of theoretical possibilities as to why teeth should wear in a concave manner on some surfaces and in a convex manner on others.

i) Differences in hardness of the mesial and distal enamel might explain such a distribution of wear. A softer surface might be expected to wear in a concave manner whilst harder surface would remain convex however there is no evidence that mesial and distal surfaces of teeth vary in this way.

ii) Since the first molar erupts before the second molar which in turn erupts before the third molar it is conceivable that the enamel of the tooth erupting first becomes more mature (Sakae and Hirai, 1982) and therefore harder at the time that the next tooth in the sequence erupts. This might explain differences in wear patterns but would be expected to result in the opposite distribution to that seen in the present material.

iii) If two surfaces of equal hardness are rotated against each other in a particular way with abrasive material between it is possible to convert one flat surface into a concave and the other into a convex shape. This is made use of in the grinding of concave telescope mirrors using a flat blank and a flat mirror at the commencement of the operation. Movement of the teeth in this fashion would depend upon relative differences in the movement of the first, second and third molars as well as the premolar teeth. It is conceivable that a tooth newly erupted would be less stable than one which had been present in the mouth for some years so that occlusal forces might in fact produce differential movements between adjacent teeth. A more likely explanation however is based upon a previous finding (Brown et al, 1977) that molar teeth especially in primitive civilisations wear occlusually in a complex helicoid manner rather than in a flat plane. It could be postulated that forces generated during this wear of the occlusal surfaces may result in differential movement of mesial and distal surfaces of teeth resulting in the incidence of concave and convex facets seen in the present material. Interactions of occlusal surfaces of this type are dependent not only upon the diet but also upon complex movements at the temporomandibular joint apparatus (Mack, 1984) and further studies of a theoretical nature are necessary before this distribution of wear can be adequately explained.

## REFERENCES


Begg, P.R. (1954). Stone age man's dentition. Amer. J. Orthod. 40: 298-312.

Brothwell, D.R. (1963). Digging up Bones. Trustees of the British Museum, London.

Brown, W.A.B., Whittaker, D.K., Fenwick, J. and Jones, D.S. (1977). Quantitative evidence for the helicoid relationship between the maxillary and mandibular occlusal surfaces. J. Oral Rehabil. 4: 91-96.

Campbell, T.D. (1925). The dentition and palate of the Australian Aboriginal. Hasselt Press, Adelaide.

Darling, A.I. and Levers, B.G.H. (1975). The pattern or eruption of some human teeth. Arch. Oral Biol. 20: 89-96.

Griffin, C.J., Powers, R. and Kruszynski, R. (1979). The incidence of osteo-arthritis of the temporomandibular joint in various cultures. Aust. Dent. J. 24: 94-106.

Gjermo, P., Bellini, H.T., Pereira Santos, V., Martins, J.G., Ferracyoli, J.R. (1984). Prevalence of bone loss in a group of Brazilian teenagers assessed on bite-wing radiographs. J. Clin. Periodont. 11: 1:4-113.

Hinton, R.J. (1982). Differences in interproximal and occlusal tooth wear among historic Tennessee Indians: Implications for masticatory function. Am. J. Phys. Anthrop. 57: 103-115.

Hull, P.S., Hillam, D.G. and Beal, J.F. (1975). A radiographic study of the prevalence of chronic periodontitis in 14 year old English schoolchildren. J. Clin. Periodont. 2: 203-210.

Latcham, N.L., Powell, R.N., Jago, J.D., Seymour, G.J., Aitken, J.F. (1983). A radiographic study of chronic periodontitis in 15 year old Queensland children. J. Clin. Periodont. 10: 37-45.

Lavelle, C.L.B. and Moore, W.J. (1969). Alveolar bone resorption in Anglo-Saxon and seventeenth century mandibles. J. Periodont Res. 4: 70-73.

Lennon, M.A. and Davies, R.M. (1974). Prevalence and distribution of alveolar bone loss in a population of 15 year old schoolchildren. J. Clin. Periodont. 1: 175-182.

Levers, B.G.H. and Darling, A.I. (1983). Continuous eruption of some adult human teeth of ancient populations. Archs. Oral Biol. 28: 401-408.

Mack, P.J. (1984). A functional explanation for the morphology of the temporomandibular joint of man. J. Dent. 12: 225-230.

Miles, A.E.W. (1962). Assessment of the ages of a population of Anglo-Saxons from their dentitions. Proc. Roy. Soc. Med. 55: 881-886.

Miles, A.E.W. (1969). The dentition of the Anglo-Saxons. Proc. Royal Soc. Med. 62: 1311-1315.

Murphy, T.R. (1964). Reduction of the dental arch by approximal attrition. Brit. Dent. J. 116: 483-488.

Newman, H.N. and Levers, B.G.H. (1979). Tooth eruption and function in an early Anglo-Saxon population. J. Roy. Soc. Med. 72: 341-350.

Poole, D.F.G. (1976). Evolution of mastication. In: Mastication, edited by Anderson, D.J. and Matthews, B. Wright, Bristol: 1-4.

Rohner, F., Cimasoni, G. and Vuagnat, P. (1983). Longitudinal radiographical study on the rate of alveolar bone loss in patients of a dental school. J. Clin. Periodont. 10: 643-651.

Sakai, T. and Hirae, G. (1982). Calcification and crystallization in bovine enamel. J. Dent. Res. 61: 57-59.

Sagnae, S. and Olsson, G. (1977). Studies of the periodontal status of a medieval population. Dento-Max. Fac. Radiol. 6: 46-52.

Shaw, J.C.M. (1931). The Teeth, the Bony Palate, and the Mandible in the Bantu Races of South Africa. Bale, Sons and Danielsson, London.

Whittaker, D.K., Molleson, T., Bennett, R.C., ap Edwards, I., Jenkins, P.R. and Llewellyn, J.H. (1981). The prevalence and distribution of dental caries in a Romano-British population. Arch. Oral Biol. 20: 237-245.

Whittaker, D.K., Parker, J.H. and Jenkins, C. (1982). Tooth attrition and continuing eruption in a Romano-British population. Archs. Oral Biol. 27: 405-409.

Wolpoff, M.H. (1971). Interstitial Wear. Amer. J. Phys. Anthrop. 34: 205-228.

Chapter 14

## DENTAL EXAMINATION OF THE ABERDEEN CARMELITE COLLECTION. LATE MEDIAEVAL 1300 - 1600

N.W. Kerr.
Department of Dental Surgery
Aberdeen Royal Infirmary
Aberdeen.

The Aberdeen Carmelite collection came to light in the winter of 1980 at a time of city centre re-development. It is presently housed in the Department of Anatomy, Marischal College, Aberdeen University.

History tells us that the site was formerly associated with the Carmelite or White Friars Order (indeed, a nearby street today still bears the name 'Carmelite Street'). The Order was forced to flee the area at about the time of the Reformation and in 1587 their lands and possessions were acquired by George Keith, 5th Earl Marischal. It seems likely the internments, which were all within the walls of the building, took place between this date and the founding of the Order in Aberdeen somewhere about the 12th or 13th century. Radiocarbon dating has since proved consistent with this estimate and the collection is dated as Late Mediaeval (1300 to 1600 A.D.).

The collection consists of approximately 200 skeletons in various states of preservation and completness. It comprises males and females with ages ranging from newborn to extremely elderly. The cranium, facial structures and dentition of only a few are completely intact (Fig. 14.1). However, some 80 adults and 20 immatures are sufficiently intact to provide a valuable nucleus for detailed dental investigations.

As far as the author is aware, this collection represents one of the largest individual Scottish Mediaeval collections available for investigation.

### PRELIMINARY PROBLEMS.

The actual examination, recording and assessment of the dental material proved to be a more complex task than the author had originally assumed. Problems included a) Precisely what was one observing? b) What was the most appropriate method of recording, storing and analysing the information? c) What was the most appropriate form in which to present the findings?

An review of the dental literature highlighted many of these problems. It was apparent there had been much subjective reporting in the past which proved to be of very little value if worthwhile comparisons were to be made. Periodontal assessment provided an example of this. In some papers it has been reported as mild, moderate or severe with no objective measurements recorded. (Tattersall, 1968; Campbell-Wilson, 1970). Other authors, (Sagne & Olsson, 1977) have observed and recorded the distance from the alveolar bone crest to the amelo-cemental junction and used this measurement

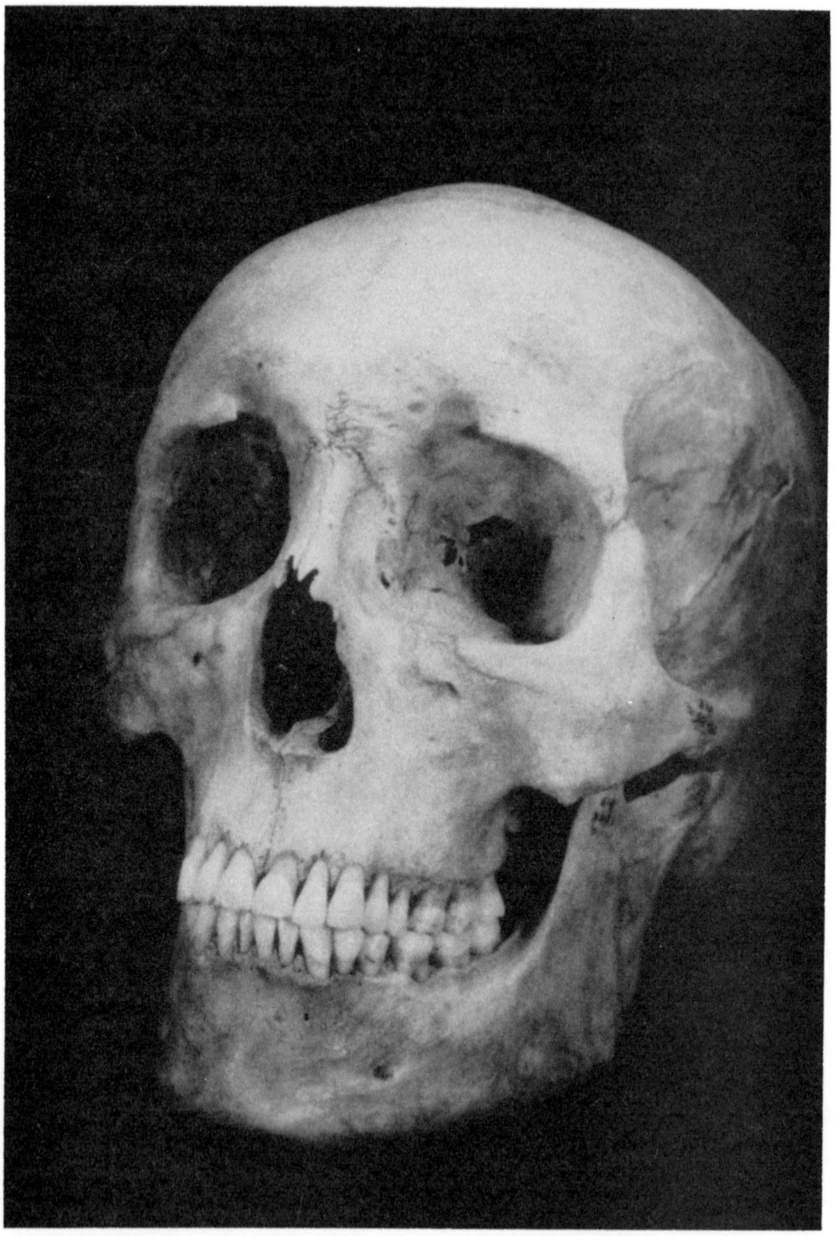

Figure 14.1. One of the better preserved skulls.

as an assessment of the severity of inflammatory bone loss. Recently, (Levers & Darling, 1983) have shown this method could be inaccurate as it fails to take into account the phenomenon of super-eruption of the teeth following excessive occlusal wear. Such wear is seen in virtually all mediaeval skeletal remains in this country and it would seem bone height measurements do not adequately observe and record the disease entity they purport to.

In research today, it is useful if findings are recorded in such a manner that they may be stored and processed by computer. The realisation of this entailed much preliminary work in searching current literature for methods of dental disease assessment that would lend themselves to data processing. An example concerning attrition is described in detail in another article in this volume (Chapter 6 by Cross, Kerr, and Bruce) whereby occlusal wear of the molar teeth is recorded on a 4-40 point ordinal scale for each tooth (Scott, 1979).

In the recording of dental caries use was made of the system for recording dental caries in prehistoric material as suggested by Moore and Corbett (1971).

Periodontal disease has been assessed using the principle suggested by Costa (1982) which takes into account altered interdental bone crest and architecture. It therefore attempts to record and quantify the actual diseased areas themselves.

For the purpose of recording and classifying the more generalised disease processes the numerical coding of the "Systematized Nomenclature of Pathology" (1965) has been adopted.

Although the intention is to make maximum use of data processing, descriptive prose must continue to hold its place in the recording and description of dental archaeological material. Garn (1977) points out some of the dangers of relying too much on numerical data and the temptation to make too many assumptions on too few cases. In this collection such a situation arose regarding the positively identified females. An effort was made to increase the number of females by employing canine size (Owsley, 1982). However, a short trial on the positively identifed females did not bear out the reliability of this method in our hands and it was discontinued. The collection has been reported as combined male and female data.

Problems in the presentation of the findings were also encountered and exemplified by such as 'caries rates' and 'caries prevalence'. Olsson & Sagne (1976) discuss many of these difficulties and the problems that ante- and post-mortem tooth loss pose when attempting to determine accurate 'caries prevalence'. Hardwick (1960) suggested a correction factor for teeth lost ante-mortem. Whittacker et al. (1981) tackled the problem by determining a caries rate for each tooth type in three different ways.

The above are just some of the problems encountered during the early stages of the investigations into the dental status of the Aberdeen Carmelite collection. However, the overriding impression still remains after some years' work that there is a need for still more objective recording methods, a need for these methods to lend themselves to data processing, and a need for more standardisation of methods on a world wide basis.

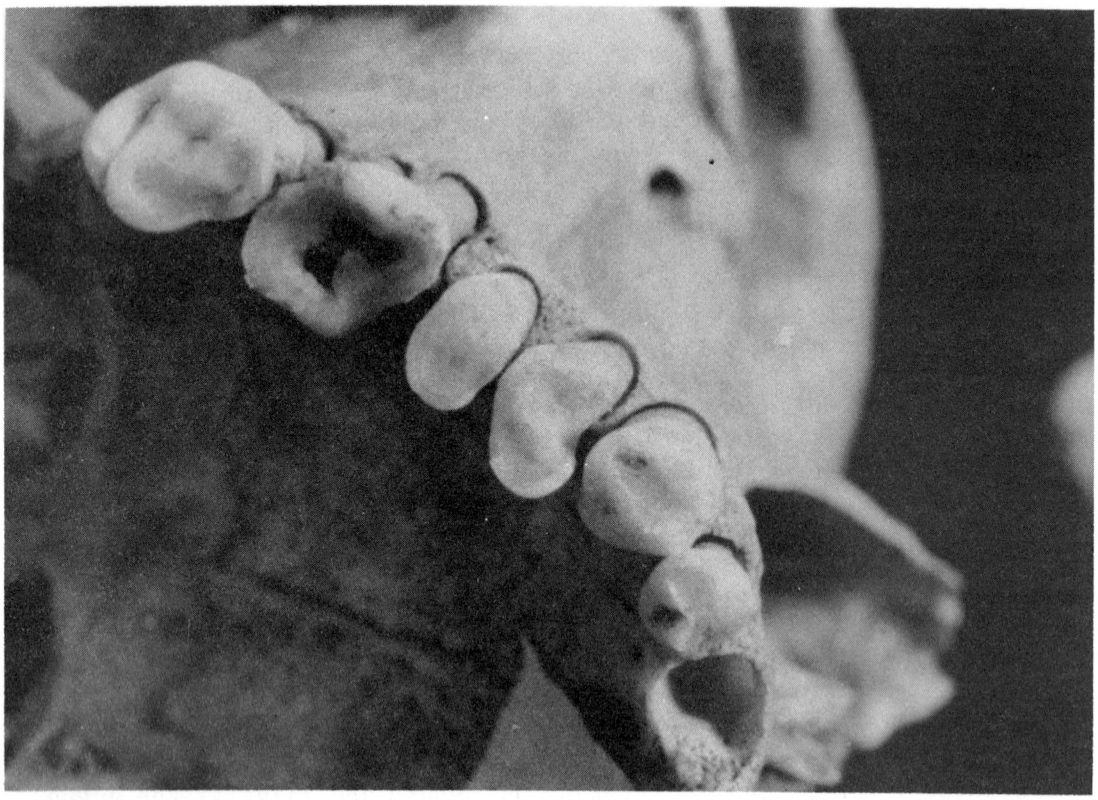

Figure 14.2. Severe attrition resulting in pulp exposure on an upper first molar.

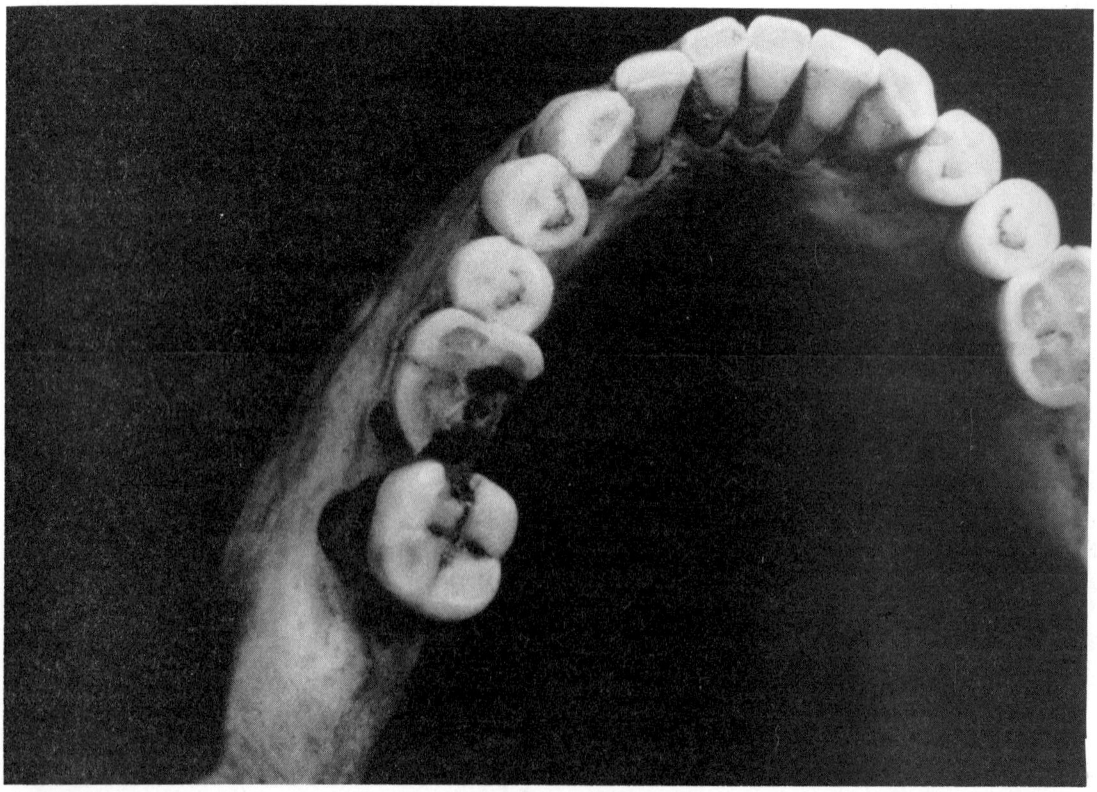

Figure 14.3. Both cervical and contact point caries on a lower left second molar tooth.

## SHORT REVIEW OF THE DENTAL STATUS OF THE ABERDEEN CARMELITE COLLECTION.

### ATTRITION.

The degree of occlusal attrition was the most obvious feature that distinguished the dentitions from those we would see in Britain today. No individual was spared. Attrition started at a very early age in the deciduous dentition and by the late twenty age group many teeth were so worn down that the pulp chamber was exposed and apical abscesses had resulted (Fig. 14.2).

The rate of attrition, provided one assumes the molar series erupts at six year intervals and diet remains constant throughout life, may be utilised to give a reasonable assessment of age at death (Miles, 1962). Our observations in this repect suggested that the average life span of an Aberdonian in Mediaeval times was something in the order of forty years.

Super-eruption of the teeth following occlusal attrition was observed and in many instances the amount of root exposure was quite extensive. In many such areas the inter-dental alveolar bone crest was healthy with intact cortical bone, thus seeming to confirm that periodontitis may not always be the principle causative factor in increasing root length exposure.

### DENTAL CARIES.

Dental caries proved to be a reasonably common disease with some 40% of adults affected. The site of the lesions was of some interest with both contact point and cervical caries observed. It has been suggested that contact-point caries is more likely to be linked with refined sugar in the diet whereas neck caries is linked with a more primitive or natural diet (Moore & Corbett, 1973). Both types were present in this collection (Fig. 14.3). It was also interesting to observe that a few individuals possessed many carious lesions whereas 60% of adults were caries free. It would seem that even in these far off days there were certain individuals who were possessed of a "sweet tooth".

From the number of dental abscesses seen there is little doubt that there were many sleepless nights in 'Old Aberdeen' as the pus pressurised its way to the exterior or else the tooth worked loose enough for it to be exfoliated or plucked from its putrid bed.

### PERIODONTITIS.

Periodontitis, measured by the degree of osteoporosity of the interdental crestal bone was a frequent finding in the older age groups and as one would expect became more widespread in the mouths with multiple toothloss. There were many individuals who had gone through the whole destructive phase and were completely edentulous, some with very severe alveolar resorption (GFig. 14.4).

### TOOTH AGENESIS AND IMPACTION.

The percentage of missing teeth were little different from what we

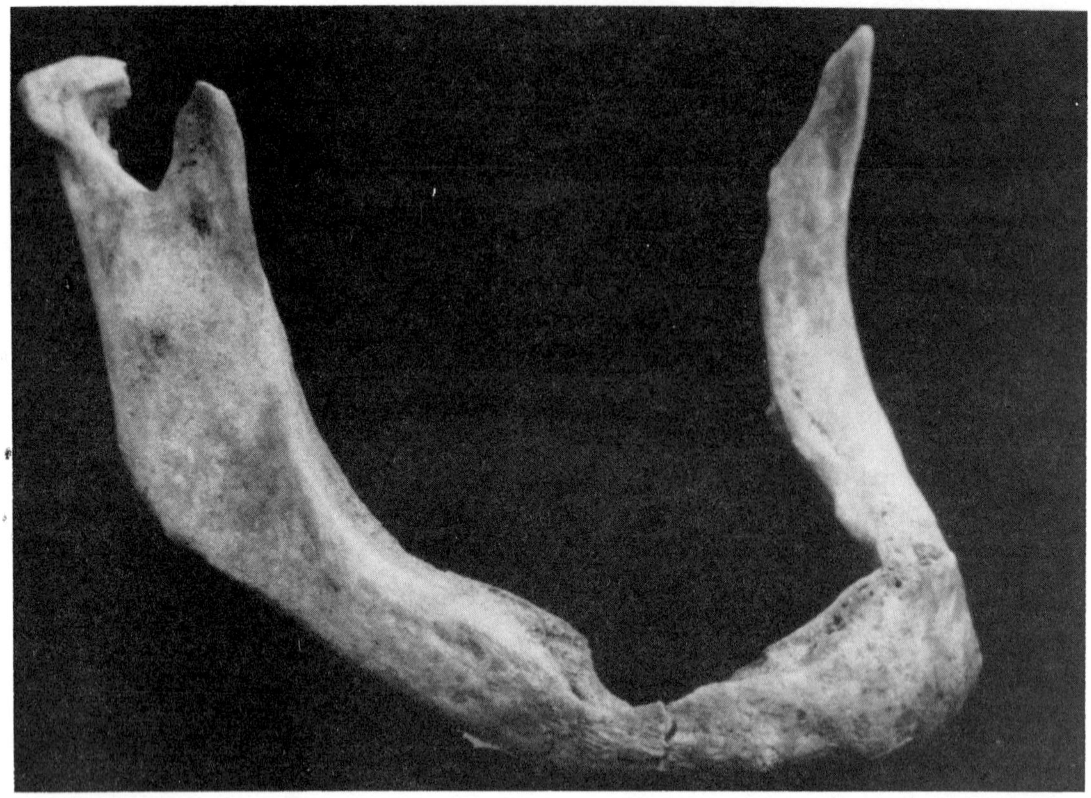

Figure 14.4. Severe alveolar resorption.

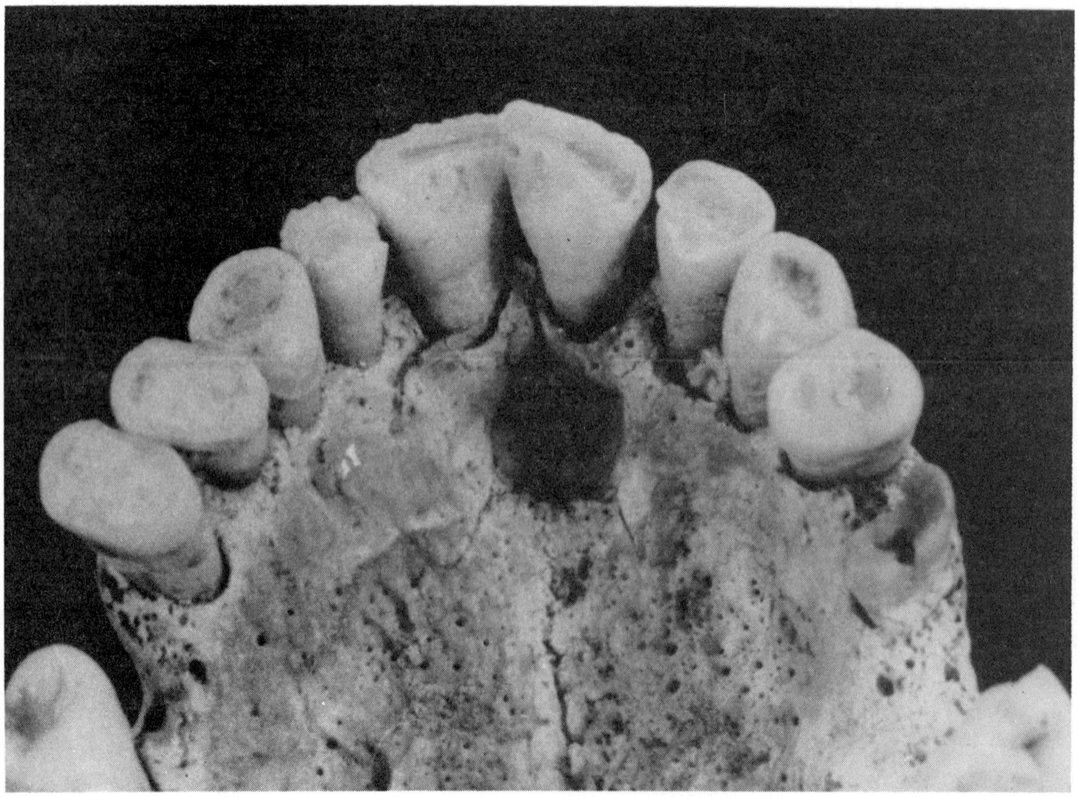

Figure 14.5. Naso-palatine cyst.

would expect today; 20% of third molars, and in addition, one specimen with both lower second premolars absent.

An interesting observation was the complete absence of any impacted wisdom teeth. It does seem as if the amount of interproximal and occlusal attrition was sufficient to allow the third molars to erupt and become functional teeth. There were, however, two cases of upper impacted canine teeth.

ENAMEL HYPOPLASIA.

Enamel hypoplasia was commonplace. It an often provide an indication of the health of an individual during the period that enamel is being laid down. It is known, for instance, that a severe generalised disturbance is lilely to cause disruption of enamel during development and leave its evidence as a linear defect on the tooth surface (Stones, 1954). Furthermore, a reasonable assessment can be made of the age of the individual when such an illness took place. Provided such defects were capable of being observed on three or more teeth and corresponded to the same age range, significance was given to them and the assumption made that a generalised systemic upset had occurred at that time (Goodman et al., 1980).

Detailed examination of the enamel using a stereo-microscope showed that hypoplastic lines were indeed extremely common throughout the collection, but in the main were of a minor nature. They did, however, suggest frequent childhood febrile illnesses and it was also interesting to observe that the ones with the more severe hypoplasias did not tend to make it through to adult life, the vast majority of the older age groups having the better formed enamel. One suspects that diseases such as rheumatic fever, bacterial endocarditis, nephritis and pulmonary infections were frequent occurrences.

ORAL PATHOLOGY.

One naso-palatine cyst was observed (Fig. 14.5). There were no instances of congenital defects such as cleft palate or other facial deformities.

No instance was seen of severe bone disturbance that would indicate an invasive tumour or severe osteomyelitis. There was one case of a deep depression on the lingual aspect at the mandible opposite to the left submandibular salivary gland and the implication must be that the gland was the site of a slowly progressive tumour such as a pleomorphic adenoma.

One individual demonstrated sound teeth on one side of the arch but decayed, periodontally involved or missing teeth on the other side. The assumption in this case must be of a severe facial palsy inhibiting the normal masticatory movements with the natural self-cleansing effects they would have in removing food debris and preventing decay and periodontal disease.

No case of jaw fracture was noted although there were one or two isntances of enamel or tooth wear that suggested the teeth might have been used in some everyday tasks.

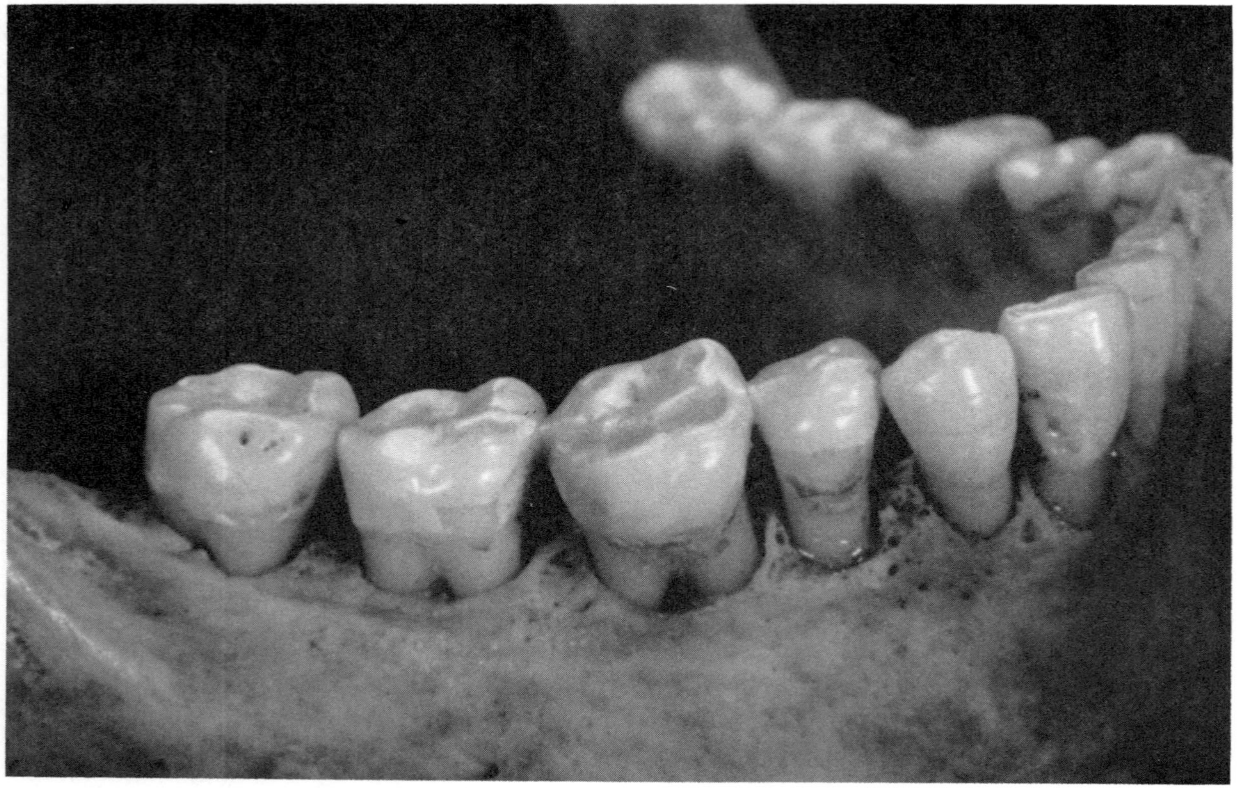

Figure 14.6. Smooth, rounded and clean buccal surfaces, suggesting personal attempts at scaling and polishing the teeth.

DENTAL TREATMENT.

There was no evidence of any dental treatment as we would know it being carried out except in the case of one or two individuals who had markedly less tartar on their teeth (especially the outer aspects), and seemed to have much smoother and rounded contours to their teeth (Fig. 14.6). These individuals may have attempted to scrape their teeth clean and used some form of abrasive powder or fluid to give a final polish or luster to their surfaces.

The above is only a brief sketch of some of the principal dental findings of the Aberdeen Collection and in the main our observations have agreed with much that has been reported in similar surveys. It is appreciated that the amount of material in this collection is small but it has been used more in the nature of a pilot study to test new methods of recording and assessing the dentition which are computer based. It is hoped to use these methods to investigate, record and analyse a much larger Scottish mediaeval collection that is presently being excavated at Linlithgow.

ACKNOWLEDGEMENTS.

The author gratefully acknowledges financial support from the Wellcome Trust and the close co-operation of the co-investigators, Juliet Cross and Margaret Bruce.

REFERENCES.

Campbell-Wilson, M. (1970). Report on the occlusions and dentitions of a group of skulls excavated at a cairn cemetery in Fife. Dent. Practit. 21: 68-71.

Costa, R.L. (1982). Periodontal Disease in the Prehistoric Ipiutak and Tigara Skeletal Remains from Point Hope, Alaska. Am. J. Phys. Anth. 59: 97-110.

Garn, S.M., Cole, P.E., Guire, K.E. (1977). The effect of Small Samples on Crown-Size Interrelationships. J. Dent. Res. 56: 1474.

Goodman, A.H., Armelagos, G.J. Rose, J.C. (1980). Enamel Hypoplasias as Indicators of Stress in Three Prehistoric Populations from Illinois. Human Biol. 52: 515-528.

Hardwick, J.L., (1960). The Incidence and Distribution of Caries Throughout the Ages in Relation to the Englishman's Diet. Brit. Dent. J. 108: 9-17.

Levers, B.G.H. & Darling, A.I. (1983). Continuous eruption of some adult human teeth of ancient populations. Archs. Oral Biol. 28: 401-408.

Miles, A.E.W. (1962). Assessment of the Ages of a Population of Anglo-Saxons from their Dentition. Proc. Roy. Soc. Med. 44: 881-886.

Moore, W.J. & Corbett, E. (1971). The Distribution of Dental Caries in Ancient British Populations. Caries Res. 5: 151-168.

Moore, W.J. & Corbett, E. (1973). The Distribution of Dental Caries in Ancient British Populations. Caries Res. 7: 139-153.

Olsson, G. & Signe, S. (1976). Studies of Caries Prevalence in a Mediaeval Population. Dentomaxillofac. Radiol. 5: 12-18.

Owsley, D.W. (1982). Dental Discriminant sexing of Arikara Skeletons. Plains Anthropologist. 27: 165-169.

Sagne, S. & Olsson, G. (1977). Studies of the Periodontal Status of a Mediaeval Population. Dentomaxillofac. Radiol. 6: 46-52.

Scott, E.C. (1979). Dental wear scoring technique. Am. J. Phys. Anth. 51: 213-218.

Stones, H.H. (1954). Oral and Dental Disease. Livingstone, Edinburgh (3rd Ed.): 149-150.

Systematized Nomenclature of Pathology. College of American Pathologists. Committee on Nomenclature and Classification of Disease. 1965.

Tattersal, I. (1968). Dental palaeopathology of mediaeval Britain. J. Hist. Med. 23: 380-385.

Whittaker, D.K., Molleson, T., Bennett, R.B., Edwards, I., Jenkins, P.R. & Llewelyn, J.H., (1981). The Prevalence and Distribution of Dental Caries in Romano-British Population. Arch. Oral Biol. 26: 237-245.

## Chapter 15

# OBSERVATIONS ON DENTAL CARIES IN PRIMARY TEETH IN SOME MEDIEVAL BRITISH SKULL MATERIAL

Sonia A. Williams
&
M.E.J. Curzon

Department of Child Dental Health
University of Leeds
Leeds, England

## INTRODUCTION

The dental condition of human skeletal material forms an important part of many archaeological studies, as teeth appear to succumb to post-mortem degeneration to a lesser extent than other skeletal remains. Many criteria for assessing dental conditions and anomalies have been described, including those by Sarnat and Schour (1941), Miles (1963), and Brothwell (1981).

The majority of reports describe the dental conditions of adults or sub-adults based on fragmentary evidence. Few researchers have the opportunity to study a series of "complete" intact dental arches, bearing a full complement of teeth, or have reported on the state of the dentition in childhood or during infancy.

### Background

The state of development or the exfoliation of deciduous teeth has been employed as a reliable and useful method of age determination in children. Although infant mortality rates even as late as the nineteenth century would suggest that a substantial proportion of British populations died before the age of 5 years, detailed reports of the condition of the teeth and jaws bearing the deciduous dentition *per se* are infrequently reported.

From the few studies involving the primary teeth it would appear that either the remains of older children and adults are better preserved or that research workers are more reluctant to report on the dental status of these younger age groups.

In addition because of the condition of dental remains, intact arches are an infrequent find, compared with the fragmented material usually excavated. Caution must be exercised in the interpretation of the findings concerning fragmentary material as isolated groups of teeth or jaws alone cannot reliably confirm the conditions of individual mouths. Such material is more useful in assessing diseases and anomalies according to the tooth types or jaws excavated (James and Miller, 1970). A particular difficulty exists in relation to the higher prevalence of post-mortem loss of certain groups of teeth, particularly those with single roots. This is even more likely to occur with primary teeth as molar teeth are more frequently retained post-mortem due to their widely divergent roots. They are also retained in the mouth in vivo for a greater duration, due to natural exfoliation at a later age. Intact arches bearing a complete deciduous dentition are unlikely to be found in an individual beyond the age of 6 years.

The present study has provided a rare opportunity to examine a number of jaws of young children, several of which were virtually intact. It was possible to observe the occlusion, and examine a number of deciduous incisors.

## Materials and Methods

An excavation at the Hirsel, near Coldstream, provided human skeletal material from a Medieval graveyard, and enabled us to examine the dentitions of 21 young children under the age of 6 years. Of these, eight infants were estimated to be less than three years old and 13 between two and five years of age. General observations concerning attrition, hypoplasia and caries have been the subject of a previous paper (Williams and Curzon, 1985). The condition of the anterior teeth and the occlusion are reported here, with special reference to the anthropological implications of these observations with respect to infant feeding practices.

The occlusal and incisor relationships between the two arches of teeth could be readily estimated in these specimens, using standard techniques (Todd, 1975). Subsequently, the anterior teeth were examined for macroscopic evidence of hypoplasia, wear and caries according to the methods described by Sarnat and Schour (1941), Brothwell (1981) and Todd (1975). Using Tessovar (Carl Zeiss) photographic microscope, photographic recording of the surface of the anterior teeth were then made (up to X 12.8).

## Results

Altogether 294 deciduous teeth were available for examination, including 44 upper and 37 lower incisors. Four children had intact upper and lower arches and a further six had fewer than five teeth missing post-mortem (i.e. 16 to 19 teeth present).

Occlusion. The occlusal relationships could be directly examined for five children and inferred from the wear facets on the teeth for another three. In the majority of children aged three to five years of age, the incisal relationship involved positive overjet values of 2 to 4 mm and usually a complete overbite. Only one slightly incomplete overbite was seen. No posterior crossbites were observed. In one more fragmentary specimen, a negative overjet was inferred from the reverse position of the incisal wear facets. No edge to edge or anterior open bite relationships were noted.

Caries. Caries was established positively as present in the maxillary deciduous incisors of three children. Interproximal cavitation was noted in two individuals; extensive and involving all four incisors in one child, and of a more limited nature affecting two adjacent teeth in another child. A third child had an extensive carious attack on the palatal surfaces of both maxillary lateral incisors. Unfortunately in this skull the central incisors were lost postmortem, but there was evidence of periapical

Table 15.1. Prevalence of Carious Cavities in primary teeth in a group of Mediaeval Infant Skulls, by tooth type.

| | Tooth Type | | | | |
|---|---|---|---|---|---|
| | Central Incisor | Lateral Incisor | Canine | First Molar | Second Molar |
| Maxilla C | 3 | 4 | 0 | 5 | 1 |
| N | 20 | 24 | 26 | 34 | 29 |
| Mandible C | 0 | 0 | 0 | 5 | 2 |
| N | 15 | 22 | 23 | 37 | 28 |

C = number of teeth with carious defect(s).
N = number of teeth examined.

pathology of these teeth in the bone of the premaxilla. The tooth type prevalence values for caries are shown in Table 15.1.

There were erosive lesions on the palatal surfaces of the primary incisors of the teeth of the two children with interproximal caries. Another two children, without definite caries, also had erosive lesions. No evidence of caries or erosive lesions were seen on the canines or lower incisors.

In those affected individuals the left side of the mouth was more severely involved than the right. The extent of cavitation varied such that in some instances only the surface enamel was affected while in other teeth the dentine was penetrated. The extent of the variation in this condition is shown in Figures 15.1 to 15.4.

Hypoplasia. The hypoplasia recorded was of the circular type (forming pits and grooves) principally affecting the labial surface of the incisor teeth. Four individuals had hypoplasia evident on the surface of the central maxillary primary incisors, all relating to periods of foetal stress between the sixth and eighth months of pregnancy. Hypoplasia was also found in other teeth in the same mouths, notably on the maxillary lateral incisors in three cases and also on the maxillary canines and first primary molars in another two cases.

Generally hypoplasias affected the maxillary lateral incisors during the perinatal period (7th foetal month to birth). In all, 12 infants had hypoplasia presenting on upper or lower canine teeth. The period of stress ranged from the sixth month of intrauterine life to seven months after birth, with a median value of three months postpartum. While contralateral teeth showed similar defects, different tooth types demonstrated systemic disturbances at different stages during life, even when the affected teeth were present in the same mouth. The data for the prevalence of hypoplasia by tooth type are given in Table 15.2.

Attrition. All erupted incisors showed some degree of wear. This was sited at, or near, the incisal edges and involved some exposure of the dentine in the two to five year old age group. These areas of wear were generally separated from the erosive lesions mentioned above.

## DISCUSSION.

This study has provided an opportunity to report on an infrequently described group of children and examine the evidence available concerning infant feeding practices and perinatal stress in a group of children who died in early infancy. However, there could be significant differences between those children who died and those that survived infancy, especially if the former succumbed after a protracted illness. Caution must therefore be used in interpreting these observations as to whether they are typical of children of that locality and historical period.

Interpretation of findings based upon skeletal remains can be difficult because postmortem changes may influence the evidence of in vivo conditions. Unfavourable soil conditions can cause some types of erosion of dental tissues, but these are usually seen as affecting all the surfaces of a

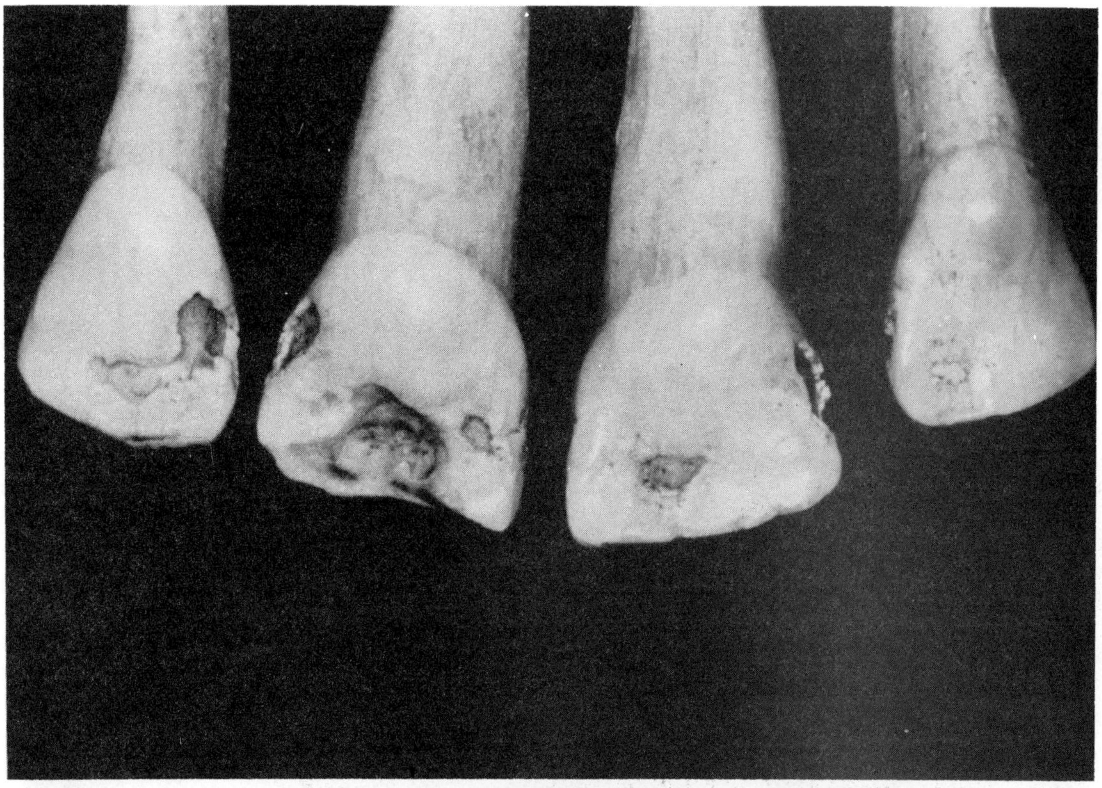

Figure 15.1. No. 82/220. Palatal aspect of maxillary primary incisors showing interproximal caries and areas of palatal erosion. Note that the area of incisal wear is separate from the area of erosion except on the left central incisor. The left side is more severely affected than the right. x 3.2.

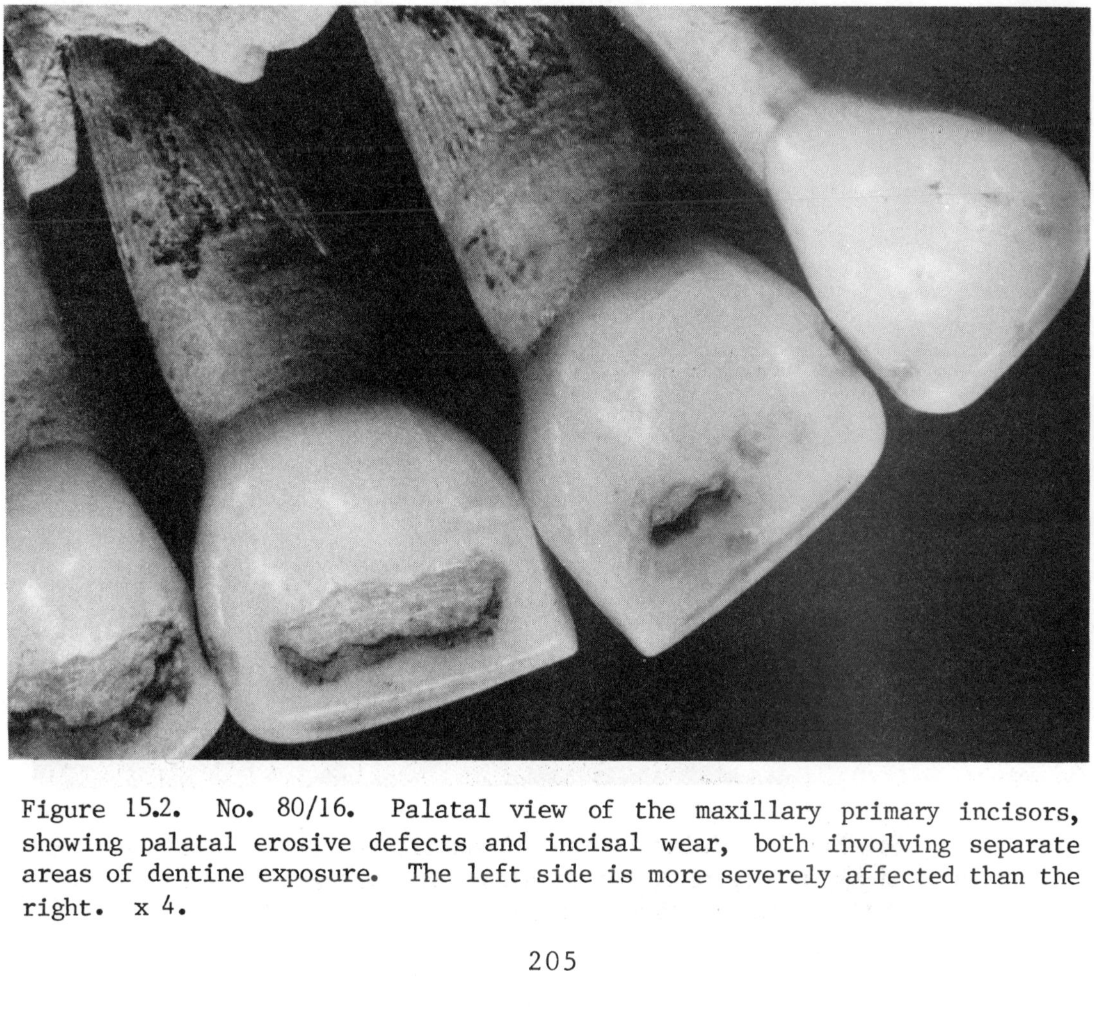

Figure 15.2. No. 80/16. Palatal view of the maxillary primary incisors, showing palatal erosive defects and incisal wear, both involving separate areas of dentine exposure. The left side is more severely affected than the right. x 4.

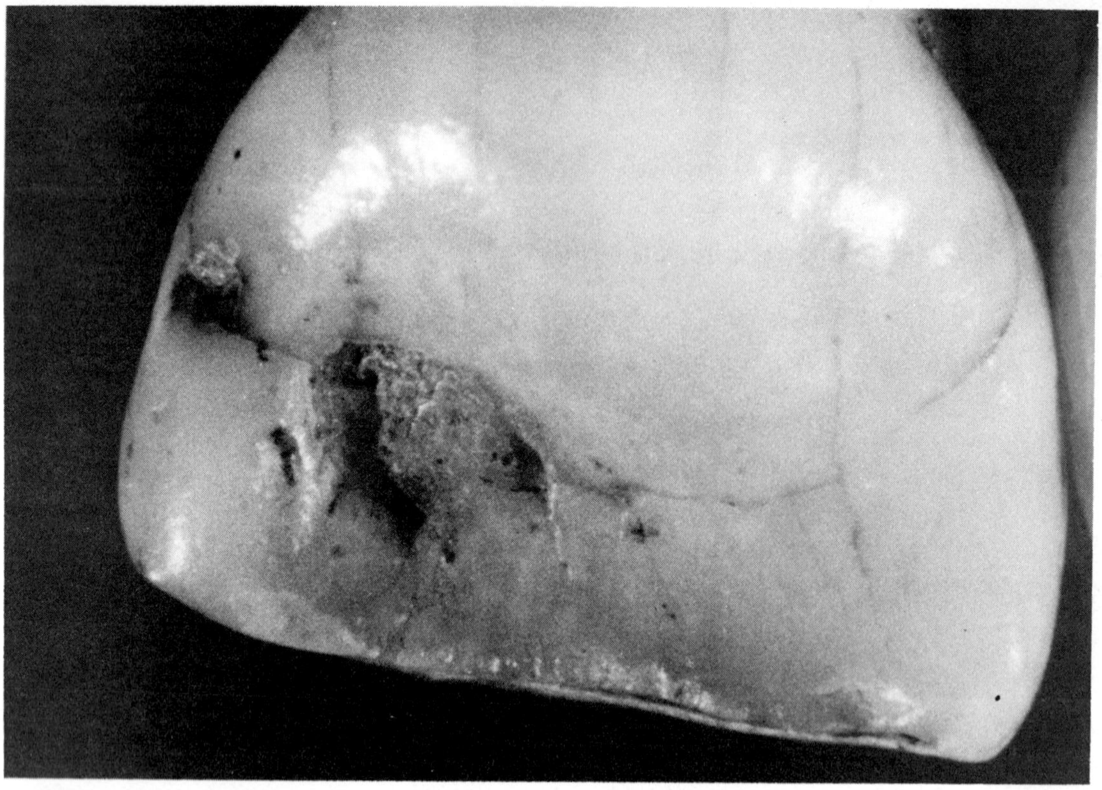

Figure 15.3. No. 81/235. Palatal view of maxillary left central incisor. The erosion and incisal attrition are separate. x 8.

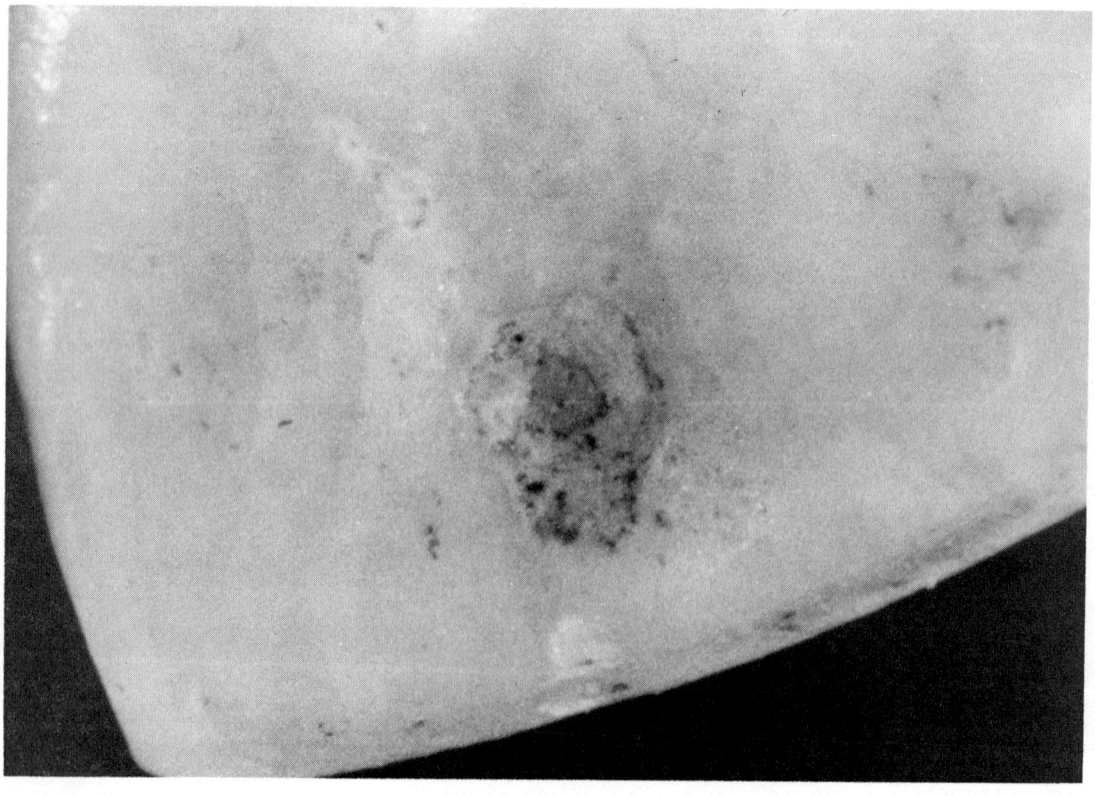

Figure 15.4. No. 81/235. Palatal view of maxillary central incisor. The same child as shown in Figure 3, but at higher magnification. Note that the defect is similar but smaller than that in the contralateral tooth. x 12.8.

Table 15.2. Prevalence of Hypoplastic defects in primary teeth in a group of Medieval Century Infant Skulls, by tooth type.

| | Tooth Type | | | | |
|---|---|---|---|---|---|
| | Central Incisor | Lateral Incisor | Canine | First Molar | Second Molar |
| Maxilla H | 5 | 8 | 12 | 5 | 1 |
| N | 20 | 24 | 26 | 34 | 29 |
| Mandible H | 1 | 2 | 8 | 5 | 1 |
| N | 15 | 22 | 23 | 37 | 28 |

H = number of teeth with hypoplastic defect(s).
N = number of teeth examined.

dentition rather than the localised effect seen here (Soggnaes, 1963; Poole and Tratman, 1978). In the present study the changes observed were quite discrete.

The children in this study did not appear to have received a diet which was substantially more abrasive during infancy than some present day British children. The gross occlusal anomalies of contemporary children relating to habitual digit, dummy and bottle sucking were not observed. However, caries of the upper anterior teeth was present.

Clinically, caries has been observed to occur readily at hypoplastic sites on teeth (Rosenzweig and Sahar, 1962; Noriforuk and Fraser, 1984). Thus hypoplasia can predispose teeth which are already poorly mineralised to carious attack, superimposing one condition on another. It is interesting to note that in the present study both conditions were seen on the same incisors in five of the seven carious teeth, indicating that two teeth were carious but not hypoplastic. However, caries and hypoplasia were only apparently present on the same surface in two teeth. Nevertheless, even in these circumstances, the development of caries requires an acidogenic diet involving fermentable carbohydrates, which would need to be a regular part of the infant's diet.

In current clinical literature, there are many reports of infant feeding practices which contribute to caries of the deciduous incisors (Winter, 1980; Johnsen et al., 1982). As in the present study, the maxillary teeth are mainly involved. The classic pattern involves a rapid destruction of more than one tooth, usually starting labially or interproximally, and extending circumferentially around the teeth involved. Ad libitum bottle feeding with sweetened milk, fruit syrups and dummies dipped in honey, are usually implicated. If the habit is stopped prior to eruption of the primary molar teeth, the latter will remain unaffected. The pattern of caries attack seen in our study suggests a less destructive form of the same condition which has failed to affect many posterior teeth either because the diet was less acidogenic or due to an early cessation of the habit.

There have been previous reports concerning dental caries in primary incisors among British children from the Medieval period (James and Miller, 1970) and in the nineteenth century (Corbett, 1975). It has been traditional to consider that caries is an affliction of advanced or civilised societies, having increased dramatically in the eighteenth and nineteenth centuries as the sugar trade developed with the removal of the sugar tax (Moore and Corbett, 1978). Bibby (1975) suggests that other carbohydrates, especially starchy baked goods, which persist around the teeth, may also be important. Thus apart from the detrimental effect of honey on infants' teeth, flour, bread and oatmeal products could also be damaging if in contact with the teeth for long periods of time.

It is interesting to speculate about the type of diet the infants in this study would have received at the time that their primary teeth were erupting. In addition to breast milk, which under certain circumstances may be cariogenic (Rugg-Gunn, 1985), animal milk could be provided using a cow's horn, as illustrated in a thirteenth century miniature (Drummond and Wilbraham, 1939). Wooden feeding bottles have also been described as in common usage in the sixteenth century, and clay or pressed leather may also have been employed (Duncum, 1947; Poynter, 1947; Tubbs, 1947; Rendle-Short, 1955; Fildes, 1981). The end to be inserted in the mouth could be covered with a soft material, such as calf's teat, sponge or cloth. It has been suggested that older infants might have drunk from these utensils when out visiting. It would have been convenient to carry them about with the children when they required an extra drink.

Pap was provided for young infants, at least as early as Elizabethen times (Fildes, 1980). It consisted of flour or bread boiled in water with flavouring added, such as spices, beer, wines, herbs or honey. Alternatively milk could be given thickened with breadcrumbs. As the infants in this study came from a more northerly part of Britain, oatmeal could have been used. This nourishment, if not a fluid consistency, may have been given using one of the artificial feeding devices as a "sucking bag".

The introduction of more solid food was suggested for infants after the eruption of their incisors, so that infants could chew (Struve, 1801; Rendle-Short, 1955; Soggnaes, 1963). In practice it seems to have occurred at any time between seven and thirty-six months, depending on the health of the child, the age of the mother and the time of the year. Teething itself was considered a hazardous problem (Hurlock, 1742), appearing on Bills of Mortality as late as 1905. Swelling of the gums and jaws, fevers, cramps, palsies and fluxes were all ascribed to teething. The child would be encouraged to chew on wood, bones, leather or rags, or sometimes on a small branch of a tree with leaves on. Lancing of the gums was often advocated (Hurlock, 1742) and one seventeenth century writer describes a young child, presumably with scurvy, who had a dark red, soft gelatenous mass protruding from the mouth "as if the child was sucking raw flesh".

An infant "sucking bag" may have been used in the cases reported here. They were first described in the German literature from 1473 (Ravn, 1974). Struve (1801) abhored the practice, claiming it to be disgusting as it often became contaminated with flies. With time the contents would go sour and the newly erupted teeth would become black, loose and fall out. The contents of the bag would include bread, milk, flour water, unfermented meal or porridge. The bags would be made from old torn up sheets, and some children slept with them. The same author remarked that it was difficult to wean children from the sucking bag after their first year, but commented that children had a propensity to suck anything and should not be permitted to suck the lips of older sickly relatives! Certainly the sucking bag may have been a useful aid in pacification during teething. It could help to initiate dental caries of the anterior teeth, being held between the upper anterior surface of the tongue and the maxillary teeth. If discontinued once the anterior teeth had erupted, then other teeth would not be affected by caries. James and Miller (1970) considered that honeycomb wrapped in linen might have been implicated in the development of large buccal cavities observed in primary teeth of the Medieval children they examined. Perhaps this was a result of placing the linen between the teeth and the cheek.

The palatal erosion seen on some of the maxillary primary incisors is difficult to explain in the present study. This finding has not been recorded previously. Although postmortem changes do modify the appearance of human teeth this is unlikely as no other teeth in the skulls were affected. The propensity for the left side to be involved to a greater degree is a curious finding. Perhaps this reflects a natural habit to favour one side of the mouth in preference to the other on inserting a feeding bottle. The descrete nature of the lesions suggest some mechnical cause due to the use of a specific object, as has been described clinically by Baden (1970). This would be in contrast to the generalised damage caused by the seepage of fermentable foods, chemicals or vomitus.

The palatal aspect of the erosion is also unusual, as objects frequently inserted into the mouth usually cause some degree of incisal edge damage. If it was due to a mechanical cause the abrasive end of a feeding device or pacifier might have been responsible. It is interesting to note that there are tooth marks on the lip of an infant's pottery feeding bottle from Greece, housed at the Ashmolean Museum in Oxford.

Children who were ill may have needed continuous pacification by various means. As the children in this study all died very young this may well have been the case. All infants anyway have a need for satisfaction from sucking far beyond the requirements to obtain nourishment. If these habits are sufficiently strong or prolonged, the oral musculature may help to create changes in the occlusal relationship of the anterior teeth. This is often seen with digit or dummy sucking, or ad libitum use of an artifical feeding bottle in children today (Winter, 1980; Peterson, 1982). As no abnormalities of the occlusion were found in the children of this study, it must be concluded that a similar practice had not occurred. The method of use of a pacifier may have avoided this type of occlusal anomaly occurring, or it could have been an earlier habit which had been discontinued and any occlusal abnormalities then spontaneously corrected.

Many studies have inferred the existence of stress factors in infancy from an examination of the permanent dentition (Huss-Ashmore et al., 1982). However, an assessment of hypoplasia in permanent teeth may provide an incomplete picture, since evidence of perinatal stress may only be obtained from an examination of the first permanent molars, and these teeth are especially prone to post eruptive influences, including attrition, which will tend to obscure the condition being studied. Realistically, clues concerning perinatal stress, (as enamel hypoplasia) and diet and infant feeding practices, (as attrition, caries and occlusal relationships), can only be obtained from an examination of complete or nearly intact deciduous dental arches.

It is helpful if the remains are examined by a researcher with clinical dental experience of young children, as relevant information might be missed by an inexperienced eye unware of the clinical implications of a minor anomaly (Haskell et al., 1985).

## CONCLUSION.

The present study reports on a number of interesting observations concerning the dental health status of some Medieval children. Dental erosion/caries of a previously unreported pattern was found on the palatal surfaces of maxillary primary incisors. This was suggested as due to feeding methods with cariogenic foods such as pap, oatmeal, honey and milk with bread. The use of feeding devices, made of pottery, cow horn or leather, may have been a factor akin to modern nursing bottles. It would be helpful to have further studies of dental remains of this age group. Archaeologists should be encouraged to retrieve even the smallest remains of teeth for further study whenever possible. A clear picture of infant welfare and dietary practices among early groups of infants could then be obtained.

ACKNOWLEDGEMENTS

We wish to thank Professor Rosemary Cramp, of the Department of Archaeology of the University of Durham, for her kind assistance in making the skeletal material available for examination, and also Dr. D. Birkett for his advice and encouragement.

REFERENCES

Baden, E. (1970). Environmental Pathology of the Teeth. In: Thoma's Oral Pathology. Vol. 1. edited by Gorlin, R.J. and Goldman, H.M. (6th edition). C.V. Mosby Co. St. Louis: 184-238.

Bibby, B.G. (1975). The Cariogenicity of Snack Food and Confections. J. Am. Dent. Assoc. 90: 121-132.

Brothwell, D.R. (1981). Digging Up Bones. British Museum (Natural History), Oxford University Press, Oxford.

Corbett, M.E. (1975). An investigation into the pattern of dental caries in nineteenth century British urban population. PhD. Thesis University of Birmingham, Birmingham, England.

Drummond, J.C. and Wilbraham, A. (1939). The Englishman's Food. Jonathan Cape Ltd., London: 77.

Duncum, B.M. (1947). Some notes on the history of Lactation. Brit. Med. Bull. 5: 253.

Fildes, V. (1980). Weaning the Elizabethan Child. Nursing Times. 76: 357-403.

Fildes, V. (1981). The early history of the infant feeding bottle. Nursing Times. 77: 128-129 and 168-170.

Haskell, B.S., Arm, R., Stroop, J.R. and Shaunessey, J. (1985). The role of the dentist in archaeologic investigation: an unusual facial fracture with healing occurring 3000 years ago. Quintessence Int. 16: 95-99.

Hurlock, J. (1742). A Practical Treatise upon Dentition; or, The Breeding of Teeth in Children. Rivington and Austen, London.

Huss-Ashmore, R., Goodman, A.H. and Armelagos, G.J. (1982). Nutritional Inferences from Paleopathology. In: Advances in Archeological Method and Theory. (Vol. 5) edited by M. Schiffer. Academic Press, New York: 395-473.

James, P.M.C. and Miller, W.A. (1970). Dental Conditions in a group of Mediaeval English children. Brit. Dent. J. 128: 391-396.

Johnson, D.C., Michel, B.C., Gerstenmaier, J.H. Parrish, S. and Schwartz, E. (1982). Characteristics and backgrounds of children with nursing caries. Pediatr. Dent. 4: 218-224.

Miles. A.E.E. (1963). Dentition in the estimation of age. J. Dent. Res. 42: 255-262.

Moore, W.J. and Corbett, M.E. (1978). Dental caries experience in man: Historical, anthropological and cultural diet-caries relationship, the English experience. In: Diet, Nutrition and Dental Caries. edited by N.H. Rowe. University of Michigan School of Dentistry: 3-19.

Nikiforuk, G. and Fraser, D. (1984). Enhanced caries susceptibility associated with neonatal enamel hypoplasia. Caries. Res. 18:185.

Petersen, J.E. (1982). Pediatric Oral habits. In: Pediatric Dentistry: Scientific Foundations and Clinical Practice. edited by R.E. Stewart et al. C.V. Mosby, London: 361-372.

Poole, D.F.G. and Tratman, E.K. (1978). Postmortem changes in human teeth from late paleolithic/mesolithic occupants on an English limestone cave. Archs. Oral. Biol. 23:1115-1120.

Poynter, F.N.L. (1947). The story of artificial infant feeding. Brit. Med. Bull. 5:254.

Ravn, J.J. (1974). The prevalence of dummy and finger sucking habits in Copenhagen children until the age of 3 years. Commun. Dent. Oral Epidemiol. 2:316-320.

Rendle-Short, J. (1955). The history of teething in infancy. Proc. Royal Soc. Med. 48:132-138.

Rosenzweig, K.A. and Sahar, M. (1962). Enamel hypoplasia and dental caries in the primary dentition of prematuri. Brit. Dent. J. 113:279-280.

Rugg-Gunn, A.J., Roberts, G.J. and Wright, W.G. (1985). Effect of human milk on plaque pH in situ and enamel dissolution in vitro compared with bovine milk, lactose and sucrose. Caries Res. 19:327-334.

Sarnat, G.B. and Schour, I. (1941). Enamel hypoplasia in relation to systemic disease; a chronological, morphological and aetiological classification. J. Am. Dent. Assoc. 29:1989-2000.

Soggnaes, R.F. (1963). Mechanisms of hard tissue destruction. Publ. No. 75, Am. Assoc. Adv. Science, Washington, DC: 120-130.

Struve, C.A. (1801). A familiar treatise on the physical education of children during the early period of their lives. Murray and Highley, London.

Todd, J.E. (1975). Childrens' Dental Health in England and Wales, 1973. H.M.S.O. London: 338-340.

Tubbs, F. (1947). Roman infant feeding bottles with particular reference to Romano-British and British Medieval vessels. Brit. Med. Bull. 5:255-256.

Williams, S.A. and Curzon, M.E.J. (1985). Dental Caries in a Scottish Medieval child population. Caries Res. 19:162.

Winter, G.B. (1980). Problems with the use of comforters. Int. Dent. J. 30:28-38.

## Chapter 16

# MEDIAEVAL DENTITIONS FROM ST. ANDREWS

DOROTHY A. LUNT

University of Glasgow Dental School
Glasgow

Until 1975, the number of Mediaeval dentitions available for study in Scotland was very small. There was a rather larger quantity of skeletal material from the immediately preceding Dark Age or Early Mediaeval phase, during which burials were characteristically made in long cists constructed of small stone slabs. For the purposes of the present paper, the period of major use of long cists will be considered to extend from the 6th to the 11th centuries AD., though it can be shown that long cists may have been used considerably later, especially in remote parts of Scotland (Stevenson, 1951-52). The Mediaeval period is considered to comprise the 12th to 16th centuries A.D.

Long cists have often been found in groups forming quite large cemeteries. In 1976 yet another long cist cemetery was discovered in St. Andrews at a site known as Hallowhill. Some 151 cists were excavated and 79 of these contained some part of a human jaw and/or dentition.

In 1980, another excavation was carried out in St. Andrews at the site of St. Mary's Church, Kirkhill, largely because burials were being exposed in the crumbling cliff-face. It was thought that this cemetery was of mediaeval date with burials perhaps ranging in date from the 11th to the 15th centuries A.D. However 14C analysis of the earliest burials has given dates of c. 685 $\pm$ 55 A.D. and c. 750 $\pm$55 A.D., and these burials are roughly contemporary with the Hallowhill cemetery. There must however be later mediaeval graves at Kirkhill, where burials in some areas were 10 layers deep, and for the purposes of the present work, the Kirkhill skeletons have been considered to date to the later Mediaeval period. Burial numbers ran up to 327, and of these 168 contained parts of the human dentition. Many of the burials had been disturbed, there was frequently evidence of more than one skeleton in the material included under a single burial number, and much of the material was fragmentary, so the total number of individuals represented is extremely difficult to assess.

Relatively large collections of skeletons from a single site, such as these collections from Hallowhill and Kirkhill, provide assemblages which are potentially more uniform than those made up by pooling small groups from widely separated areas. Although the burials may be spread over several centuries, at least the genetic background and environmental conditions of the population are likely to show less variation. It is possible to study such a population group by itself and compare the results with the pooled data collected from smaller sites scattered randomly over the country.

Study of the dentition is particularly valuable in assessing individual ages at death, such assessment being based upon the stage of tooth development in juveniles and upon the degree of dental attrition in adults (Brothwell, 1981). With burial groups of reasonable size such as those from

Table 16.1. Age Distribution of dentitions from sites at Hallowhill and Kirkhill, St. Andrews.

| | HALLOWHILL | | KIRKHILL | |
|---|---|---|---|---|
| Age group | No. | % | No. | % |
| 0 - 6 | 5 | 7.25 | 27 | 12.68 |
| 6 - 14 | 6 | 8.70 | 16 | 7.51 |
| 15 - 19 | 9 | 13.04 | 9 | 4.22 |
| 20 - 25 | 13 | 18.84 | 25 | 11.74 |
| 25 - 35 | 16 | 23.19 | 56 | 26.29 |
| 35 - 45 | 9 | 13.04 | 57 | 26.76 |
| 45 + | 11 | 15.94 | 23 | 10.80 |
| Total | 69 | 100.00 | 213 | 100.00 |

Hallowhill and Kirkhill, it is possible to examine the proportions of different age groups present in the skeletal material.

Table 16.1 shows the distribution of individuals by age in the Hallowhill and Kirkhill groups. Children between 6 and 14, and adults aged 25-35 form similar proportions of both groups. There are higher proportions of adolescents, adults aged 20-25 and adults aged more than 45 in the Hallowhill group, and higher proportions of children aged from birth to 6 years, and adults aged 35-45 in the Kirkhill group.

These age distributions may be compared with the data obtained (Lunt, 1974) from the relatively small numbers of skeletons studied prior to 1974 (Table 16.2).

A striking feature of such a comparison is the high proportion of children and juveniles in the Hallowhill group. Individuals aged up to 19 years make up almost 30% of the population, compared with 15% of skeletal material from other long cist sites. By contrast, the proportion of children and juveniles in the Kirkhill group (24%) is only slightly higher than that recorded from other Mediaeval sites (20%).

The age distribution of the Kirkhill population is thus very similar to the age distribution of a random collection of Mediaeval skeletons, while the Hallowhill population is markedly different in age distribution from other long cist material. One can only speculate as to why there seem to be so many more children and juveniles in the Hallowhill cemetery. This could represent a real difference in average age at death, perhaps due to particularly severe epidemics of childhood fevers affecting the Hallowhill people. Against this interpretation is the fact that enamel hypoplasia is very rare in the Hallowhill dentitions: this developmental abnormality of enamel is often thought to be caused by environmental stress (Coodman et al., 1980; 1984) which may include the exanthematous fevers (Kreshover & Clough, 1953; Rose et al. 1978) and if severe epidemics of these fevers had occurred, one would expect to see evidence of hypoplasia in the survivors. However, the connection between the exanthemata and hypoplasia has not been proved conclusively, and there could have been an unusually high death rate at Hallowhill as the result of diseases which are not associated with enamel hypoplasia.

But the relatively high proportion of children and juveniles at Hallowhill may be due to variations in soil conditions, which at other sites might militate against the preservation of the more delicate juvenile skulls; or it may be due to chance, or to variations in archaeological technique: some fragmentary juvenile material may not have been recovered by the earlier excavators.

The prevalence of dental caries is another aspect of the dentition which is of considerable interest. In dealing with fragmentary skeletal material, the only really accurate way of calculating caries prevalence is to express the number of teeth with carious lesions as a percentage of the total number of teeth which had erupted and were therefore at risk. When some of the dentitions are incomplete, it is impossible to make accurate calculations of the number of individuals who had experienced dental caries.

A comparison of the figures for caries prevalence in the permanent dentition of the Hallowhill and Kirkhill populations with the results obtained for Dark Age and Mediaeval material available prior to 1974 (Lunt,

Table 16.2. Age Distribution of dentitions in Scottish Dark Age and Mediaeval skeletal groups.

| | Children 0 - 14 | Juveniles 15 - 19 | Adults 20 - 45 | Elderly 45 + |
|---|---|---|---|---|
| Dark Age | 6.2 | 9.4 | 70.3 | 14.1 |
| Hallowhill | 16.0 | 13.0 | 55.1 | 15.9 |
| Medieval | 13.8 | 6.9 | 69.0 | 10.3 |
| Kirkhill | 20.2 | 4.2 | 64.8 | 10.8 |

Table 16.3. Caries Prevalence in Permanent Teeth in Scottish Dark Age and Mediaeval Skeletal Groups.

| Population group | No. teeth present | No. teeth carious | % teeth carious |
|---|---|---|---|
| Long cist | 1041 | 45 | 4.32 |
| Hallowhill | 1162 | 33 | 2.84 |
| Medieval | 400 | 24 | 6.00 |
| Kirkhill | 2864 | 196 | 6.84 |

1974) is shown in Table 16.3. The Hallowhill dentitions show a rather lower prevalence of dental caries than those of the long cist population in general, whereas the Kirkhill skeletons have a slightly higher prevalence of dental caries than that of the small Mediaeval group.

When the original study of caries prevalence in prehistoric and mediaeval Scottish dentitions was carried out, it became clear that caries prevalence was related to age, caries being unknown in children and juveniles, rare in young adults, and becoming more common only in the older adults. The lower caries prevalence in the Hallowhill population could therefore be due to the higher proportion of juveniles, which has already been mentioned. There was a slightly increased proportion of older adults in the Kirkhill group, which could account for its slightly higher caries prevalence.

This hypothesis may be tested by examining caries prevalence by age group in the two populations from St. Andrews. The data for the Hallowhill dentitions are shown in Table 16.4. Children and adolescents (no permanent teeth are at risk in children below the age of 6) show no caries, while the younger adults show a low caries prevalence and there is a much higher prevalence of caries in the older adults.

The same pattern is repeated in the figures for the Kirkhill group (Table 16.5). But the actual prevalence figures for both adult groups are higher in the Kirkhill than in the Hallowhill population: thus between the period of the long cists and the mediaeval period in the same geographical area, there was an increase in dental caries. The prevalence figure for the younger adults from Kirkhill had increased more than that for the older adults, and this suggests an earlier onset of the disease.

In previous studies of the deciduous dentition, dental caries was not observed in deciduous teeth from long cist burials, but was seen in a few dentitions from the mediaeval period (Lunt, 1972). These findings are borne out by the St. Andrews skeletal material, in that the Hallowhill deciduous teeth show no evidence of dental caries, whereas caries does appear in deciduous teeth from Kirkhill (Table 16.6). The caries prevalence is very low in children below 5 years of age but is much higher in the 6-12 year age group. It is interesting that the presence of carious deciduous teeth does not seem to have led to the development of caries in the permanent dentition of these individuals.

In summary, a comparison between the Hallowhill dentitions and those of other long cist burials shows that at Hallowhill there was a higher proportion of children and juveniles, and a lower prevalence of dental caries. The dentitions from the mediaeval cemetery at Kirkhill indicate a considerable degree of similarity in age distribution and in caries prevalence to mediaeval skeletal material from other sites in Scotland.

Table 16.4. Caries Prevalence in Permanent Teeth from Hallowhill, St. Andrews.

| Age group | No. teeth present | No. teeth carious | % teeth carious |
|---|---|---|---|
| 6 - 19 | 197 | 0 | 0 |
| 20 - 35 | 595 | 9 | 1.51 |
| OVER 35 | 328 | 21 | 6.40 |
| Total | 1120 | 30 | 2.68 |

Note: The totals in this table are slightly lower than in Table 3, because a few specimens could not be aged.

Table 16.5. Caries Prevalence in Permanent Teeth from Kirkhill, St. Andrews.

| Age group | No. teeth present | No. teeth carious | % teeth carious |
|---|---|---|---|
| 6 - 19 | 250 | 0 | 0 |
| 20 - 35 | 1120 | 60 | 5.36 |
| over 35 | 1319 | 116 | 8.79 |
| Total | 2689 | 176 | 6.55 |

Note: The totals in this table are slightly lower than in Table 3, because a few specimens could not be aged.

Table 16.6. Caries Prevalence in Deciduous Teeth from Kirkhill, St. Andrews.

| Age group | No. teeth present | No. teeth carious | % teeth carious |
|---|---|---|---|
| 0 - 5 | 148 | 1 | 0.68 |
| 6 - 12 | 83 | 9 | 10.84 |
| Total | 231 | 10 | 4.33 |

Acknowledgements

I should like to thank Mrs. E.V.W. Proudfoot and Mr. J. Wordsworth for allowing me to study the Hallowhill and Kirkhill collections respectively, and for their kind permission to publish the results of this study.

References

Brothwell, D.R. (1981). Digging up Bones. British Museum (Natural History), London.

Goodman, A.H., Armelagos, G.J. and Rose, J.C. (1980). Enamel hypoplasias as indicators of stress in three prehistoric populations from Illinois. Hum. Biol. 52: 515-528.

Goodman, A.H., Armelagos, G.J. and Rose, J.C. (1984). The chronological distribution of enamel hypoplasia from prehistoric Dickson Mounds populations. Am. J. Phys. Anthrop. 65: 259-266.

Kreshover, S.J. & Clough, O.W. (1953). Prenatal influences on tooth development. II Artificially induced fever in rats. J. Dent. Res. 32: 565-577.

Lunt, D.A. (1972). The dentition in a group of mediaeval Scottish children. Br. Dent. J. 132: 443-446.

Lunt, D.A. (1974). The prevalence of dental caries in the permanent dentition of Scottish prehistoric and mediaeval populations. Archs. Oral Biol. 19: 431-437.

Rose, J.C., Armelagos, G.J. and Lallo, J.W. (1978). Histological enamel indicator of childhood stress in prehistoric skeletal samples. Am. J. Phys. Anthrop. 49: 511-516.

Stevenson, R.B.K. (1951-52). Long cist burials, particularly those at Galson (Lewis) and Gairloch (Wester Ross), with a symbol stone at Gairloch. Proc. Soc. Antiq. Scot. 86: 106.

Chapter 17

# TRACE ELEMENTS IN TEETH OF EGYPTIANS AND NUBIANS

M.V. Stack

MRC Dental Unit
University of Bristol Dental School

## Material and Method.

Impressions of the nutritional status of the more privileged amongst those who lived in ancient Egypt may be gained by determining levels of various trace elements in bones and teeth. In addition, when such analyses are applied to toxic, non-essential trace elements, such as lead and cadmium, they may afford 'baseline' data with which findings in modern surveys can be compared.

The teeth providing the original objective of this study were from the recently studied 'Bristol mummy', identified as that of Horemkenesi, a necropolis supervisor in the Valley of the Tombs of the Kings during the XXIst Dynasty. He was in his mid-fifties; his teeth were worn so severely that the tips of the roots were thought most likely to provide suitable material for analysis. A few other ancient Egyptian and Nubian tooth specimens were supplied (see acknowledgements) for comparison with the original tooth fragments.

Root tips were analysed by atomic absorption spectrometry, with volatilisation of elements by electrothermal atomisation, following brief chemical 'cleaning' by exposure to dilute nitric acid. Samples were dissolved in concentrated nitric acid (30 - 50 milligrams/0.15 - 0.25 millilitres acid) and the digests diluted first to provide stock solutions and further as required for analysis. Standard volumes of 0.01 ml were injected into the graphite furnace of the Pye Unicam SP9 instrument, in which the atomic vapours were generated at specific temperatures after controlled drying and ashing programmes.

The 'method of standard additions' was used to calibrate analyses. These were also monitored by analysing a 'reference material' for which analyses have been reported by a number of investigators. This material was an animal bone prepartion (H-5, International Atomic Energy Agency, Vienna), for which results for intercomparison analyses are given in Table 17.1.

## Results and Discussion

The trace metals cadmium, copper, iron, lead, strontium, zinc and the minor element magnesium were analysed in six Egyptian teeth (two from Horemkenesi, giving similar values) and in four Nubian teeth, as listed in Table 17.2. Molybdenum, in Egyptian teeth only, was determined because this element has been discussed more frequently in relation to dental caries than any other element except fluorine.

Table 17.1. Trace metal concentrations[a] in reference bone material H-5 (International Atomic Agency, Vienna: Intercomparison.)

| | Cadmium (Cd) | Copper (Cu) | Iron (Fe) | Lead (Pb) | Strontium (Sr) | Zinc (Zn) | Magnesium (Mg) |
|---|---|---|---|---|---|---|---|
| Number of laboratories[b] | 8 | 16 | 30 | 18 | 13 | 44 | 24 |
| Laboratory mean values reported | 23 | 0.64 | 80 | 3.0 | 105 | 90 | 3.53 |

[a] Units Cd - micrograms/kg; Cu ... Zn - micrograms/g; Mg - micrograms/mg
[b] Laboratories reporting 'acceptable' values (8/13 in the case of Cd).

Table 17.2. Trace metal concentrations[a] in Egyptian and Nubian teeth.

| Age[b] in millenia | Cadmium (Cd) | Copper (Cu) | Iron (Fe) | Lead (Pb) | Strontium (Sr) | Zinc (Zn) | Magnesium (Mg) |
|---|---|---|---|---|---|---|---|
| 3.05[c] | 20 | 30 | 22 | 1.4 | 80 | 130 | 4.5 |
| 2.8 | (0) | 0.5 | 13 | 0.6 | 105 | 90 | 3.5 |
| 5.0 | 10 | 0.35 | 115 | 0.5 | 370 | 95 | 4.6 |
| 5 | 40 | 0.3 | 26 | (0) | 85 | 120 | 4.8 |
| 3 | 25 | 0.3 | 23 | 4.0 | 80 | 120 | 5.0 |
| 2.9[d] | 105 | 8.6 | 25 | 2.8 | 510 | 120 | 2.6 |
| 2.6 | 10 | 7.0 | 17 | 1.6 | 90 | 235 | 12 |
| 2 | 30 | 4.1 | 24 | 0.4 | 110 | 110 | 3.4 |
| 4 | 15 | 2.4 | 10 | 0.8 | 90 | 220 | 4.2 |

A units as footnote to Table 1

b Ages correspond to XXIst, XXIInd, Ist, pre-Ist, and XXIst Dynasty for the Egyptian specimens, and XXIInd, XXVIth, post-XXXIIIrd, and 'Old/Middle Kingdom' for the group of Nubian specimens.

c Egyptian teeth (5): first listed is one of two from Horemkenesi; molybdenum levels 0.7, 0.4, 10.5, 0.35, 0.4 resp.

d Nubian teeth (4)

Cadmium levels were low, but comparable with those of the reference sample, and the median represented a proportion of one part to fifty million parts of specimen.

Copper levels in the Nubian teeth and in the teeth of Horemkenesi were typical of recent specimens, those for the other four Egyptian teeth being much lower.

Iron levels were, with one exception, so low as to suggest the possibility of a deficiency state during tooth formation.

Lead levels were less in the three oldest teeth than in the more recent teeth of this small group. One value, as was the case with cadmium, could not be distinguished from the background level due to the solvent. Cadmium and lead were present at very much lower concentrations than are found currently (Table 17.3).

Strontium levels were typically low, but one Egyptian and one Nubian specimen showed relatively high values.

Zinc levels were within modern limits, the highest value being 2½ times the lowest, as was the case with all but one of the iron values. Only two strontium:zinc ratios were suggestive of a vegetarian diet (see, e.g., Edward et al, 1984).

Molybdenum levels ranged from 0.4 to 1 microgram/gram, within the very wide range reported for teeth (Curzon & Cutress, 1983, p. 153).

Other evidence on the concentration of lead in Egyptian and Nubian mummies suggests typical values in the microgram/gram range (Shapiro et al. 1975; Grandjean, Nielsen & Shapiro, 1979; Shapiro, et al. 1980). The more recent references account for lead in bone and tooth specimens and the authors suggested that 'background' values were represented by the oldest material. However, some lead technology was used in the area after the fifth millenium before present. Drasch (1982) suggested lower minimum levels in bone specimens. The present limited study shows such levels in the oldest teeth.

The use of the reference bone material in standardising analyses was particularly advantageous, for concentrations of Cd, Mo, Sr, Zn and Mg were comparable with median values for these elements in the Egyptian and Nubian root apex specimens. Values for lead and iron were less in the teeth than in reference bone material. For copper the value was above the four lowest values for Egyptian teeth but much less than those for the Nubian teeth. In Figure 17.1, a logarithmic scale is used in order to show concentration of magnesium and the trace metals together. The expected widening of the range for accepted means reported in the intercomparison study of the bone material can be seen at the low concentration values. Open bars in this Figure show extreme values. Consensus values for trace metals in modern teeth are also shown, that for lead being the most distant from the range of values now reported.

## Summary

Trace metals were determined in root apex portions of teeth of the "Bristol mummy" (Horemkenesi, H7386), from four other artificially mummified

Table 17.3. Trace metal concentrations[a] in dentine: major population surveys (Data from Curzon & Cutress, 1983, Table 3.14).

| | Cadmium (Cd) | Copper (Cu) | Iron (Fe) | Lead (Pb) | Strontium (Sr) | Zinc (Zn) | Magnesium (Mg) |
|---|---|---|---|---|---|---|---|
| Data in order | 0.08 | 1 | 43 | 33 | 67 | 175 | 7.4 |
| of magnitude | 0.43 | 6 | 80 | 37 | 120 | 180 | 8.5 |
| (mean values) | 0.61 | 7 | 110 | 43 | 180 | 180 | 8.7 |

a Units as footnote a to Tables 1 & 2.
b Curzon & Cutress (1983), Table 21.3: tooth data.

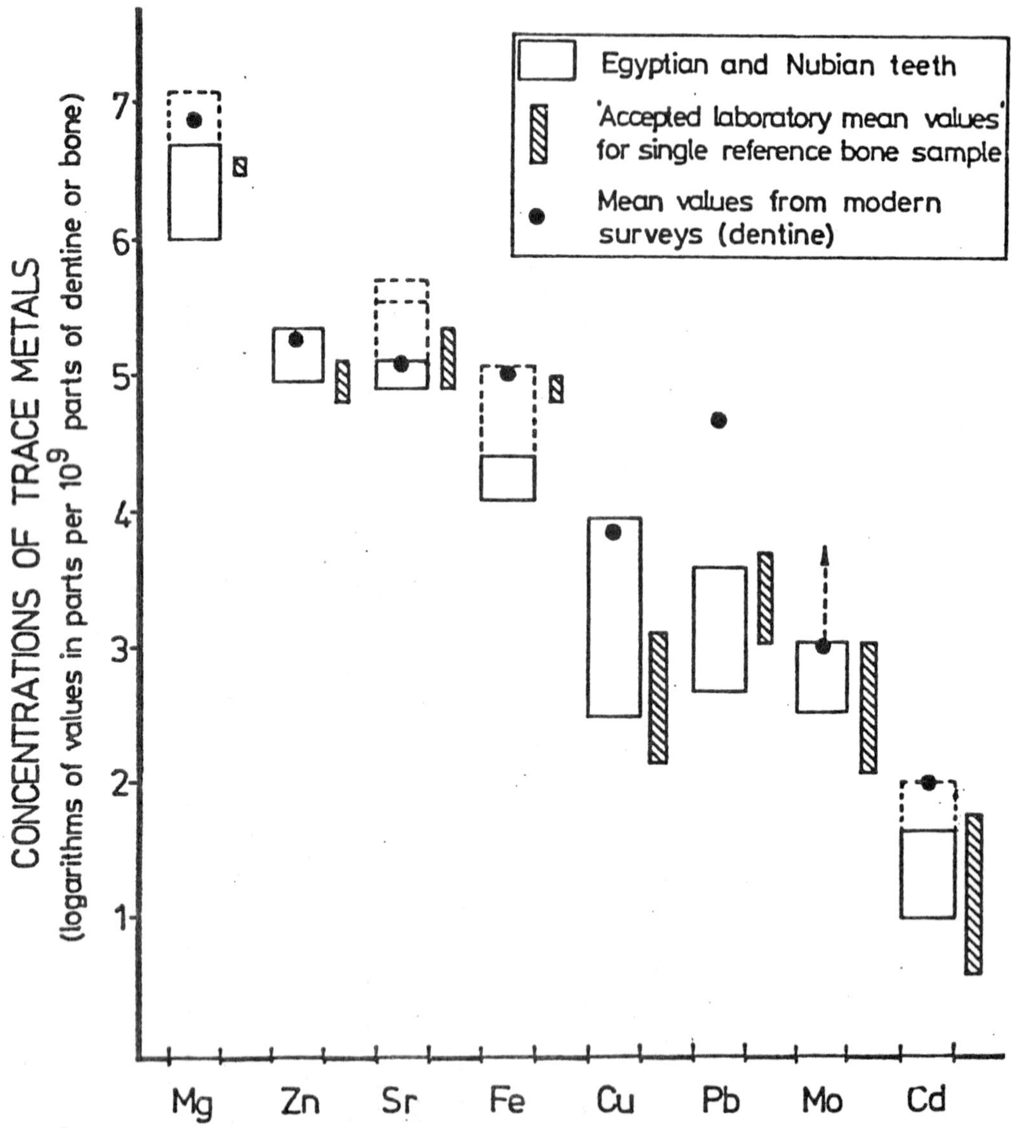


Figure 17.1. Trace metal concentration ranges in Egyptian and Nubian teeth.

Egyptians, and from four naturally mummified Nubians dated 2 - 5 millenia ago. Median values for eight metals were: cadmium 0.02, copper 2.4, iron 23, lead 0.8, molybdenum 0.4, strontium 90, zinc 120 and magnesium, a minor element, 4500 micrograms/gram. Copper values in the Nubian teeth exceeded those in the additional Egyptian teeth.


## Acknowledgements

Teeth were denoted by F.F. Leek (Manchester Mummy Team), T.I. Molleson (British Museum Sub-Department of Anthropology) and D. Dawson (Archaeology Curator, Bristol City Museum & Art Gallery). R.P. Fletcher (MRC Dental Unit) operated the analytical system and R.M. Parr (I.A.E.A., Vienna) provided the reference bone material H-5 and a report collating values for trace elements analysed by collaborating laboratories.


## References


Curzon, M.E.J. Cutress, T.W. (1983). Trace Elements and Dental Disease (eds) Postgrad Dent Hbdk Ser, Vol. 9. Wright. PSG Inc. Bristol & Boston.

Drasch, G.A. 1983. Sci. Total Environ. 24: 199-231.

Edward, J., Fossey, J.M., Yaffe, L. 1984. J. Field Archaeol. 11: 37-46.

Grandjean, P., Nielson, O.V., Shapiro, I.M. 1979. J. Environ. Pathol. Toxicol. 2: 781-787.

Shapiro, I.M., Grandjean, P., Nielson, O.V. 1980. In: Needleman HL (ed) Low Level Lead Exposure (Symp) Raven Press.

Shapiro, I.M., Mitchell, G., Davidson, I., Katz, S.H. 1975. Archs. Environ. Health 30: 483-486.

Stack, M.V. 1984. In: Metals in Bone (CEC & EULEP Symp) p. 405-406.